Basic ICD-9-CM Coding
2006 Edition

Lou Ann Schraffenberger, MBA, RHIA, CCS, CCS-P

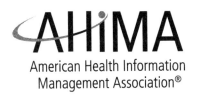

American Health Information
Management Association®

This book includes ICD-9-CM changes announced in the CMS Hospital Inpatient Prospective Payment Systems Proposed Rules, as published in the May 4, 2005 *Federal Register* available at http://www.access.gpo.gov/su_docs/fedreg/a050504c.html. Any additional changes to these codes may be obtained at the CMS Web site or in the Final Rule for IPPS in the *Federal Register* when it is available (usually in August). The official ICD-9-CM addenda are available at: http://www.cdc.gov/nchs/datawh/ftpserv/ftpicd9/ftpicd9.htm#guidelines.

Material quoted in this book from ICD-9-CM Official Guidelines for Coding and Reporting is taken from the April 2005 updated version.

First edition 1993, revised annually

ISBN 1-58426-150-1

AHIMA Product No. AC200505 (without answers)
AHIMA Product No. AC200505K (with answers)

Ann Zeisset, RHIT, CCS, CCS-P, Reviewer
Marcia Loellbach, MS, Project Editor
Melissa Ulbricht, Editorial/Production Coordinator

AHIMA strives to recognize the value of people from every racial and ethnic background as well as all genders, age groups, and sexual orientations by building its membership and leadership resources to reflect the rich diversity of the American population. AHIMA encourages the celebration and promotion of human diversity through education, mentoring, recognition, leadership, and other programs.

American Health Information Management Association
233 North Michigan Avenue, Suite 2150
Chicago, Illinois 60601-5800

http://www.ahima.org

Contents

Contents

About the Author

Lou Ann Schraffenberger, MBA, RHIA, CCS, CCS-P, is the manager of clinical data in the Center for Health Information Services of Advocate Health Care in Oak Brook, Illinois. Her position is dedicated to systemwide health information management and clinical data projects, clinical coding education, chargemaster, and coding compliance issues. Prior to her current position, Lou Ann served as director of hospital health record departments, director of AHIMA's Professional Practice Division, and a faculty member at the University of Illinois at Chicago. An experienced seminar leader, Lou Ann continues to serve as adjunct faculty and a continuing education instructor in the health information technology and coding certificate program at Moraine Valley Community College. She has also contributed her knowledge and skills as a consultant for clinical coding projects with hospitals, ambulatory care facilities, physicians, and medical group practices. Lou Ann has been active in national, state, and local HIM associations. In 1997, Lou Ann was awarded the first AHIMA Volunteer Award. She has served as chair of the Society for Clinical Coding (2000), and she is a former member of the AHIMA Council on Certification and former chair of the Certified Coding Specialist (CCS) Examination Construction Committee.

Acknowledgments

This book was originally published in 1993 under the authorship of Toula Nicholas, RHIT, CCS, and Linda Ertl Bank, RHIA, CCS.

Preface

The coding process requires a range of skills that combines knowledge and practice. *Basic ICD-9-CM Coding* was designed to provide a comprehensive text for students. It introduces the basic principles and conventions of ICD-9-CM coding and illustrates the application of coding principles with examples and exercises based on actual case documentation.

Organization of the Book

The twenty-three chapters of *Basic ICD-9-CM Coding* are organized to cover each section of *ICD-9-CM*. The coding self-test, index, and appendices at the back of the book make information readily accessible and provide additional resources for students.

Basic ICD-9-CM Coding is available with answers or without answers. Please contact the publisher directly if you need a copy of the answer key.

Information Updates

This book must be used with the 2006 edition of *ICD-9-CM* (code changes effective October 1, 2005). It includes the code updates listed in the CMS Hospital Inpatient Prospective Payment Systems Proposed Rules, May 4, 2005 *Federal Register* available at http://www.access.gpo.gov/su_docs/fedreg/a050504c.html.

Every effort has been made to include the most current coding information in this textbook. Because coding is so dynamic, there are continuous changes. In order to keep you informed about some of them, the following information is provided to you.

Coding Guidelines

The ICD-9-CM Official Guidelines for Coding and Reporting, effective April 2005, are included as appendix I of this book. Additional information and updates to current coding guidelines can be found on the following Web site: www.cdc.gov/nchs/icd9.htm.

Classification of Death and Injury Resulting from Terrorism

Because of the events of September 11, 2001, there is a need to be able to classify, report, and analyze injuries and deaths associated with terrorism. Codes have been developed for both ICD-10 and ICD-9-CM. These codes, which were published in the *Federal Register* in May 2002 and became effective October 1, 2002, are available at www.cdc.gov/nchs/about/otheract/icd9/terrorism-_code.htm.

ICD-9-CM Procedure Codes

In order to provide an expedited process for the approval of procedure codes, the Centers for Medicare and Medicaid Services (CMS) now allows procedures approved at the spring Coordination and Maintenance Committee meeting to fast-track with the codes effective October 1 of each year. Because they are not discussed until the spring, these codes are not included in the final codes listed in the May *Federal Register*. The codes listed in the May 4, 2005 *Federal Register* are included in this updated textbook. They are available at http://www.access.gpo.gov/su_docs/fedreg/a050504c.html. Additional procedure codes that are effective October 1, 2005, may be listed in the August Final Rule, which will be published in the *Federal Register*.

Additional Practice

AHIMA's publication *Clinical Coding Workout* is an excellent follow-up resource after the coder completes *Basic ICD-9-CM Coding*. Containing beginning, intermediate, and advanced exercises, it is also a perfect teaching tool for coders wanting to sharpen their ability to make critical coding decisions. The book is made up entirely of case studies that help students and coders alike understand what they need to know when it comes to correct coding practices and procedures. The case studies in the book require users to make the kinds of decisions that coding professionals must make every day on the job.

Chapter 1

Introduction to ICD-9-CM

What Is Coding?

In its simplest form, coding is the transformation of verbal descriptions into numbers. We are all very familiar with this task because we use codes every day to carry out simple business and personal transactions. For example, when we use a zip code in addressing a letter, we are transforming a street address into numbers.

In the healthcare arena, specific codes describe diseases, injuries, and procedures. Whereas assigning a zip code is a rather simple activity, the assignment of diagnostic and procedural codes requires a detailed thought process that is supported by a thorough knowledge of medical terminology, anatomy, and pathophysiology.

How Are Codes Assigned, and What System Is Used?

Hospitals and other healthcare facilities index healthcare data by referring and adhering to a classification system published by the U.S. Department of Health and Human Services: *International Classification of Diseases, 9th Revision, Clinical Modification (ICD-9-CM).* As the title states, ICD-9-CM has been revised nine times, giving evidence to the fact that the system has been in use for many years.

The notion of employing classification systems can be traced back to the time of the ancient Greeks. In the seventeenth century, English statistician John Graunt developed the London Bills of Mortality, which provided the first documentation of the proportion of children who died before reaching age six. In 1838, William Farr, the registrar general of England, developed a system to classify deaths. In 1893, a French physician, Jacques Bertillon, introduced the Bertillon Classification of Causes of Death at the International Statistical Institute in Chicago.

Several countries subsequently adopted Dr. Bertillon's system; and in 1898, the American Public Health Association (APHA) recommended that the registrars of Canada, Mexico, and the United States also adopt it. In addition, APHA recommended revising the system every ten years so as to remain current with medical practice. As a result, the first international conference to revise the International Classification of Causes of Death convened in 1900; subsequent revisions occurred every ten years. At that time, the classification system was contained in one book, which included an Alphabetic Index as well as a Tabular List. The book was quite small compared with current coding texts.

The revisions that followed contained minor changes; however, the sixth revision of the classification system brought drastic changes, as well as an expansion into two volumes. The sixth revision included morbidity and mortality conditions, and its title was modified to reflect these changes: *Manual of International Statistical Classification of Diseases, Injuries and Causes of Death (ICD)*. Prior to the sixth revision, responsibility for ICD revisions fell to the Mixed Commission, a group composed of representatives from the International Statistical Institute and the Health Organization of the League of Nations. In 1948, the World Health Organization (WHO), with headquarters in Geneva, Switzerland, assumed responsibility for preparing and publishing the revisions to ICD every ten years. WHO sponsored the seventh and eighth revisions in 1957 and 1968, respectively.

The entire history of coding emphasizes the determination of many people to provide an international classification system for compiling and presenting statistical data. ICD now has become the most widely used statistical classification system in the world. Although some countries found ICD sufficient for hospital indexing purposes, many others felt that it did not provide adequate detail for diagnostic indexing. In addition, the original revisions of ICD did not provide for classification of operative and diagnostic procedures. As a result, interested persons in the United States began to develop their own adaptation of ICD for use in this country.

In 1959, the U.S. Public Health Service published *The International Classification of Diseases, Adapted for Indexing of Hospital Records and Operation Classification (ICDA)*. Completed in 1962, a revision of this adaptation—considered to be the seventh revision of ICD—expanded a number of areas to more completely meet the indexing needs of hospitals. The U.S. Public Health Service later published the *Eighth Revision, International Classification of Diseases, Adapted for Use in the United States*. Commonly referred to as ICDA-8, this classification system fulfilled its purpose to code diagnostic and operative procedural data for official morbidity and mortality statistics in the United States.

WHO published the ninth revision of ICD (ICD-9) in 1978. The U.S. Public Health Service modified ICD-9 to meet the needs of American hospitals and called it *International Classification of Diseases, Ninth Revision, Clinical Modification (ICD-9-CM)*. The ninth revision expanded the book to three volumes and introduced a fifth-digit subclassification.

ICD-10-CM and ICD-10-PCS

The National Center for Health Statistics (NCHS), the federal agency responsible for the use of the *International Statistical Classification of Diseases and Related Health Problems, 10th Revision (ICD-10)* in the United States, has developed a clinical modification of the classification for morbidity purposes. The new ICD-10-CM would be used for the reporting of diseases and conditions of patients treated in the United States healthcare system. For the coding of death certificates (mortality data), ICD-10 replaced ICD-9 as of January 1, 1999. ICD-10-CM is intended to be the replacement for ICD-9-CM, volumes 1 and 2.

ICD-10 is copyrighted by the World Health Organization (WHO), which owns and publishes the classification. WHO authorized the development of the adaption of ICD-10 for use in the United States. All modifications to ICD-10 must conform to WHO conventions for ICD.

ICD-10-CM was developed following a thorough evaluation by a Technical Advisory Panel and extensive additional consultation with physician groups, clinical coders, and others to ensure clinical accuracy and utility. NCHS believes the clinical modification represents a significant improvement over ICD-9-CM and ICD-10.

The current draft of ICD-10-CM contains significantly more codes than exist in ICD-9-CM and offers many additional advantages. Some of these features include:

- ICD-10-CM has the same hierarchical structure as ICD-9-CM, but the codes are all alphanumeric and all letters except U are used.

- The codes corresponding to ICD-9-CM V and E codes are incorporated into the main classification and are not separated into supplementary classifications as in ICD-9-CM.

- New diseases and conditions not uniquely identified in ICD-9-CM have been given codes. In addition, conditions with newly discovered etiology or treatment protocols have been reclassified to a more appropriate chapter.

- Injuries are grouped by body part instead of by categories of injury.

- Excludes notes are expanded to provide guidance on the hierarchy of chapters and to clarify priority of code assignment.

- Combination codes have been created, such as arteriosclerotic heart disease with angina.

- The concept of laterality (right–left) has been added.

- The codes for postoperative complications have been expanded, and a distinction has been made between intraoperative complications and postprocedural disorders.

- The obstetric codes indicate which trimester the patient is in and no longer identify whether the patient has delivered.

- The diabetes codes indicate insulin-requiring and non-insulin-requiring types.

- Information relevant to ambulatory and managed care encounters has been added.

- In general, the classification allows greater specificity in code assignment.

The draft revision of ICD-10-CM is available on the NCHS Web site, Classifications of Diseases and Functioning and Disability home page, at www.cdc.gov/nchs/about/otheract/icd9/abticd10.htm. The codes in ICD-10-CM are not currently valid for any purpose or use. Testing of ICD-10-CM will continue, based on the draft version. It is anticipated that updates to the draft will occur prior to implementation of ICD-10-CM.

As of early 2005, there is no anticipated implementation date for ICD-10-CM. For ICD-10-CM to be implemented, it must be recommended by the Secretary of Health and Human Services as a replacement for the ICD-9-CM diagnosis code set national standard. Once this is done, implementation will be based on the process for adoption of standards under the Health Insurance Portability and Accountability Act of 1996 (HIPAA). There will be at least a two-year implementation window once the final notice to implement has been published in the *Federal Register*. This notice is anticipated to propose naming ICD-10-CM for diagnoses in all healthcare settings and ICD-10-PCS to replace volume 3 of ICD-9-CM for procedures in the hospital inpatient setting only.

ICD-10-PCS has been under development by the Centers for Medicare and Medicaid Services (CMS) for a number of years. It is intended to replace ICD-9-CM, volume 3, for the reporting of hospital inpatient procedures. It is believed to be a significant improvement over ICD-9-CM, volume 3, in terms of its comprehensiveness and expandability.

ICD-10-PCS has a multiaxial, seven-character, alphanumeric code structure, which provides a unique code for all substantially different procedures and allows new procedures to be easily incorporated as new codes. Procedures in ICD-10-PCS are divided into sections that relate to the general type of procedure. The first character of the procedure codes always specifies the section or type of procedure. The second through seventh characters have a standard meaning within each section but may have a different meaning across sections. In ICD-10-PCS, the term *procedure* is used to refer to the complete specification of the seven characters. All terminology in ICD-10-PCS is precisely defined, with a specific meaning attached to all terms used in the system.

ICD-10-PCS continues to be refined and updated awaiting the final decision from the Department of Health and Human Services on whether it will propose adoption of ICD-10-CM and ICD-10-PCS as a HIPAA standard. The previous training manual has been updated by a new reference manual that includes definitions for PCS terms, root operations and approaches, and draft PCS coding guidelines. Plans for 2006 include completion of the ICD-9-CM to ICD-10-PCS crosswalk and work on the task of converting the DRGs into ICD-10-CM and PCS. The goal is to complete a prototype of the DRGs in the new code sets by the end of 2005. The latest updates are available on the CMS Web site at http://cms.hhs.gov/paymentsystems/icd9/icd10.asp

Although it is likely that the new coding system will require coders to have more knowledge of anatomy and physiology, as well as requiring complete documentation of a procedure to be available prior to coding, ICD-10-PCS appears to provide more complete and accurate descriptions of the procedures performed than does ICD-9-CM, volume 3. All procedures on a particular body part, by a particular approach, or by another characteristic can be easily retrieved using ICD-10-PCS data. The codes will provide very specific information about a particular procedure.

Additional readings on ICD-10-CM and ICD-10-PCS can be found in appendix G of this book. A description of ICD-10 can be found at the Web site for the World Health Organization (WHO) (www.who.int/whosis/icd10/index.html). For more information on the versions that will be implemented in the United States, watch the Web sites for NCHS (www.cdc.gov/nchs) and CMS (www.CMS.gov), in addition to AHIMA's site (www.ahima.org).

Proposals to consider the new coding systems (ICD-10-CM and ICD-10-PCS) as national standards must take place within the federal government's administrative simplification process. The administrative simplification requirements of the Health Insurance Portability and Accountability Act (HIPAA), Public Law 104-191, require the establishment of national standards for code sets. HIPAA requires a proposed and final notice establishing initial national code sets. The initial code sets will become the national standards at least two years after publication of the final notice. No notices have been published regarding ICD-10-CM and ICD-10-PCS.

HIPAA Electronic Transactions and Coding Standards Rule

On August 17, 2000, the U.S. Department of Health and Human Services (DHHS) published the final regulations for electronic transactions and coding standards as established under HIPAA in the *Federal Register* (65 FR 50312). The final rule designated five medical code standards to be used initially under the HIPAA rule. These included:

- *International Classification of Diseases, 9th Edition, Clinical Modification (ICD-9-CM),* Volumes 1 and 2

- *International Classification of Diseases, 9th Edition, Clinical Modification (ICD-9-CM),* Volume 3

- *Current Procedural Terminology, 4th Edition (CPT-4)*

- *Healthcare Common Procedure Coding System (HCPCS)*

- *Code on Dental Procedures and Nomenclatures, 2nd Edition (CDT-2)*

- *National Drug Codes (NDC)*

On February 20, 2003, the DHHS published a final rule in the *Federal Register* (68 FR 8381) that repealed the adoption of the *National Drug Codes (NDC)* for institutional and professional claims. It did allow the NDC to remain the standard medical data code set for reporting drugs and biologics for retail pharmacy claims. The intent of this decision was to give covered entities the choice in determining which code set to use with respect to payment of claims, including HCPCS and NDC codes. Hospitals and physicians are likely to continue using HCPCS. As a result of this repeal, there is no identified standard medical data code set in place for reporting drugs and biologics on non–retail pharmacy transactions. Covered entities could use HCPCS or NDC as the preferred and agreed-upon code set with their trading partners.

The ICD-9-CM Official Guidelines for Coding and Reporting were named as a required component of the ICD-9-CM code set in the final rule for electronic transactions and coding standards (65 FR 50323). This makes adherence to the ICD-9-CM guidelines a requirement for compliance with the rule. No other set of coding guidelines was specified in the coding standards.

The original deadline for compliance with the electronic transactions rule was October 16, 2002, for all covered entities except small health plans, which by law had an additional year. However, in January 2002, in the Administrative Simplification Compliance Act, Congress authorized a one-year extension, to October 16, 2003, for those covered entities required to comply in 2002.

As noted above, the final rule identified five medical code sets. Although it is true that most of the code sets adopted are in current use, some changes have been made regarding their use and context. It is important to note that, upon implementation, these medical code sets will become the rule for nearly all insurance payers.

ICD-9-CM, volumes 1 and 2, will cover diseases, injuries, impairments, and other health problems and their manifestations, as well as causes of injury and disease impairment. Essentially, this part of the rule maintains the status quo.

ICD-9-CM, volume 3, Procedures, has been limited to procedures or other actions taken for diseases, injuries, and impairments of hospital *inpatients* reported by hospitals and related to prevention, diagnosis, treatment, and management. This means that nonacute facilities will no longer be able to use volume 3 to report procedures and will, instead, have to use CPT-4 or HCPCS codes as appropriate.

The combination of HCPCS and CPT-4 will continue to be used for physicians and other healthcare services, such as hospital outpatient services. These services include, but are not limited to, physician services, physical and occupational therapy services, radiological services, clinical laboratory tests, other medical diagnostic procedures, hearing and vision services, and transportation services, including ambulances.

The rule makes it clear that the use of ICD-9-CM procedure codes is restricted to the reporting of inpatient procedures by hospitals and that the combination of CPT-4 and HCPCS Level 2 codes will be used by physicians and other healthcare services. There is no clear commitment to resolve duplication and overlap between CPT-4 and HCPCS Level 2 codes, such as the G codes in HCPCS that duplicate services described by CPT-4.

More information about the medical code sets and other facts about the HIPAA transactions and code sets final rule can be found on the AHIMA Web site (www.ahima.org) or in the published final rule in the August 17, 2000 *Federal Register* (volume 65, number 160, pages 50312–50372). The *Federal Register* may be accessed from the Government Printing Office Web site at www.access.gpo.gov/su_docs/fedreg/a000817c.html.

Medicare Prescription Drug, Improvement, and Modernization Act of 2003

The Medicare Prescription Drug, Improvement, and Modernization Act (MMA) was signed into law by President George W. Bush on December 8, 2003. Section 503 of the bill includes language concerning the timeliness of data collection and contains the following clause, which affects the updating of ICD-9-CM:

> Sec. 503 Recognition of New Medical Technology Under Inpatient Hospital Prospective Payment System, (a) Improving Timeliness of Data Collection, (vii) Under the mechanism of this new subparagraph, the Secretary shall provide for the addition of new diagnosis and procedure codes in April 1 of each year, but the addition of such codes shall not require the Secretary to adjust the payment (or diagnosis-related group classification) under this subsection until the fiscal year that begins after such date.

This means that, beginning in 2005, ICD-9-CM diagnosis and procedure codes could be issued to be effective twice a year, April 1 and October 1. The DRG software and Medicare Code Editor will have to be updated twice a year, as will all the coding software vendor products and healthcare providers' information systems for capturing data and processing information.

The Centers for Medicare and Medicaid Services (CMS) discussed a proposal to accomplish this new congressional requirement in the Notice of Proposed and Final Rulemaking for the Hospital Inpatient Payment System. Information on this April 1 update process can be found in the Final Rule published August 11, 2004 (69 FR 48954), beginning on page 48954. In general, new diagnosis and procedure codes will be implemented on October 1 as has been the standard practice. However, consideration will be given to implementing new codes on April 1 if a strong and convincing case is made by the requestor at the ICD-9-CM Coordination and Maintenance Committee meeting that the new code is needed to describe new technologies. Otherwise, the codes will be considered for the next October 1 implementation. A number of organizations have expressed concerns about the impact of the April 1 ICD-9-CM coding update on providers. There were no requests for an ICD-9-CM code to be implemented April 1, 2005.

Official Addendum to ICD-9-CM

ICD-9-CM represents the most current and comprehensive statistical classification system of its kind. Compared with international ICD updates that occur approximately every ten years, ICD-9-CM undergoes annual updates in the United States to remain current. Codes may be added, revised, or deleted. An *Official Authorized Addendum* documents the changes, which are effective October 1 of each year. CMS and NCHS publish the addenda with the approval of WHO. NCHS is responsible for maintaining the diagnosis classification—volumes 1 and 2; CMS is responsible for maintaining the procedure classification—volume 3. The American Health

Information Management Association (AHIMA) and the American Hospital Association (AHA) give advice and assistance, as do HIM practitioners, physicians, and other users of ICD-9-CM.

A point to remember: To ensure accurate coding, all ICD-9-CM coding books *must* be updated yearly with ICD-9-CM revisions. In addition, all coding software (encoders) must be updated. As a general rule, new ICD-9-CM codes are effective October 1 of each year.

Characteristics of ICD-9-CM

As it has since the October 1991 publication by the U.S. Department of Health and Human Services, the single, official ICD-9-CM codebook currently comprises three volumes:

Volume 1: Tabular List of Diseases and Injuries
Volume 2: Alphabetic Index to Diseases
Volume 3: Tabular List and Alphabetic Index to Procedures

The official ICD-9-CM is available only on CD-ROM from the U.S. Government Printing Office in Washington, DC ([800] 512-1800).

A copyright of ICD-9-CM does not exist, so many versions of the codebook appear on the market. Although each book may offer special features, the ICD-9-CM codes themselves remain the same. This workbook, *Basic ICD-9-CM Coding,* refers to the official ICD-9-CM codebook throughout its text.

Because ICD-9-CM is reviewed annually, it is important to remember that all ICD-9-CM codebooks must be kept current to reflect the revisions, deletions, and additions of codes that are generally implemented in the United States on October 1 of each year.

Volume 1: Tabular List of Diseases and Injuries

The Tabular List of Diseases and Injuries (volume 1) contains the following major subdivisions:

Classification of Diseases and Injuries
Supplementary Classifications (V Codes and E Codes)
Appendices

Classification of Diseases and Injuries

Volume 1, Classification of Diseases and Injuries, contains seventeen chapters that classify conditions according to etiology (cause of disease) or by specific anatomical (body) system.

> **EXAMPLE:** Chapter 1, Infectious and Parasitic Diseases, represents classification by etiology or cause of disease.
>
> Chapter 7, Diseases of the Circulatory System, represents classification by anatomical system.

The Tabular List contains the following seventeen chapters:

Chapter Titles	Categories
1. Infectious and Parasitic Diseases	001–139
2. Neoplasms	140–239
3. Endocrine, Nutritional and Metabolic Diseases, and Immunity Disorders	240–279
4. Diseases of the Blood and Blood-Forming Organs	280–289
5. Mental Disorders	290–319
6. Diseases of the Nervous System and Sense Organs	320–389
7. Diseases of the Circulatory System	390–459
8. Diseases of the Respiratory System	460–519
9. Diseases of the Digestive System	520–579
10. Diseases of the Genitourinary System	580–629
11. Complications of Pregnancy, Childbirth, and the Puerperium	630–677
12. Diseases of the Skin and Subcutaneous Tissue	680–709
13. Diseases of the Musculoskeletal System and Connective Tissue	710–739
14. Congenital Anomalies	740–759
15. Certain Conditions Originating in the Perinatal Period	760–779
16. Symptoms, Signs, and Ill-Defined Conditions	780–799
17. Injury and Poisoning	800–999

Format

Each chapter of volume 1 is structured into the following subdivisions: sections, categories, and subcategories.

Sections

A section consists of a group of three-digit categories that represent a single disease entity, or a group of similar or closely related conditions.

DISORDERS OF THE THYROID GLAND (240–246)

Categories

A three-digit category represents a single disease entity, or a group of similar or closely related conditions.

520   Disorders of tooth development and eruption

Subcategories

The fourth-digit subcategory provides more specificity or information regarding the etiology (cause of a disease or illness), site (location), or manifestation (display of characteristic signs, symptoms, or secondary processes of a disease or illness). Fourth-digit subcategories are collapsible to the three-digit level.

A three-digit code cannot be assigned if a category has been subdivided and fourth digits are available.

---

476 Chronic laryngitis and laryngotracheitis

   476.0 Chronic laryngitis
      Laryngitis:
         catarrhal
         hypertrophic
         sicca
   476.1 Chronic laryngotracheitis
      Laryngitis, chronic, with tracheitis (chronic)
      Tracheitis, chronic, with laryngitis

Exercise 1.1

Turn to code 055, Measles, in volume 1 (Tabular List) to answer the following questions:

1.   Is code 055 a category or a subcategory?

   category

2.   What is the subcategory code for measles without complications?

   _055.9_

3.   What do the subcategory codes represent?   *existance of complications and uncomplications of measles*

   more specificity or information

4.   Are the subcategories manifestations, sites, or causes of the disease?

   manifestations

5.   In what chapter and section is code 055 located?

   Chapter 1 - Infectious and Parasitic Diseases
   Section - (001-139)

Fifth-Digit Subclassifications

In some cases, fourth-digit subcategories have been expanded to the fifth-digit level to provide even greater specificity. Fifth-digit assignments and instructions can appear at the beginning of a chapter, a section, a three-digit category, or a fourth-digit category, as illustrated below.

At the chapter level: An instruction at the beginning of chapter 13, Diseases of the Musculoskeletal System and Connective Tissue (710–739), states that certain categories must be assigned a fifth digit to describe the affected body site. Fifth-digit assignments and instructions appearing at the beginning of this chapter are shown in the following illustration:

13. DISEASES OF THE MUSCULOSKELETAL SYSTEM AND CONNECTIVE TISSUE (710–739)

The following fifth-digit subclassification is for use with categories 711–712, 715–716, 718–719, and 730:

0 site unspecified

1 shoulder region
  Acromioclavicular
  Glenohumeral
  Sternoclavicular   Joint(s)
  Clavicle
  Scapula

2 upper arm
  Elbow joint   Humerus

3 forearm
  Radius   Wrist joint
  Ulna

4 hand
  Carpus   Phalanges [fingers]
  Metacarpus

5 pelvic region and thigh
  Buttock   Hip (joint)
  Femur

6 lower leg
  Fibula   Patella
  Knee joint   Tibia

7 ankle and foot
  Ankle joint   Phalanges, foot
  Digits [toes]   Tarsus
  Metatarsus   Other joints in foot

8 other specified sites
  Head   Skull
  Neck   Trunk
  Ribs   Vertebral column

9 multiple sites

At the section level: Information at the beginning of section 200–208, Malignant Neoplasm of Lymphatic and Hematopoietic Tissue, notes that a fifth digit must be assigned to categories 200 through 202 to describe the site of the lymph nodes involved. Fifth-digit assignments and instructions appearing at the beginning of this section are shown in the following illustration:

MALIGNANT NEOPLASM OF LYMPHATIC AND HEMATOPOIETIC TISSUE (200–208)

Excludes:	secondary neoplasm of:

> secondary neoplasm of:
>   bone marrow (198.5)
>   spleen (197.8)
> secondary and unspecified neoplasm of
>   lymph nodes (196.0–196.9)

The following fifth-digit subclassification is for use with categories 200–202:

0   **unspecified site, extranodal and solid organ sites**
1   **lymph nodes of head, face, and neck**
2   **intrathoracic lymph nodes**
3   **intra-abdominal lymph nodes**
4   **lymph nodes of axilla and upper limb**
5   **lymph nodes of inguinal region and lower limb**
6   **intrapelvic lymph nodes**
7   **spleen**
8   **lymph nodes of multiple sites**

At the three-digit category level: An instruction from the beginning of category 250, Diabetes mellitus, states that a fifth digit should be assigned to describe the type of diabetes mellitus. Fifth-digit assignments and instructions appearing at the beginning of this three-digit category are shown in the following illustration:

250   Diabetes mellitus

Excludes:	gestational diabetes (648.8)

> gestational diabetes (648.8)
> hyperglycemia, NOS (790.6)
> neonatal diabetes mellitus (775.1)
> nonclinical diabetes (790.29)

The following fifth-digit subclassification is for use with category 250:

0   **type II or unspecified type, not stated as uncontrolled**

    Fifth-digit 0 is for use for type II patients, even if the patient requires insulin

    Use additional code, if applicable, for associated long-term (current) insulin use, V58.67

1   **type I [juvenile type], not stated as uncontrolled**

2   **type II or unspecified type, uncontrolled**

    Fifth-digit 2 is for use for type II patients, even if the patient requires insulin

    Use additional code, if applicable, for associated long-term (current) insulin use, V58.67

3   **type I [juvenile type], uncontrolled**

At the fourth-digit subcategory level: The fourth-digit subcategory 786.5, Chest pain, is further subdivided to the fifth-digit level to describe specific types of chest pain. Fifth-digit assignments and instructions appearing at the beginning of this fourth-digit subcategory are shown in the following illustration:

786.5	**Chest pain**	
	786.50	**Chest pain, unspecified**
	786.51	**Precordial pain**
	786.52	**Painful respiration**

Pain:
    anterior chest wall
    pleuritic
Pleurodynia

Excludes:	epidemic pleurodynia (074.1)

	786.59	**Other**

Discomfort
Pressure   } in chest
Tightness

Excludes:	pain in breast (611.71)

A point to remember: The use of fifth digits is *not* optional. Fifth digits are quite easy to overlook. To remember to assign fifth digits, it is helpful to highlight all the fourth-digit subcategories requiring a fifth-digit subclassification in volume 1 of ICD-9-CM. Many publishers include special symbols and/or color highlighting to identify codes requiring fourth and/or fifth digits.

Exercise 1.2

In volume 1 (Tabular List) of ICD-9-CM, turn to the section titled "Malignant Neoplasm of Lymphatic and Hematopoietic Tissue," which begins with code 200, to answer questions 1 through 3. Then turn to category code 820, Fracture of neck of femur, to answer questions 4 and 5.

1. Identify the correct fifth digit for a patient with Hodgkin's sarcoma (201.2) with involvement of the intrapelvic lymph nodes. _201.26_

2. Identify the correct fifth digit for a patient with Burkitt's tumor (200.2) of the intra-abdominal lymph nodes. _200.23_

3. Identify the correct fifth digit for a patient with nodular lymphoma (202.0) with involvement of lymph nodes of multiple sites. _202.08_

4. Identify the code for a patient with a closed transcervical fracture of the epiphysis. _820.01_

5. Identify the code for a patient with an open fracture of the neck of the femur, with the actual site unspecified. _820.09_

Residual Subcategories

Residual subcategories are codes with titles of "other" and "unspecified." They were developed to classify conditions not assigned a separate subcategory, thus ensuring that every disease always has a code. Residual subcategories titled "other" are easily distinguished because the fourth digit is often the number 8. Those codes describing "unspecified" conditions are usually assigned a fourth digit of 9.

003.8	**Other specified salmonella infections**
003.9	**Salmonella infection, unspecified**

In the preceding example, code 003.8 would include all other specified types of salmonella infections, excluding those listed in codes 003.0 through 003.29. But code 003.9 is assigned when the physician documents a diagnosis of salmonella infection without further specification.

However, in a few instances, fourth digit 9 is assigned for both "other" and "unspecified" because digits 0 through 8 have been used.

478.9   Other and unspecified diseases of upper respiratory tract

Abscess ⎱
Cicatrix ⎰ of trachea

Codes 478.0 through 478.8 are used to describe specific upper respiratory tract diseases. However, code 478.9 includes both unspecified diseases and other diseases not classified in subcategories 478.0 through 478.8.

Supplementary Classifications

Two supplementary classifications exist in addition to the main classification for diseases and injuries. Unlike the numeric codes in the disease classification, the supplementary classifications contain alphanumeric codes.

Supplementary Classification of Factors Influencing Health Status and Contact with Health Services (V01–V84)—V Codes

V codes consist of the alphabetic character V followed by two numeric digits, a decimal point, a fourth digit, and, where applicable, a fifth digit.

V64		**Persons encountering health services for specific procedures, not carried out**
	V64.0	Vaccination not carried out because of contraindication
	V64.1	Surgical or other procedure not carried out because of contraindication
	V64.2	Surgical or other procedure not carried out because of patient's decision
	V64.3	Procedure not carried out for other reasons
	V64.41	Laparoscopic surgical procedure converted to open procedure
	V64.42	Thoracoscopic surgical procedure converted to open procedure
	V64.43	Arthroscopic surgical procedure converted to open procedure

Supplementary Classification of External Causes of Injury and Poisoning (E800–E999)—E Codes

E codes consist of the alphabetic character E followed by three numeric digits, a decimal point, and a fourth digit.

E953	**Suicide and self-inflicted injury by hanging, strangulation, and suffocation**
E953.0	**Hanging**
E953.1	**Suffocation by plastic bag**
E953.8	**Other specified means**
E953.9	**Unspecified means**

Both supplementary classifications (E codes and V codes) are discussed in detail later in this book. E codes are discussed in chapter 21; V codes are discussed in chapter 23.

Appendices

Volume 1 of ICD-9-CM has traditionally included five appendices. Changes in the mental disorders codes, as described below, have resulted in the deletion of appendix B in October 2004 and subsequent publications.

Appendix A: Morphology of Neoplasms

Appendix A includes a listing of all morphology types with the appropriate morphology, or M code. Chapter 5 of this book describes morphology codes, or M codes, in greater detail.

Appendix B: Glossary of Mental Disorders (Deleted)

In 2003 and prior years, the Glossary of Mental Disorders included definitions for the psychiatric terms found in chapter 5, Mental Disorders, of ICD-9-CM. However, this appendix was not maintained for many years and was considered to contain many inaccuracies. In response to a request from the American Psychiatric Association, the Glossary of Mental Disorders was removed from the official government (CD-ROM) version of ICD-9-CM, effective with the October 1, 2004 update. Coders should refer to the *Diagnostic and Statistical Manual of Mental Disorders, Fourth Edition, Text Revision (DSM-IV-TR)*, published by the American Psychiatric Association, for definitions of the mental disorders classified in chapter 5 of ICD-9-CM.

Appendix C: Classification of Drugs by the American Hospital Formulary Service List

The classification of drugs by the American Hospital Formulary Service (AHFS) list is published by the American Society of Hospital Pharmacists. It categorizes drugs to family-related groups. When coders must locate the category of a new drug or cannot find a new drug in the Table of Drugs and Chemicals, they turn to the AHFS list as a helpful reference. The Table of Drugs and Chemicals lists the AHFS number under the main term "Drug." Appendix C of ICD-9-CM includes a listing of the AHFS categories and the appropriate ICD-9-CM code.

Appendix D: Classification of Industrial Accidents according to Agency

Appendix D classifies industrial accidents according to agency (machines, equipment, radiation, and so forth), as adopted by the Tenth International Conference of Labor Statisticians on October 12, 1962.

Appendix E: List of Three-Digit Categories

Appendix E includes a listing of each three-digit category in ICD-9-CM, along with the appropriate title of each.

Volume 2: Alphabetic Index to Diseases

Volume 2 contains the following major sections:

Index to Diseases and Injuries
Table of Drugs and Chemicals
Alphabetic Index to External Causes of Injury and Poisoning (E Codes)

Index to Diseases and Injuries

The Index to Diseases and Injuries includes the terminology for all the codes appearing in volume 1 (Tabular List) of ICD-9-CM. The Alphabetic Index employs three levels of indentations:

Main terms
Subterms
Carryover lines

Main Terms

Printed in boldface type, main terms are set flush with the left margin of each column for easy reference. They may represent the following:

- Diseases: influenza, bronchitis

- Conditions: fatigue, fracture, injury

- Nouns: disease, disturbance, syndrome

- Adjectives: double, large, kink

Instead of a listing of subterms or codes, ICD-9-CM provides anatomical terms with a cross-reference that directs the coder to reference the condition. For example, bronchial asthma is found under the disease term "asthma" rather than the site "bronchial."

A point to remember: Many conditions are found in more than one place in the Alphabetic Index; for example:

- Complications of medical or surgical care are indexed under the name of the condition, as well as the main term "Complications."

- Obstetrical conditions are found under the name of the condition and/or under main terms such as "Delivery," "Labor," "Pregnancy," and "Puerperal" (after delivery).

- Conditions that include the term *disease* or *syndrome* in their titles or descriptions may be found under "Disease" or "Syndrome," as well as under the disease or syndrome's name. For example, chronic obstructive lung disease may be found in the Alphabetic Index under "Obstructive," as well as under "Disease."

Exercise 1.3

Using the Alphabetic Index, underline the main term in each of the following:

1. Breast <u>mass</u>

2. Primary <u>hydronephrosis</u>

3. <u>Deviated</u> nasal septum

4. <u>Inguinal adenopathy</u>

5. <u>Arteriosclerotic</u> heart disease

Subterms

Some main terms are followed by a list of indented subterms (modifiers) that affect the selection of an appropriate code for a given diagnosis. The subterms form individual line entries arranged in alphabetical order and printed in regular type beginning with a lowercase letter. Subterms are indented one standard indentation to the right under the main term. They describe essential differences in site, cause, or clinical type. More specific subterms are indented farther to the right, as needed; indented one standard indentation after the preceding subterm; and listed in alphabetical order.

Prior to selecting a code, all subentries following the main term should be reviewed to determine the appropriate code. Note that the terms *with* and *without* are listed at the beginning of all the subterms, rather than in alphabetical order.

Incontinence 788.30	← **Main Term**
without sensory awareness 788.34	
anal sphincter 787.6	← **Site**
continuous leakage 788.37	
feces 787.6	
due to hysteria 300.11	
nonorganic origin 307.7	
hysterical 300.11	
mixed (male) (female) (urge and stress) 788.33	
overflow 788.39	
paradoxical 788.39	
rectal 787.6	
specified NEC 788.39	
stress (female) 625.6	← **Cause**
male NEC 788.32	
urethral sphincter 599.84	
urge 788.31	
and stress (male) (female) 788.33	
urine 788.30	
active 788.30	← **Clinical Type**
male 788.30	
stress 788.32	
and urge 788.33	
neurogenic 788.39	
nonorganic origin 307.6	
stress (female) 625.6	
male NEC 788.32	
urge 788.31	
and stress 788.33	

Carryover Lines

Carryover lines are needed because the number of words that can fit on a single line of print in the Alphabetic Index is limited. They are indented two indents from the preceding line. Coders must be careful to avoid confusing carryover lines with subterm entries. Careful reading is essential.

Rubella (German measles) 056.9
    complicating pregnancy, childbirth, or puerperium 647.5

Exercise 1.4

Using the Alphabetic Index only, assign codes to the following:

1. Tension headache

   _307.81_

2. Suppurative pancreatitis

   _577.0_

3. Neonatal tooth eruption

   _520.6_

4. Infectious endocarditis

   _421.0_

5. Mitral endocarditis with active aortic disease

   _391.1_

Nonessential Modifiers

Nonessential modifiers are a series of terms in parentheses that sometimes directly follow main terms, as well as subterms. The presence or absence of these parenthetical terms in the diagnosis has no effect on the selection of the code listed for that main term or subterm.

Pneumonia (acute) (Alpenstich) (benign) (bilateral) (brain) (cerebral) (circumscribed) (congestive) (creeping) (delayed resolution) (double) (epidemic) (fever) (flash) (fulminant) (fungoid) (granulomatous) (hemorrhagic) (incipient) (infantile) (infectious) (infiltration) (insular) (intermittent) (latent) (lobe) (migratory) (newborn) (organized) (overwhelming) (primary) (progressive) (pseudolobar) (purulent) (resolved) (secondary) (senile) (septic) (suppurative) (terminal) (true) (unresolved) (vesicular) **486**

EXAMPLE:
    1. Mike Rogers was seen by Dr. Moore and diagnosed with congestive pneumonia. The appropriate code assignment is 486. ("Congestive" is a nonessential modifier.)

    2. Cindy Stevens was seen by Dr. Smith and diagnosed with pneumonia. The appropriate code assignment is 486. (Nonessential modifier is not stated.)

In the preceding patient examples, the presence or absence of a nonessential modifier in the diagnostic statement did not affect the code that was selected.

Exercise 1.5

Using the Alphabetic Index only, underline the term that is the nonessential modifier in each of the following diagnostic statements and then assign a code to each condition:

1. Congenital distortion of chest wall _756.3_

2. Ruptured diverticula of cecum _562.10_

3. Bleeding external hemorrhoids of rectum _455.5_

4. Surgical menopausal syndrome _627.4_

5. Acute urethritis _597.80_

Eponyms

Many diseases and operations carry the name of a person, or an eponym. An eponym is defined by *Stedman's Medical Dictionary* as: "The name of a disease, structure, operation, or procedure, usually derived from the name of the person who discovered or described it first" (Stedman 2000, 611). The main terms for eponyms are located in the Alphabetic Index as follows:

1. Under the eponym itself

> **Alzheimer's**
>   disease or sclerosis 331.0

2. Under main terms such as disease, syndrome, and disorder

> **Disease . . .**
>   Alzheimer's—*see* Alzheimer's

3. With description of the disease or syndrome, usually enclosed in parentheses, but sometimes following the eponym

> **Chiari's**
>   disease or syndrome (hepatic vein thrombosis) 453.0

Exercise 1.6

Using the Alphabetic Index only, assign codes to the following:

1. Briquet's disorder

    _____300.81_____

2. Lou Gehrig's disease

    _____335.20_____

3. Stokes-Adams syndrome

    _____426.9_____

4. Sprengel's deformity

    _____755.52_____

5. Erb's disease

    _____359.1_____

Terms Not Listed in the Tabular List

Occasionally, a diagnostic or procedure term located in the Alphabetic Index is not included in the Tabular List. In these situations, only similar terms are listed and the guidance of the Alphabetic Index should be trusted.

EXAMPLE: The condition *listlessness* is included in the Alphabetic Index with a code assignment of 780.79. In reviewing the Tabular List to verify the accuracy of the code, the following is noted:

780.7	**Malaise and fatigue**
Excludes:	*debility, unspecified (799.3)*
	fatigue (during):
	combat (308.0–308.9)
	heat (992.6)
	pregnancy (646.8)
	neurasthenia (300.5)
	senile asthenia (797)
780.71	**Chronic fatigue syndrome**
780.79	**Other malaise and fatigue**
	Asthenia NOS
	Lethargy
	Postviral (asthenic) syndrome
	Tiredness

Although the Alphabetic Index assigns 780.79 as the code for listlessness, that particular term is not included in the Tabular List description, but similar terms are given. Always trust the guidance of the Alphabetic Index in such cases.

Index Tables

The following main entries in the Alphabetic Index to Diseases have subterms arranged in tables:

- Hypertension
- Neoplasm

Using tables for these terms simplifies access to complex combinations of subterms. These index tables are discussed in detail in other chapters of this book.

Conventions in ICD-9-CM

To assign diagnostic and procedure codes accurately, a thorough understanding of ICD-9-CM conventions is necessary. All three volumes of ICD-9-CM adhere to most of the conventions addressed next, with the exception of volume 3 where slight variations occur. (Chapter 2 in *Basic ICD-9-CM Coding* discusses these variations.)

Cross-Reference Terms

Cross-references are used in the Alphabetic Index as directions to look elsewhere in the code-book before assigning a code. Three types of cross-reference terms appear in the Alphabetic Index: *see, see also,* and *see category.*

See

The *see* cross-reference points to an alternative term. This mandatory instruction must be followed to ensure accurate ICD-9-CM code assignment.

> **Hemorrhage . . .**
>   ulcer—*see* Ulcer, by site, with hemorrhage

In the preceding example, a code cannot be assigned until the instruction that has been provided is followed. The codes under the main term "Ulcer" must be reviewed.

Often the cross-reference *see* is found under the anatomical site, directing the coder to the condition or disease affecting that site.

> **Aorta, aortic**—*see* condition

In the preceding example, the main term "Aorta" offers the instruction to "*see* condition." Therefore, a condition affecting the aorta, such as arteriosclerosis, should be sought out. The *see* instruction also is used when a condition is indexed under more than one main term.

> **Metrorrhexis**—*see* Rupture, uterus

In the preceding example, the direction is to "*see* Rupture, uterus," for a listing of codes.

See Also

The second type of cross-reference direction is *see also*. This instruction requires the review of another main term in the index if all the needed information cannot be found under the first main term.

EXAMPLE: Patient's diagnosis is osteoarthritis, localized to the hip.

Osteoarthritis (*see also* Osteoarthrosis) 715.9
　　distal interphalangeal 715.9
　　hyperplastic 731.2
　　interspinalis (*see also* Spondylosis) 721.90
　　spine, spinal NEC (*see also* Spondylosis) 721.90
Osteoarthrosis (degenerative) (hypertrophic)
　　　(rheumatoid) 715.9

> *Note — Use the following fifth-digit subclassification with category 715:*
>
> *0　site unspecified*
> *1　shoulder region*
> *2　upper arm*
> *3　forearm*
> *4　hand*
> *5　pelvic region and thigh*
> *6　lower leg*
> *7　ankle and foot*
> *8　other specified sites except spine*
> *9　multiple sites*

　　deformans alkaptonuria 270.2
　　generalized 715.09
　　juvenilis (Kohler's) 732.5
　　localized 715.3

In the preceding example, the coder is instructed to "*see also* Osteoarthrosis." But first, the subterms under osteoarthritis would have to be reviewed to find an entry titled "localized." If that subterm were found, the code provided after it would be assigned. When the subterm is not found—as is the case in the preceding example—the next step is to turn to the main term "Osteoarthrosis" in the index and review its subterms to find an entry of "localized." When that entry is found, code 715.3 can be selected. The boxed note appearing under the main term "Osteoarthrosis" reminds the coder that a fifth digit is required. The final code assignment is 715.35.

See Category

The *see category* is the least-used cross-reference in the Alphabetic Index. It is an instruction to consult a specific category in volume 1 (Tabular List).

> Late—*see also* condition
>   effect(s) (of)—*see also* condition
>   abscess
>   intracranial or intraspinal (conditions
>   classifiable to 324)—*see* category 326

The *see category* instruction in the preceding example refers to category 326, which provides additional information on the coding of late effects of intracranial abscess or pyogenic infection.

Exercise 1.7

Review each diagnostic statement and underline the appropriate main term. Locate the main term in the Alphabetic Index and follow all cross-references. Confirm the code in the Tabular List and enter it on the line provided.

1. Acute <u>endomyometritis</u>

    _____615.0_____

2. <u>Metrorrhexis</u>, nontraumatic

    _____621.8_____

3. Localized <u>osteoarthritis</u>, shoulder

    _____715.31_____

4. Cervical <u>intervertebral disc</u> prolapse

?   _____722.71_____722.0_____

5. <u>Stenosis</u> of endocervical os

    _____622.4_____

Instructional Notations

Occasionally, instructional notations appear throughout the Tabular List to clarify information or provide additional information. The following subsections describe the various types of instructional notes.

Includes Notes

Inclusion (or includes) notes are used throughout the Tabular List to further define or provide an example of a category or section. The conditions may be synonyms or similar conditions that may be classifiable to the same code. It is important to note that inclusion notes are not exhaustive; that is, not every synonym or similar condition may be listed. The notes usually list other common phrases used to describe the same condition.

Inclusion notes can appear at the beginning of a chapter or section, or directly below a category or subcategory code.

At the beginning of a chapter or section: The instructions apply to all the codes within that chapter or section.

The following inclusion note appears at the beginning of a chapter:

> ## INFECTIOUS AND PARASITIC DISEASES (001–139)
> Includes: diseases generally recognized as communicable or transmissible
>   as well as a few diseases of unknown, but possibly infectious, origin

The following inclusion note appears at the beginning of a section:

> ## ISCHEMIC HEART DISEASE (410–414)
> Includes: that with mention of hypertension

Directly below a category or a subcategory code: The instructions in the inclusion note apply to all codes within that range.

The following inclusion note appears below a category:

> **461   Acute sinusitis**
>
> Includes: abscess
>   empyema
>   infection   acute, of sinus
>   inflammation (accessory) (nasal)
>   suppuration

A point to remember: Because the inclusion note is not repeated, the coder must look back to the beginning of the subcategory, category, section, or chapter to ensure that important instructions are not missed.

Excludes Notes

The exclusion (or excludes) notes found in the Tabular List are hard to miss on review because the word *Excludes* appears in italicized print with a box around it. Exclusion notes can appear at the beginning of a chapter or section, or below a category, subcategory, or subclassification. Essentially, exclusion notes should be interpreted as a direction to code the particular condition listed elsewhere, usually with the code listed in the exclusion note.

Exclusion terms have three different meanings:

1. The most common exclusion note indicates that the code under consideration cannot be assigned if the associated condition specified in the exclusion note is present. Rather, the code specified in the exclusion note is assigned to fully identify the condition.

> **424.3   Pulmonary valve disorders**
>
>   Pulmonic: Pulmonic:
>   incompetence NOS   regurgitation NOS
>   insufficiency NOS   stenosis NOS
>
> | *Excludes:* | *that specified as rheumatic (397.1)*

The exclusion note indicates that code 397.1, rather than code 424.3, should be assigned if the pulmonary valve disorder is specified as rheumatic.

2. The second type of exclusion note indicates that the condition may have to be coded elsewhere. The etiology of the condition determines whether the code under review or the code suggested in the exclusion note should be assigned. One or the other code is used, but not both.

---

603   Hydrocele

Includes: hydrocele of spermatic cord, testis, or tunica vaginalis

Excludes: *congenital (778.6)*

The exclusion note indicates that a code from category 603, Hydrocele, should not be assigned if the hydrocele is congenital. Instead, code 778.6, Congenital hydrocele, is assigned.

3. The third type of exclusion note indicates that an additional code may be required to fully explain the condition. This note specifies conditions that are not included in the code under review. Should the condition specified in the exclusion note be present, the additional code should be assigned.

---

4. DISEASES OF THE BLOOD AND BLOOD-FORMING ORGANS (280–289)

Excludes: *anemia complicating pregnancy or the puerperium (648.2)*

The exclusion note indicates that two codes should be assigned to code an anemia that occurs during pregnancy or the puerperium: code 648.2x, Anemia in the mother classifiable elsewhere but complicating pregnancy, childbirth, or the puerperium, to indicate that the anemia is occurring during pregnancy; and a code from chapter 4, Diseases of the Blood and Blood-Forming Organs (280–289), to indicate the specific type of anemia.

Exercise 1.8

Answer the following questions:

1. Identify the site that is excluded from code 213.0.

    lower jaw bone

2. According to the inclusion note in category 555, what conditions are included in codes 555.0–555.9?

    Crohn's disease + Granulomatous enteritis

3. According to the exclusion note in category 558, what condition is assigned codes 009.2–009.3?

    Infectious

4. According to the inclusion note in category 056, what condition is included in codes 056.0–056.9?

    German measles

5. According to the exclusion note in category 056, what condition is assigned code 771.0?

    Congenital rubella

Notes

Notes appear in the Tabular List and the Alphabetic Index in all three volumes of ICD-9-CM. Some notes carry an instruction to assign a fifth digit.

---

831   Dislocation of shoulder

Excludes:	*sternoclavicular joint (839.61, 839.71)*
	sternum (839.61, 839.71)

The following fifth-digit subclassification is for use with category 831:

0   shoulder, unspecified
    Humerus NOS
1   anterior dislocation of humerus
2   posterior dislocation of humerus
3   inferior dislocation of humerus
4   acromioclavicular (joint)
    Clavicle
9   other
    Scapula

Other notes provide additional coding instruction and also define terms.

Injury 959.9

Note—For abrasion, insect bite (nonvenomous), blister, or scratch, see Injury, superficial.

For laceration, traumatic rupture, tear, or penetrating wound of internal organs, such as heart, lung, liver, kidney, pelvic organs, whether or not accompanied by open wound in the same region, see Injury, internal.

For nerve injury, see Injury, nerve.

For late effect of injuries, classifiable to 850–854, 860–869, 900–919, 950–959, see Late, effect, injury, by type.

---

326   Late effects of intracranial abscess or pyogenic infection

Note: This category is to be used to indicate conditions whose primary classification is to 320–325 [excluding 320.7, 321.0–321.8, 323.0–323.4, 323.6–323.7] as the cause of late effects, themselves classifiable elsewhere. The "late effects" include conditions specified as such, or as sequelae, which may occur at any time after the resolution of the causal condition.

Use additional code to identify condition, as:
    hydrocephalus (331.4)
    paralysis (342.0–342.9, 344.0–344.9)

765.0   Extreme immaturity

Note: Usually implies a birthweight of less than 1,000 grams. Use additional code for weeks of gestation (765.20–765.29).

A point to remember: The appearance of a note differs, depending on the volume of ICD-9-CM in which it is located. Alphabetic Index notes are boxed and set in italic type; Tabular List notes are located at various levels of the classification system and are not boxed.

Exercise 1.9

Use the Tabular List and Alphabetic Index to answer the following questions:

1. According to the note under code 766.0, what is considered an exceptionally large baby?

   A Birthweight of 4500 grams or more

2. What do the fifth digits in category 832 indicate?

   site of elbow dislocation

3. Use the Alphabetic Index and the note following the main term "Fracture" to answer this question: Is a greenstick fracture open or closed?

   closed

4. Turn to category 250, Diabetes mellitus. What is the appropriate fifth digit for uncontrolled type I diabetes?

   250.13

5. Use the Alphabetic Index and the note following the main term "Injury" to answer this question: What main term and subterm should be indexed to code the diagnosis of nonvenomous insect bite?

   Injury, superficial 919.4

Multiple Coding

In ICD-9-CM, it often is necessary to use more than one code number to fully identify a given condition. A diagnostic statement that includes phrases such as "due to," "secondary to," or "with" may require multiple codes. The coder should follow the directions in the Tabular List for the use of additional codes. The Alphabetic Index may refer the coder to a combination code through the use of connecting terms. When no combination codes are available, multiple codes should be assigned to fully describe the condition.

Mandatory Multiple Coding

Certain conditions require mandatory multiple coding. In such cases, one code describes the underlying condition (cause or etiology of the condition) and the other identifies the manifestation(s). Mandatory multiple coding is identified in the Alphabetic Index with the second code listed in brackets. The first code identifies the underlying condition, and the second code identifies the manifestations or other conditions that occur as a result of the underlying condition. In such cases, both codes must be assigned and sequenced in the order listed in the Alphabetic Index.

In the Tabular List, mandatory multiple coding is indicated by the phrase "use additional code" and the code for the underlying condition. The manifestation code acknowledges the need for multiple codes with the phrase "code first underlying condition." The manifestation codes and the titles are listed in italic print. The codes in italic print can never be designated as principal diagnoses and always require a code for the underlying condition to be listed first.

Indiscriminate Multiple Coding

Multiple codes should not be used to code irrelevant medical information, such as certain signs and symptoms that are integral to a condition. The signs and symptoms that are characteristic of an illness are not coded when the causes of the signs or symptoms are known. For example, abdominal pain is integral to acute appendicitis and thus is not coded.

Indiscriminate coding of conditions listed in diagnostic test reports should be avoided. When a laboratory test, x-ray, EKG (electrocardiogram), or other diagnostic test includes a finding, that condition is not coded unless the diagnosis is confirmed by the physician.

Coders should follow the Uniform Hospital Discharge Data Set (UHDDS) criteria when reporting additional diagnoses. Often diagnostic reports mention conditions such as atelectasis, hiatal hernias, or nonspecific cardiac arrhythmias with no other information in the record as to treatment or evaluation. Assigning a code for such conditions would be inappropriate without first consulting with the physician.

Finally, coding both an unspecified and a specified type of condition is usually not done to describe the same general condition. For example, a patient with chronic maxillary sinusitis would not be identified with both codes 473.0, Chronic sinusitis, maxillary, and 473.9, Unspecified sinusitis (chronic). Code 473.0 is more specific, fully describing the patient's condition, and should be assigned.

Use Additional Code

The instructional notation "Use additional code" is found in the Tabular List of ICD-9-CM. This notation indicates that use of an additional code may provide a more complete picture of the diagnosis or procedure. The additional code should always be assigned if the health record provides supportive documentation.

If this instruction appears at the beginning of a chapter, it applies to all the codes in that chapter.

---

8. DISEASES OF THE RESPIRATORY SYSTEM (460–519)

Use additional code to identify infectious organism.

Sometimes it appears at the beginning of a section.

INFLAMMATORY DISEASE OF FEMALE PELVIC ORGANS (614–616)

Use additional code to identify organism such as Staphylococcus (041.1),
    or Streptococcus (041.0).

Finally, it also may appear in a subcategory.

530.2 **Ulcer of esophagus**

Ulcer of esophagus: Ulcer of esophagus due to ingestion of:
    fungal   aspirin
    peptic   chemicals
                            medicines

Use additional E code to identify cause, if induced by chemical or drug

---

Code First Underlying Disease

The instruction "Code first underlying disease" is found in the Tabular List for categories in which primary tabulation is not intended. (See the subsection on mandatory multiple coding.) The code, title, and instructions are set in italic type to serve as a red flag not to assign that code as a principal diagnosis. The note requires listing, first, the code for the underlying disease (etiology) and, second, the code for the manifestation. Though the note will suggest underlying diseases in most instances, it is not all-inclusive because the physician may identify other causes not included in the list.

366.4 **Cataract associated with other disorders**

366.41 *Diabetic cataract*
    Code first diabetes (250.5)
366.42 *Tetanic cataract*
    Code first underlying disease, as:
        calcinosis (275.4)
        hypoparathyroidism (252.1)
366.43 *Myotonic cataract*
    Code first underlying disorder (359.2)
366.44 *Cataract associated with other syndromes*
    Code first underlying condition, as:
        craniofacial dysostosis (756.0)
        galactosemia (271.1)
366.45 **Toxic cataract**
    Drug-induced cataract
    Use additional E code to identify drug or other
        toxic substance
366.46 **Cataract associated with radiation and other**
    physical influences
    Use additional E code to identify cause

Connecting Words

Connecting words are subterms that indicate a relationship between the main term and an associated condition or etiology in the Alphabetic Index. Following are examples of these subterms:

Associated with	During	Secondary to
Complicated (by)	Following	With
Due to	In	With mention of
Of	Without	

A point to remember: The connecting words "with" and "without" are sequenced before all other subterms. Other connecting words are listed in alphabetical order.

ICD-9-CM assumes a causal relationship between some combinations of conditions, even though the diagnostic statement may not make such a distinction.

> **EXAMPLE:** Mitral valve stenosis is assumed to be rheumatic in origin and is assigned code 394.0, Mitral stenosis, from the chronic rheumatic heart disease section.

For cases where conditions often occur together, ICD-9-CM developed combination codes to identify both the etiology and the manifestation.

> **EXAMPLE:** Streptococcal infection occurs often in the throat resulting in streptococcal sore throat. Therefore, code 034.0, Streptococcal sore throat, incorporates both the underlying disease, the streptococcal infection, and the manifestation—the sore throat.

Exercise 1.10

Using the Tabular List and Alphabetic Index, assign codes to the following:

1. Bleeding esophageal varices in liver cirrhosis

   _571.5, 456.20_

2. Urinary tract infection due to Escherichia coli

   _599.0, 041.4_

3. Acute duodenal ulcer with hemorrhage and obstruction

   _532.01_

4. Anemia of prematurity

   _776.6_

5. Rheumatic chorea without mention of heart involvement

   _392.9_

Symbols, Punctuation, and Abbreviations

ICD-9-CM uses numerous symbols, punctuation marks, and abbreviations to facilitate the coding process.

Abbreviations

Two abbreviations are used in ICD-9-CM:

- NEC: Not elsewhere classifiable

- NOS: Not otherwise specified

NEC: Not Elsewhere Classifiable

NEC serves two purposes. First, it can be used with ill-defined terms listed in the Tabular List to warn the user that specified forms of the condition are classified differently. The codes given for such terms should be used only if more precise information is unavailable.

459.0   Hemorrhage, unspecified
Rupture of blood vessel, not otherwise specified (NOS)
Spontaneous hemorrhage, not elsewhere classified (NEC)

Excludes:	*hemorrhage:*

gastrointestinal NOS (578.9)
in newborn NOS (772.9)
secondary or recurrent following trauma (958.2)
traumatic rupture of blood vessel (900.0–904.9)

The material in the preceding example advises to assign code 459.0 only if no other information is available. Furthermore, the exclusion note indicates that other forms of hemorrhage, such as gastrointestinal hemorrhage, NOS (578.9), are classified elsewhere.

Second, NEC can be used with terms for which a more specific code is unavailable, even though the diagnostic statement is very specific.

008.67   Enteritis due to Enterovirus NEC
Coxsackie virus
Echovirus

Excludes:	*poliovirus (045.0–045.9)*

In this example, code 008.67 is reported even if a specific enterovirus such as echovirus has been identified because ICD-9-CM does not provide a specific code for it.

NOS: Not Otherwise Specified

NOS is the equivalent of "unspecified." It is used only in the Tabular Lists for both diseases and procedures. Codes describing "not otherwise specified" conditions or procedures are assigned only when the diagnostic or procedural statement, as well as the health record, does not provide enough information.

382.9   Unspecified otitis media
Otitis media:
NOS
acute NOS
chronic NOS

In the preceding example, code 382.9 is the appropriate code assignment because the diagnostic statement and/or the health record lack(s) additional information, such as purulent or serous.

Symbols

The official ICD-9-CM uses two symbols:

§   Section Mark

□   Lozenge

Section Mark §

In ICD-9-CM, a section mark symbol precedes codes in the Tabular Lists of both procedures and diseases. It indicates the presence of a footnote at the bottom of the page or references an instructional note located earlier in the section. A section mark symbol preceding a category applies to all subdivisions in that category.

---

§656   **Other fetal and placental problems affecting management of mother**

The section mark symbol preceding category 656 indicates that a footnote with an instruction to assign fifth digits printed on a previous page can be found at the bottom of the page.

A point to remember: Some publishers of ICD-9-CM have elected not to use the section mark symbol in their versions of the official coding manual, opting instead for some other symbol as an alert of special instructions.

Lozenge □

Found immediately preceding a four-digit code in volume 1, the lozenge symbol identifies the code as unique to the clinical modification of ICD-9 (or ICD-9-CM, the system used in the United States). However, this symbol does not correlate directly with ICD-9. Although researchers may find this information helpful, coders ignore it because it has no significance to their tasks. Many publishers of ICD-9-CM codebooks have eliminated this symbol from their editions.

---

§851   **Cerebral laceration and contusion**

    □ **851.0 Cortex (cerebral) contusion without mention of open intracranial wound**

    □ **851.1 Cortex (cerebral) contusion with open intracranial wound**

    □ **851.2 Cortex (cerebral) laceration without mention of open intracranial wound**

    □ **851.3 Cortex (cerebral) laceration with open intracranial wound**

    □ **851.4 Cerebellar or brain stem contusion without mention of open intracranial wound**

    □ **851.5 Cerebellar or brain stem contusion with open intracranial wound**

    □ **851.6 Cerebellar or brain stem laceration without mention of open intracranial wound**

    □ **851.7 Cerebellar or brain stem laceration with open intracranial wound**

    □ **851.8 Other and unspecified cerebral laceration and contusion, without mention of open intracranial wound**

    □ **851.9 Other and unspecified cerebral laceration and contusion, with open intracranial wound**

Punctuation Marks

ICD-9-CM contains five punctuation marks with specialized meanings.

A point to remember: Some publishers of ICD-9-CM have elected not to use certain punctuation marks.

Parentheses ( )

Parentheses enclose supplementary words or explanatory information that may or may not be present in the statement of a diagnosis or procedure. They do not affect the code number assigned to the case. Terms in parentheses are considered nonessential modifiers, and all three volumes of ICD-9-CM use them.

---

494   Bronchiectasis
      Bronchiectasis (fusiform) (postinfectious) (recurrent)
      Bronchiolectasis

      | *Excludes:* | *congenital (748.61)*
                        tuberculous bronchiectasis
                           (current disease) (011.5)

In the preceding example, category 494 includes three nonessential modifiers enclosed in parentheses: fusiform, postinfectious, and recurrent. The presence or absence of these modifiers in the diagnostic statement has no bearing on the assignment of code 494.

Square Brackets [ ]

Square brackets are used to enclose synonyms, alternative wordings, abbreviations, and explanatory phrases. In effect, they are similar to parentheses in that they are not required as part of the diagnostic or procedural statement. Square brackets are used for both diseases and procedures, but only in the Tabular Lists.

427.0   Paroxysmal supraventricular tachycardia
      Paroxysmal tachycardia:
         atrial [PAT]
         atrioventricular [AV]
         junctional
            nodal

Because they are abbreviations, PAT (paroxysmal atrial tachycardia) and AV (atrioventricular) are enclosed in brackets.

---

460   Acute nasopharyngitis [common cold]
      Coryza (acute)
      Nasal catarrh, acute
      Nasopharyngitis:
         NOS
         Acute
         Infective, NOS
      Rhinitis:
         acute
         infective

In the preceding example, the phrase "common cold" is a synonym for acute nasopharyngitis and is enclosed in brackets.

Slanted Brackets [ ]

Slanted, or italicized, brackets are found only in the Alphabetic Index. They enclose a code number that must be used in conjunction with a code immediately preceding it. Thus, the code in the slanted brackets is always sequenced second.

In the Alphabetic Index to Diseases, the first code represents the underlying condition and the second code, enclosed in italicized brackets, is the manifestation.

Retinitis (*see also* Chorioretinitis) 363.20
    diabetic 250.5 *[362.01]*

The sequencing of the preceding example is as follows:

250.5x   Diabetes with ophthalmic manifestations
362.01   Background diabetic retinopathy

Colon :

The colon is used in the Tabular List after an incomplete term that needs one or more modifiers in order to be assigned to a given category or code.

---

204 Lymphoid leukemia
    Includes: leukemia: leukemia:
                    lymphatic   lymphocytic
                    lymphoblastic   lymphogenous

In the preceding example, the colon indicates that the type of leukemia must be lymphatic, lymphoblastic, lymphocytic, or lymphogenous to be assigned a code from category 204.

Brace }

Braces simplify tabular entries and save printing space by reducing repetitive wording. They connect a series of terms on the left or right with a statement on the other side of the brace. A term from the left must be associated with the term on the right before the code under consideration can be assigned.

INTERNAL INJURY OF THORAX, ABDOMEN, AND PELVIS (860–869)

Includes: blast injuries
                blunt trauma
                bruise
                concussion injuries
                    (except cerebral)
                crushing   } of internal organs
                hematoma
                laceration
                puncture
                tear
                traumatic rupture

Without the brace, the narrative would take up space and prove hard to read, as shown below:

blast injuries of internal organs
blunt trauma of internal organs
bruise of internal organs
concussion injuries (except cerebral) of internal organs,
and so forth

Exercise 1.11

Using the Tabular List and Alphabetic Index, assign codes to the following:

1. Anterolateral wall myocardial infarction, initial episode

   _410.01_

2. Angiodysplasia of stomach and duodenum, no hemorrhage noted

   _537.82_

3. Tuberculous iritis

   _017.30, 364.11_

4. Primary malignant neoplasm of the spleen

   _159.1_

5. Fifth disease

   _057.0_

Basic Steps in ICD-9-CM Coding

To code each disease or condition completely and accurately, the coder should:

1. Identify all main terms included in the diagnostic statement.

2. Locate each main term in the Alphabetic Index.

3. Refer to any subterms indented under the main term. The subterms form individual line entries and describe essential differences by site, etiology, or clinical type.

4. Follow cross-reference instructions if the needed code is not located under the first main entry consulted.

5. Verify the code selected in the Tabular List.

6. Read and be guided by any instructional terms in the Tabular List.

7. Assign codes to their highest level of specificity.

   —Assign three-digit codes only when no four-digit codes appear within the category.

   —Assign a fifth digit for any subcategory where a fifth-digit subclassification is provided.

8. Continue coding the diagnostic statement until all the component elements are fully identified.

Review Exercise: Chapter 1

Using the instructions and conventions introduced in chapter 1, assign the appropriate codes to the following:

1. Acute appendicitis with perforation

   _540.0_

2. Streptococcal pneumonia

   _482.30_

3. Chest pain, originating in chest wall

   _786.52_

4. Acute cor pulmonale

   _415.0_

5. Osteoarthrosis, localized, primary of ankle

   _715.17_

6. Toxic nodular goiter with crisis

   _242.31_

7. Extra thyroid gland

   _759.2_

   7 Email

8. Angiodysplasia of the colon with hemorrhage

   _569.85_   _596.85_

9. Acute tracheobronchitis with bronchospasm

   _466.0_

10. Arteriosclerotic heart disease of native coronary artery with angina

    _414.01, 413.9_

11. Nephrotic syndrome secondary to systemic lupus erythematosus

    _710.0, 581.81_

12. Prenatal care, normal first pregnancy

    _V22.0_

13. Comminuted fracture of femur involving the subtrochanteric section

    _820.22_

14. Prostatitis due to Trichomonas

    _131.03_

15. Carotid artery occlusion with cerebral infarction; essential hypertension

    _433.11 401.9_

Chapter 2

Procedures

Volume 3

ICD-9-CM classifies procedures in volume 3, which includes both an Alphabetic Index and a Tabular List. The classification of procedures in volume 3 follows much of the same format, organization, and conventions as the classification of diseases in volumes 1 and 2 of ICD-9-CM. The few variations are discussed in this chapter. Specific procedures are discussed in other chapters of this book.

ICD-9-CM procedure classification is used to code hospital inpatient procedures. Hospital inpatient procedures are consistently coded when performed in the range of procedure code categories 00–86. ICD-9-CM, Volume 3, chapter 16, Miscellaneous Diagnostic and Therapeutic Procedures (87–99), may be used selectively for inpatient procedure coding. For example, subcategory 88.5, Angiocardiography using contrast material, would definitely be assigned when the procedure was performed on an inpatient. However, Diagnostic ultrasound, subcategory 88.7, is less likely to be used for any inpatient coding. Because facility policies may vary, coders should follow the hospital or facility coding policy concerning the coding of procedures in categories 87–99 for miscellaneous diagnostic and therapeutic procedures for inpatient services.

Hospital outpatient departments and other ambulatory facilities are required to use *Current Procedural Terminology, Fourth Edition (CPT)*, as well as *Healthcare Common Procedure Coding System (HCPCS)* to code outpatient procedures. Likewise, physician practices are required to use CPT and HCPCS to report services and procedures. Because of this fact, publishers of ICD-9-CM market books with only volumes 1 and 2 to physician practices.

Tabular List

Volume 3 contains the following seventeen chapters:

	Chapter Titles	Categories
0.	Procedures and Interventions, Not Elsewhere Classified	00
1.	Operations on the Nervous System	01–05
2.	Operations on the Endocrine System	06–07
3.	Operations on the Eye	08–16
4.	Operations on the Ear	18–20
5.	Operations on the Nose, Mouth, and Pharynx	21–29
6.	Operations on the Respiratory System	30–34

Almost all the chapters classify data by anatomical system. Chapter 13 classifies procedures performed for obstetrical purposes, and chapter 16 classifies diagnostic and therapeutic procedures that are not generally considered surgical in nature. A chapter was added to volume 3, effective October 1, 2002, titled Procedures and Interventions, Not Elsewhere Classified. Codes begin with digits 00 in this chapter, which is intended to capture new technology. This category includes the following subcategories:

- 00.0, Therapeutic ultrasound

- 00.1, Pharmaceuticals

- 00.4, Adjunct vascular system procedures

- 00.5, Other cardiovascular procedures

Format of the Tabular List

Volume 3 of ICD-9-CM uses numeric codes only. Procedure codes consist of three or four digits, with two digits preceding a decimal point and one or two following it. Three-digit codes cannot be used if four-digit codes are available. The third and fourth digits provide further information about the site, procedure, or diagnosis.

---

53 Repair of hernia
Code also any application or administration
   of an adhesion barrier substance (99.77)
   Includes: hernioplasty
               herniorrhaphy
               herniotomy

   Excludes: *manual reduction of hernia (96.27)*

   53.0 Unilateral repair of inguinal hernia
   53.00 Unilateral repair of inguinal hernia, not otherwise specified
         Inguinal herniorrhaphy NOS
   53.01 Repair of direct inguinal hernia
   53.02 Repair of indirect inguinal hernia
   53.03 Repair of direct inguinal hernia with graft or prosthesis
   53.04 Repair of indirect inguinal hernia with graft or prosthesis
   53.05 Repair of inguinal hernia with graft or prosthesis, not otherwise specified

---

In the preceding example, repair of hernia is assigned to category 53. At the third-digit level, the codes describe whether the hernia repair was unilateral or bilateral. At the fourth-digit level, they describe the clinical type of hernia, direct or indirect.

Alphabetic Index

The Alphabetic Index to Procedures contains a listing of procedures, studies, tests, operations, surgeries, therapies, and so forth. It contains many procedures that the text of the Tabular List may not include.

A point to remember: Always trust the Alphabetic Index. The terms listed in the Tabular List are examples of the contents of the category, whereas the entries in the Alphabetic Index are much more comprehensive.

> **EXAMPLE:**   In Tabular List—**93.53 Application of other cast**
> In Alphabetic Index—**Application**
>   Unna's paste boot 93.53

By trusting the Alphabetic Index, code 93.53 is assigned for Unna's paste boot because the narrative of the code in the Tabular List does not include Unna's paste boot.

Main Terms

The structure of the Alphabetic Index to Procedures is similar to that of the Alphabetic Index to Diseases. The main terms are set in boldface type and identify the type of procedure performed, with the subterms indented in alphabetical order.

Main terms can include:

- Operations, such as cholecystectomy, duodenostomy, Dorrance operation

- Procedures or tests, such as bronchogram, audiometry, physical therapy, scan

- Nouns, such as examination, operation, pacemaker

- Verbs, such as clipping, cooling, repair

Exercise 2.1

Using the Alphabetic Index, underline the main term(s) in the following statements:

1. Anorectal myectomy

2. Bilateral repair of inguinal hernia

3. Removal of intrauterine contraceptive device

4. Transurethral biopsy of bladder

5. Dilation and curettage of uterus

6. Irwin operation   *Either*

7. Mohs' chemosurgery   *Either*

8. Chest wall suture,

9. Activities of daily living (ADL) training   *Either*

10. Stomach anastomosis takedown
          or

Subterms

The subterms listed under the main term in the Alphabetic Index have a definitive effect on the selection of the appropriate code for a given procedure. They form individual line entries and describe essential differences in site, diagnosis, or surgical technique. Subterms can be indented farther and farther to the right, with each indentation amounting to two spaces.

The appropriate main term should be located in the Alphabetic Index first, then the subterm that leads to the correct code. All entries must be verified in the Tabular List.

> **EXAMPLE:**   Removal . . .
>
>   prosthesis . . .
>
>   joint structures 80.00
>
>   ankle 80.07
>
>   elbow 80.02
>
>   foot and toe 80.08
>
>   hand and finger 80.04
>
>   hip 80.05
>
>   knee 80.06
>
>   shoulder 80.01
>
>   specified site NEC 80.09
>
>   spine 80.09
>
>   wrist 80.03

Connecting Words

Because they are considered connecting words, subterms beginning with the words *as*, *by*, and *with* immediately follow the main term or subterm, instead of appearing in the usual alphabetical sequence.

> **Laminectomy** (decompression) (for
>   exploration) 03.09
>   as operative approach—*omit code*
>   with
>   excision of herniated intervertebral
>   disc (nucleus pulposus) 80.51
>   excision of other intraspinal lesion
>   (tumor) 03.4
>   reopening of site 03.02

In this example, *as* and *with* are indented before the subterm "reopening of site," indicating that these terms are being used as connecting words.

Exercise 2.2

Assign procedure codes to the following:

1. Arthrodesis of ankle

    _81.11_

2. Percutaneous needle biopsy of breast

    _85.11_

3. Control of epistaxis by anterior nasal packing

    _21.01_

4. Myotomy of the hand with division

    _82.19_

5. Phlebectomy with thoracic graft replacement

    _38.45_

Eponyms

Surgical procedures that are identified by eponyms (named for their originators) are indexed in the following three ways:

1. Under the eponym

McDonald operation (encirclement suture, cervix) 67.59

2. Under the main term "Operation" or "Procedure"

Operation . . .
    McDonald (encirclement suture, cervix) 67.59

3. Under a main term or subterm describing the operation

Suture . . .
    cervix . . .
        internal os, encirclement 67.59

Exercise 2.3

Assign procedure codes to the following:

1. Marshall-Marchetti-Krantz operation

   _59.5_

2. Nissen's fundoplication

   _44.66_

3. Shirodkar operation

   _67.59_

4. Mayo operation—bunionectomy

   _77.59_

5. Maxillary sinusotomy, Caldwell-Luc approach

   _22.39_

ICD-9-CM Conventions in Volume 3

Most of the principles concerning ICD-9-CM conventions discussed in chapter 1 of *Basic ICD-9-CM Coding* also apply to volume 3 of ICD-9-CM. The few exceptions are discussed below.

Code Also

In volume 3, the phrase "code also" serves as a reminder to code additional procedures only when they have actually been performed. The instruction is used for two purposes:

1. To code each individual component of an operation or two procedures that are often performed together

> **46.2 Ileostomy**
> Code also any synchronous resection (45.34, 45.61–45.63)

In the above example, the "code also" statement serves as a reminder to assign an additional code for any synchronous resection performed in conjunction with an ileostomy.

> **13.5 Other extracapsular extraction of lens**
> Code also any synchronous insertion of pseudophakos (13.71)

This example directs the coder to assign a code for synchronous insertion of pseudophakos, along with the code for the extracapsular extraction of the lens.

2. To code the use of special adjunctive procedures or equipment

---

35.6   Repair of atrial and ventricular septa with tissue graft
Code also cardiopulmonary bypass [extracorporeal circulation]
[heart-lung machine] (39.61)

Again, in this example, the reminder is to code also cardiopulmonary bypass, if performed with repair of atrial and ventricular septa with tissue graft.

Effective with the changes for October 1, 2002, multiple references to "code also" have been added to the procedure section. The reference states: Code also any application or administration of an adhesion barrier substance (99.77).

The first mention is with category 03, Operations on spinal cord and spinal canal structures. There are multiple references throughout the abdominal surgery sections starting with category 41 and ending with 71.

New code 99.77, Application or administration of an adhesion barrier substance, was added to classify this technique. This barrier is used in the prevention of postoperative adhesions following procedures. The adhesion barrier is a temporary bioresorbable membrane used during the primary surgical procedure. It is used to reduce the incidence, extent, and severity of postoperative adhesions between organs, such as the abdominal wall and the underlying viscera (omentum, small bowel, bladder, and stomach), and between the uterus and surrounding structures (tubes and ovaries, large intestine, and bladder).

The procedure for placing the adhesion barrier prior to closure requires a significant change in operative technique. The product is customized to fit the desired application site, and once the application is prepared, it is necessary to retract the abdominal wall and organs from the desired site of application. The product is placed at the site of trauma, and the average procedure requires the preparation and placement of multiple adhesion barriers.

Omit Code and Coding Operative Approach

The convention *omit code* is found only in volume 3 of ICD-9-CM, in both the Tabular List and the Alphabetic Index. This instruction indicates that no code is to be assigned and usually applies to the following procedures:

- An exploratory procedure incidental to the procedure carried out

- The usual surgical approaches of a given procedure

- Blunt, digital, manual, or mechanical lysis of adhesions

- The closure portion of a procedure

Laparotomy   NEC 54.19
as operative approach—*omit code*
exploratory (pelvic) 54.11
reopening of recent operative site
(for control of hemorrhage) (for exploration) (for incision of hematoma) 54.12

The Alphabetic Index advises the coder to omit the code if the laparotomy is the operative approach or the surgical entry into the body. For example, in an open appendectomy, the laparotomy would not be assigned because it is the operative approach. The abdominal wall must be incised to perform the removal.

When a definitive procedure (therapeutic or diagnostic) is performed, the operative approach is considered part of the procedure and is not coded. The Alphabetic Index and Tabular List frequently indicate when a code should be omitted. However, some procedures that constitute an operative approach are listed in the Alphabetic Index or Tabular List without the instruction to omit code. In such cases, the coder's knowledge of operative techniques is essential. Regardless of the presence or lack of instruction, if the procedure itself serves as the operative approach, it is not coded. For example, the title of the procedure describes an exploratory laparotomy and an open cholecystectomy. Only the open cholecystectomy would be coded because the laparotomy is the approach and the exploration is incidental to the definitive procedure.

When only a diagnostic procedure is performed, the operative approach, such as opening a body cavity, is coded. For example, an exploratory thoracotomy is performed to remove a mediastinal tumor. On entering the cavity, the surgeon determines the tumor is far too extensive to remove. Instead, the surgeon takes a biopsy of the mediastinum and closes the incision. In this case, the exploratory thoracotomy is sequenced first, with an additional code for the open biopsy.

Codes for Procedures Involving a Laparoscope, Thoracoscope, or Endoscope

Numerous procedures that once required an incision into a cavity or a joint, typically referred to as open procedures, now are performed through a less invasive procedure. A laparoscope or thoracoscope allows the removal of organs or tissue through small incisions under videoscopic guidance. ICD-9-CM provides a unique code for some laparoscopic and thoracoscopic procedures. When a separate code is unavailable, the open procedure code is assigned. In this instance, no code is assigned for procedures using a laparoscope, thoracoscope, arthroscope, or laryngoscope.

If the laparoscopic approach is unsuccessful, the surgeon may elect to perform an open approach to complete the procedure. When the procedure is converted to an open approach, only the open approach is coded. The fact that the laparoscopic approach was first used is indicated by the supplementary V code, V64.41, Laparoscopic surgical procedure converted to open procedure. V codes are discussed in lesson 23 of this book. In the Alphabetic Index to Diseases, the main term "Conversion" is used to locate the code that describes the conversion of a laparoscopic procedure to an open procedure.

The main term "Endoscopy" may be used in the Alphabetic Index to locate a variety of endoscopic procedures. More precise terms describing endoscopic procedures also may be referenced, for example, bronchoscopy, colonoscopy, or cystoscopy. When an endoscope is passed through more than one body cavity, the code for the endoscope should identify the most distant site. For example, an esophagogastroduodenoscopy is assigned code 45.13, Other endoscopy of small intestine, to reflect the fact that the duodenum or small bowel was visualized.

Exercise 2.4

Assign procedure codes to the following:

1. Thoracotomy with total lobectomy of left lung

   _____32.4_____

2. Craniotomy with excision of meningeal cyst

   _____01.51_____

3. Partial resection of colon with end-to-end anastomosis

   _____45.79_____

4. Injection of cortisone into hip joint

   _____81.92, 99.23_____

5. Intracapsular extraction of lens by temporal inferior route with insertion of pseudophakos

   _____13.11_____13.71_____

6. Laparoscopic cholecystectomy

   _____51.23_____

7. Transpleural thoracoscopy

   _____34.21_____

8. Cystoscopy with biopsy

   _____57.33_____

9. Arthroscopy of knee

   _____80.26_____

10. Arthroscopic meniscectomy

   _____80.6_____

Slanted Brackets [ ]

The requirement to assign two codes for closely related procedures is indicated in the Alphabetic Index or the Tabular List by slanted brackets enclosing the second code. This convention means both codes must be used and sequenced as listed.

> **Aneurysmectomy** . . .
> with
> graft replacement (interposition) 38.40
> aorta (arch) (ascending) (descending thoracic)
> abdominal 38.44
> thoracic 38.45
> thoracoabdominal 38.45 [38.44]

Therefore, to fully describe a thoracoabdominal aneurysmectomy, code 38.45 is sequenced first, followed by code 38.44.

Coding Canceled Surgery or Procedure

If a surgical procedure was started, but not completed due to unforeseen circumstances, review the operative report carefully and code the procedure to the extent it was performed. For example:

- If a cavity or space was entered, assign a code describing the exploratory procedure for that site.

    EXAMPLE: Cholecystectomy canceled secondary to tachycardia after the abdomen was entered.

    The cholecystectomy is not coded because it was not performed; however, code 54.11, Exploratory laparotomy, is assigned to describe the extent of the procedure. Diagnostic codes include the reasons for the surgery and the tachycardia, and the appropriate V code for the canceled procedure.

    Although the procedure was not performed as planned, the principal diagnosis does not change. If the patient's diagnosis was acute cholecystitis with cholelithiasis, the diagnostic code assigned is 574.00.

- If an incision was made, assign a code describing the incision for that site.

    EXAMPLE: Patient admitted for cardiac catheterization. Upon incision into a vein in the upper limb, the patient experienced an anxiety attack and blood pressure became elevated. Procedure was canceled and rescheduled for a later time.

    Code 38.03, Incision of upper limb vessels, is assigned to describe the extent of the surgery.

- If a closed fracture reduction was attempted and aborted, no procedure code is available. Code V64.1, Surgical or other procedure not carried out because of contraindication, should be assigned as an additional diagnostic code. In the Alphabetic Index to Diseases, the main term used to locate the V64 code is "Procedure (surgical) not done."

- In some cases, a procedure is canceled before it begins. Often cancellation is due to contraindications such as infections or other illnesses. Other reasons for canceled surgery include unavailability of the surgeon, patient's decision, or malfunctioning equipment. As an additional diagnostic code, a code should be assigned from category V64, Persons encountering health services for specific procedures, not carried out.

    EXAMPLE: Patient is admitted to outpatient surgery department with hypertrophy of tonsils and adenoids and is scheduled for tonsillectomy and adenoidectomy. The nurse notes the patient has a runny nose and cough, and a diagnosis of upper respiratory infection is made. The physician cancels the surgery until the infection has cleared.

    The following codes are assigned: 474.10, Hypertrophy of tonsils with adenoids; 465.9, Acute upper respiratory infection; and V64.1, Surgical or other procedure not carried out because of contraindication. No procedure code is assigned.

Coding Incomplete Procedures

ICD-9-CM generally does not include codes for procedures that are not completed. The one exception is code 73.3, Failed forceps, in chapter 13, Obstetrical Procedures. When a planned procedure is started, but not completed, it is coded according to the following principles:

- When a cavity or space is entered, code exploration of the site.

- When an endoscopic approach is used, but the definitive procedure could not be carried out, code the endoscopy only.

- When only an incision is made, code the incision of the site.

- When the procedure does not involve an incision, no procedure code is assigned. Instead, a code from the V64 category is used to indicate why the planned procedure was not carried out.

> EXAMPLE: A patient was scheduled for a cholecystectomy, but shortly after the abdominal incision was made, the patient developed a severe bradycardia. The procedure was stopped and the incision closed.
>
> Only code 54.0, Incision of the abdominal wall, should be assigned.

> EXAMPLE: A patient was scheduled for a resection of a mediastinal tumor. After entering the thoracic cavity, the surgeon determined the tumor was unresectable.
>
> Only code 34.02, Exploratory thoracotomy, should be assigned.

> EXAMPLE: A patient was scheduled for a colonoscopic biopsy of a tumor in the large intestine. The tumor could not be reached with the colonoscope, and no biopsy was obtained.
>
> Only code 45.23, Colonoscopy, should be assigned.

Coding Failed Procedures

Some procedures are considered to have failed. This means that either not every objective of the procedure was secured or the procedure did not achieve the desired result. In such a situation, the procedure is coded as performed.

> EXAMPLE: A patient underwent a percutaneous coronary angioplasty for an occluded coronary artery. Immediately after the procedure, the coronary artery became occluded again.
>
> Because the procedure was performed, it should be coded 36.01, even though the desired result, an open coronary artery, was not achieved.

> EXAMPLE: A patient suffering from a severe epistaxis came to the emergency department. An anterior nasal packing was performed. A few hours later, the patient returned to the emergency department complaining that the hemorrhage had not stopped. The first packing was removed and another anterior nasal packing was performed.
>
> Both the first and second anterior packing should be coded 21.01, even though the first packing seemed to have failed to control the hemorrhage.

Codes for Biopsy with Extensive Surgical Procedure

When a biopsy is performed and then followed by a more extensive surgery, code the surgical procedure first, followed by the biopsy. Typically, these are open biopsies followed by definitive procedures. An open biopsy is performed by means of an incision with removal of tissue for microscopic examination. When an open biopsy is performed by incision, the incision is implicit in the code.

> **EXAMPLE:** Open biopsy of the breast with frozen section and unilateral radical mastectomy
>
> 85.45, Unilateral radical mastectomy
> 85.12, Open biopsy of breast

> **EXAMPLE:** Open biopsy of pancreas via laparotomy
>
> 52.12, Open biopsy of pancreas

Codes for Closed-Biopsy Procedure

A closed biopsy may be performed percutaneously, endoscopically, or through use of a needle. When a needle or percutaneous biopsy is performed via an open procedure, such as a laparotomy, code both the open procedure and the needle biopsy. Another type of closed biopsy is a brush biopsy. In a brush biopsy, tissue is removed by using a brush or bristle-type instrument to collect cells for cytological examination.

The following guidelines apply for coding endoscopic biopsies:

1. When ICD-9-CM provides one code to identify both the biopsy and the endoscopy, assign that code.

   > **EXAMPLE:** 45.16, Esophagogastroduodenoscopy [EGD] with closed biopsy

2. When ICD-9-CM does not provide a code to identify both the biopsy and the endoscopy, assign two separate codes. The principal procedure is the endoscopy code.

   > **EXAMPLE:** 34.22, Mediastinoscopy
   >
   > 34.25, Closed [percutaneous] [needle] biopsy of mediastinum

Bilateral Procedure Coding

In some cases, ICD-9-CM provides a single code to identify that a bilateral procedure was performed. In these cases, that code is listed only once.

> **EXAMPLE:** 53.10, Bilateral inguinal hernia repair

When the same procedure is performed bilaterally, and ICD-9-CM does not identify it as being performed bilaterally, assign the code of the procedure twice.

> **EXAMPLE:** 79.04 and 79.04, Closed reduction of two finger fractures

HIPAA Standard Code Sets

HIPAA is the acronym for the Health Insurance Portability and Accountability Act of 1996. The Administrative Simplification provisions of HIPAA require the Department of Health and Human Services to establish national standards for electronic healthcare transactions and national identifiers for providers, health plans, and employers. Part of this requirement is the designation of code sets for the reporting of diagnoses and procedures on health claims. A code set means any set of codes used to encode data elements, such as medical diagnostic codes or medical procedure codes. A code set includes the codes and the descriptors of the codes. The rules of the law concerning code sets are found in 45 CFR, part 162, Administrative Requirements, Subpart J-Code Sets, sections 162.1000, 162.1002, and 162.1011.

The Transactions and Code Sets regulations state that ICD-9-CM procedure codes are the adopted standard code set for hospital inpatient services. *Healthcare Common Procedure Coding System (HCPCS)* with *Current Procedural Terminology, Fourth Edition (CPT-4)*, was designated as the code set for reporting procedures performed by physicians and for procedures performed in other healthcare settings, including hospital outpatient departments.

As of October 2003, hospitals were required to be HIPAA compliant by reporting ICD-9-CM procedure codes for hospital inpatient procedures only. The ICD-9-CM procedure codes were not named as a HIPAA standard for procedures in other settings such as hospital outpatient services or other types of ambulatory services. Hospitals may capture the ICD-9-CM procedure codes for internally tracking or monitoring hospital outpatient services; but when conducting standard transactions, hospitals must use HCPCS/CPT codes to report outpatient services at the service-line level and at the claim level on the uniform bill (UB-92) claim form. In other words, ICD-9-CM procedure codes should not appear on a hospital UB-92 claim form to report outpatient procedures performed. If the hospital wants to continue to assign ICD-9-CM procedure codes for all patients, inpatients and outpatients, the hospital must have a mechanism in place to remove the ICD-9-CM procedure codes from the UB-92 claim form prior to submitting it to the insurance or other payer.

Selection of Principal and Secondary Procedure Codes

The Uniform Hospital Discharge Data Set (UHDDS) requires that all significant procedures be reported. The principal procedure is defined as "that which was performed for definitive treatment rather than for diagnostic or exploratory purposes or for treatment of a complication." When more than one procedure meets the criteria for principal procedure, the one most closely related to the principal diagnosis should be selected.

Additional significant procedures also should be coded, including those that are surgical in nature, as well as those that carry a procedural or anesthetic risk or that require specialized training. The Uniform Bill-92 (UB-92) provides space for six procedures to be reported with ICD-9-CM codes. When the patient has more than six procedures performed, all the therapeutic procedures, especially those related to the principal diagnosis or secondary diagnoses, should be reported. Other diagnostic or nonsurgical procedures may be reported as space permits, according to hospital coding policies.

Basic Instructions for Procedural Coding

To code procedures performed for a patient completely and accurately, the coder must:

1. Identify all main terms included in the procedural statement.

2. Locate each main term in the Alphabetic Index.

3. Refer to any subterms indented under the main term.

4. Follow cross-reference instructions when the needed code is not located under the first main entry consulted.

5. Verify the code selected from the index in the Tabular List.

6. Read and be guided by any instructional terms in the Tabular List.

7. Continue coding the procedural statement until all the component elements are fully identified.

A point to remember: Each healthcare facility should specify in its coding policies the procedures that will be assigned codes in that particular facility. Some healthcare facilities do not assign codes to many diagnostic and nonsurgical procedures, such as radiology procedures, cardiovascular monitoring, blood transfusions, and suture removal.

Additional Exercises

Additional exercises for coding surgical and other procedures can be found in other chapters in this book. Chapters 9–16, 19, 20, 23, and the self-test contain other procedural statements to be coded with answers found within the respective answer key.

Review Exercise: Chapter 2

Assign procedure codes and diagnosis codes (when applicable) to the following:

1. Ventral herniorrhaphy canceled after beginning laparotomy

   54.11

2. Appendectomy with drainage of appendiceal abscess

   47.09

3. Removal of leg cast

   97.88

4. Alcoholism counseling

   94.46

5. Coronary artery bypass graft of three coronary arteries with cardiopulmonary bypass

   36.13   39.61

6. Esophagoscopy with removal of chicken bone   ?

   42.23   98.02

7. Colostomy takedown

   46.52

8. Surgical removal of impacted tooth

   23.19

9. Open biopsy of liver via laparotomy

   50.12

10. Gill arthrodesis, shoulder

    81.23

11. Ovarian cyst; oophorectomy planned, but canceled due to patient's upper respiratory infection

    620.2 , 465.9, V64.1

12. Open reduction of femur fracture with internal fixation

    79.35

13. Tarsoplasty with skin graft

    08.61

14. Turbinectomy with frontal and maxillary sinusectomy   22.42, 22.62

    22.60, 22.42

15. Percutaneous biopsy of the prostate

    60.11

Chapter 3

Introduction to the Prospective Payment System and the Uniform Hospital Discharge Data Set

Uniform Hospital Discharge Data Set

The Uniform Hospital Discharge Data Set (UHDDS) was promulgated by the U.S. Department of Health, Education, and Welfare in 1974 as a minimum, common core of data on individual acute care, short-term hospital discharges in Medicare and Medicaid programs. It sought to improve the uniformity and comparability of hospital discharge data.

In 1985, the data set was revised to improve the original version in light of timely needs and developments. These data elements and their definitions can be found in the July 31, 1985 *Federal Register* (Vol. 50, No. 147), pp.31038–31040. Since that time, the application of the UHDDS definitions has been expanded to include all nonoutpatient settings (acute care, short-term, long-term care, and psychiatric hospitals; home health agencies; rehab facilities; nursing homes; and so forth).

Part of the current UHDDS includes the following specific items pertaining to patients and their episodes of care:

- **Personal identification:** The unique number assigned to each patient that distinguishes the patient and his or her health record from all others

- **Date of birth**

- **Sex**

- **Race**

- **Ethnicity**

- **Residence:** The zip code or code for foreign residence

- **Hospital identification:** The unique number assigned to each institution

- **Admission and discharge dates**

- **Physician identification:** The unique number assigned to each physician within the hospital (the attending physician and the operating physician [if applicable] are to be identified)

- **Disposition of patient:** The way in which the patient left the hospital—discharged to home, left against medical advice, discharged to another short-term hospital, discharged to a long-term care institution, died, or other

- **Expected payer for most of the bill:** The single major source expected by the patient to pay for this bill (for example, Blue Cross/Blue Shield, Medicare, Medicaid, Workers' Compensation)

In keeping with UHDDS standards, medical data items for the following diagnoses and procedures also are reported:

- **Diagnoses:** All diagnoses affecting the current hospital stay must be reported as part of the UHDDS.

- **Principal diagnosis:** The principal diagnosis is designated and defined as the condition established after study to be chiefly responsible for occasioning the admission of the patient to the hospital for care.

- **Other diagnoses:** These are designated and defined as all conditions that coexist at the time of admission, that develop subsequently, or that affect treatment received and/or length of stay (LOS). Diagnoses are to be excluded that relate to an earlier episode that has no bearing on the current hospital stay. Within the Medicare Acute Care Prospective Payment System, *other diagnoses* may qualify as a complication or comorbidity, although the terms *complication* and *comorbidity* are not part of the UHDDS definition set but developed as part of the DRG system. The presence of the complication or comorbidity may influence the diagnosis-related group (DRG) assignment and produce a higher-valued DRG with a high payment for the hospital.

- **Complication:** This is defined as an *additional* diagnosis that describes a condition arising after the beginning of hospital observation and treatment and then modifying the course of the patient's illness or the medical care required. The patient's LOS is prolonged by at least one day in 75 percent of such cases.

- **Comorbidity:** This is defined as a *preexisting* condition that, because of its presence with a specific principal diagnosis, will cause an increase in the patient's LOS by at least one day in 75 percent of such cases.

- **Procedures and dates:** All significant procedures are to be reported. For significant procedures, both the identity (by unique number within the hospital) of the person performing the procedure and the date of the procedure must be reported.

- **Significant procedure:** A procedure is identified as significant when it:

  —Is surgical in nature

  —Carries a procedural risk

  —Carries an anesthetic risk

  —Requires specialized training

- **Principal procedure:** This type of procedure is performed for definitive treatment rather than for diagnostic or exploratory purposes, or when it is necessary to take care of a complication. If two procedures appear to be principal, the one most related to the principal diagnosis should be selected as the principal procedure.

Uniform Bill-92

In 1975, the National Uniform Billing Committee (NUBC) was established with the goal of developing an acceptable, uniform bill that would consolidate the numerous billing forms hospitals were required to use. In 1982, the Uniform Bill-82 (UB-82), also known as the CMS-1450 form, was implemented for use in billing services to Medicare fiscal intermediaries and other third-party payers. In 1988, the NUBC began preparations for a revised uniform bill. The resulting Uniform Bill-92 (UB-92) was implemented in October 1993 and provided for the collection of additional statistical data, including clinical information.

The revised UB-92 currently in use allows hospitals to report eleven diagnosis codes (one admitting diagnosis field, nine diagnosis fields, and one E code field) and six procedure codes. (See appendix D for a sample UB-92 form.) Although the billing office collects data for the billing form, the health information department supplies the clinical data placed on the form and thus must ensure the data's accuracy.

Selection of Principal Diagnosis

As the UHDDS definition states, a principal diagnosis is the condition "established after study to be chiefly responsible for occasioning the admission of the patient to the hospital for care." Selecting the principal diagnosis depends on the circumstances of the admission, or why the patient was admitted. The admitting diagnosis has to be worked up through diagnostic tests and studies. Therefore, the words "after study" serve as an integral part of this definition. During the course of hospitalization, the admitting diagnosis, which may be a symptom or ill-defined condition, could change substantially based on the results of "further study."

> **EXAMPLE:** Patient was admitted through the emergency department with an admitting diagnosis of seizure disorder. During hospitalization, diagnostic tests and studies revealed carcinoma of the brain, which explained the seizures.
>
> The principal diagnosis was the carcinoma of the brain, which was the condition determined after study.

At times, however, it may be difficult to distinguish between the *principal* diagnosis and the *most significant* diagnosis. The most significant diagnosis is defined as the condition having the most impact on the patient's health, LOS, resource consumption, and the like. However, the most significant diagnosis may or may not be the principal diagnosis.

In determining principal diagnosis, the coding conventions in ICD-9-CM, volumes 1 and 2, take precedence over the Official Coding Guidelines. (See Section I.A., Conventions for the ICD-9-CM.)

> **EXAMPLE:** Patient was admitted with a fractured hip due to an accident. The fracture was reduced and the patient discharged home.
>
> In this case, the principal diagnosis was fracture of the hip.

> **EXAMPLE:** Patient was admitted with a fractured hip due to an accident. While hospitalized, the patient suffered a myocardial infarction.
>
> In this case, the principal diagnosis was still the fracture of the hip, with the myocardial infarction coded as an additional diagnosis. Although the myocardial infarction may be the most significant diagnosis in terms of the patient's health and resource consumption, it was not the reason, after study, for the admission; therefore, it was not the principal diagnosis.

ICD-9-CM Official Guidelines for Coding and Reporting

The ICD-9-CM Official Guidelines for Coding and Reporting is available from the Centers for Disease Control and Prevention (http://www.cdc.gov/nchs/datawh/ftpserv/ftpicd9/ftpicd9.htm); in *Coding Clinic for ICD-9-CM,* published by the American Hospital Association; and on the CD-ROM containing the official government version, available through the Government Printing Office. All coding students are strongly encouraged to read the guidelines and become familiar with the rules in order to put them into practice. The application of the guidelines in everyday practice helps to ensure data accuracy in both coding and reporting for all healthcare encounters.

Selecting Principal Diagnosis for Inpatient Care

The following information on selecting the principal diagnosis and additional diagnoses should be reviewed carefully to ensure appropriate coding and reporting of hospital claims.

The circumstances of inpatient admission always govern selection of the principal diagnosis in keeping with the UHDDS definition of the term as the condition determined after study to be chiefly responsible for bringing about the admission of the patient to the hospital for care. In determining the principal diagnosis, the coding directives in ICD-9-CM, volumes 1, 2, and 3, take precedence over all other guidelines. General guidelines related to the selection of the principal diagnosis follow. Disease-specific guidelines are discussed in later chapters. Guidelines throughout this section are titled and numbered as presented in the ICD-9-CM Official Guidelines for Coding and Reporting.

Guideline II.A. Codes for symptoms, signs, and ill-defined conditions: Codes for symptoms, signs, and ill-defined conditions from chapter 16 are not to be used as the principal diagnosis when a related definitive diagnosis has been established.

> **EXAMPLE:** Patient was admitted to the hospital with chest pain to rule out myocardial infarction. After study, myocardial infarction was ruled out; the cause of the chest pain was undetermined.
>
> Code 786.50, Chest pain, unspecified, was assigned. Although the code for chest pain (786.50) is located in chapter 16, a definitive diagnosis could not be made, so chest pain was coded as the principal diagnosis.
>
> **EXAMPLE:** Patient was admitted to the hospital with dysphagia secondary to malignant neoplasm of the mouth. A PEG tube was inserted.
>
> Code 145.9, Malignant neoplasm of the mouth, unspecified, was selected as the principal diagnosis, with code 787.2 as an additional diagnosis to describe the dysphagia. Because the dysphagia was related to the malignancy and code 787.2 is from chapter 16, the principal diagnosis was the definitive diagnosis rather than the symptom.

Guideline II.B. Two or more interrelated conditions, each potentially meeting the definition for principal diagnosis: When there are two or more interrelated conditions (such as diseases in the same ICD-9-CM chapter, or manifestations characteristically associated with a certain disease) potentially meeting the definition of principal diagnosis, either condition may be sequenced first, unless the circumstances of the admission, the therapy provided, the Tabular List, or the Alphabetic Index indicates otherwise.

EXAMPLE: Patient was admitted with closed fracture of the femur and tibia of the right leg. The fractures were reduced.

The following codes were assigned: 821.00, Fracture of unspecified part of femur, closed; 823.80, Fracture of unspecified part of tibia, closed; 79.05, Closed reduction of fracture of femur without internal fixation; and 79.06, Closed reduction of fracture of tibia and fibula without internal fixation. Both fractures potentially met the definition of principal diagnosis; therefore, either code 821.00 or code 823.80 could be sequenced first.

Guideline II.C. Two or more diagnoses that equally meet the definition for principal diagnosis: In the unusual instance when two or more diagnoses equally meet the criteria for principal diagnosis, as determined by the circumstances of admission, diagnostic workup, and/or the therapy provided, and the Alphabetic Index, Tabular List, or another coding guideline does not provide sequencing direction in such cases, any one of the diagnoses may be sequenced first.

EXAMPLE: Patient was admitted for elective surgery. A lesion on the lip was excised and revealed squamous cell carcinoma. In addition, a right recurrent inguinal hernia was repaired.

The following codes were assigned: 140.9, Malignant neoplasm of lip, unspecified, vermilion border; 550.91, Inguinal hernia, without mention of obstruction or gangrene, unilateral or unspecified, recurrent; 27.43, Other excision of lesion or tissue of lip; 53.00, Unilateral repair of inguinal hernia, not otherwise specified. Both the squamous cell carcinoma of the lip and the right recurrent inguinal hernia met the criteria for principal diagnosis; therefore, either condition could be selected as the principal diagnosis.

Guideline II.D. Two or more comparative or contrasting conditions: In those rare instances when two or more contrasting or comparative diagnoses are documented as "either/or" (or similar terminology), they are coded as if confirmed and sequenced according to the circumstances of the admission. If no further determination can be made as to which diagnosis is principal, either diagnosis may be sequenced first.

EXAMPLE: Diverticulosis of colon versus angiodysplasia of intestine

Codes 562.10, Diverticulosis of colon (without mention of hemorrhage), and 569.84, Angiodysplasia of intestine (without mention of hemorrhage), are assigned.

Either unconfirmed diagnosis, diverticulosis of colon or angiodysplasia of intestine, may be sequenced as the principal diagnosis.

Note: Guidelines II.A through II.D reveal that designation of the principal diagnosis is not always an exact and easy task. At times, more than one condition may have occasioned the admission. In such cases, the actual circumstances of the case dictate designation of the principal diagnosis.

Guideline II.E. A symptom(s) followed by contrasting/comparative diagnoses: When a symptom(s) is (are) followed by contrasting or comparative diagnoses, the symptom code is sequenced first. All the contrasting or comparative diagnoses should be coded as additional diagnoses.

EXAMPLE: Patient was admitted with symptoms of periodic diarrhea and constipation during the previous three weeks. Following workup, physician documented the following diagnostic statement: Constipation and diarrhea due to either irritable bowel syndrome or diverticulitis.

The following codes were assigned: 564.00, Constipation; 787.91, Diarrhea; 564.1, Irritable bowel syndrome; and 562.11, Diverticulitis of colon (without mention of hemorrhage).

Guideline II.F. Original treatment plan not carried out: Sequence as the principal diagnosis the condition that after study occasioned the admission to the hospital, even if treatment may not have been carried out due to unforeseen circumstances.

EXAMPLE: Patient with ulcerated internal hemorrhoids was admitted for hemorrhoidectomy. Prior to the beginning of surgery, the patient developed bradycardia and the surgery was canceled.

The following codes were assigned: 455.2, Internal hemorrhoids with other complication; 427.89, Other specified cardiac dysrhythmias; and V64.1, Surgical or other procedure not carried out because of contraindication. The code for ulcerated internal hemorrhoids (455.2) was listed as the principal diagnosis because it was the reason for admission. An additional code for sinus bradycardia (427.89) was reported, as well as code V64.1, Surgical or other procedure not carried out because of contraindication, to indicate that the procedure was not carried out due to the complication of sinus bradycardia.

Guideline II.G. Complications of surgery and other medical care: When the admission is for treatment of a complication resulting from surgery or other medical care, the complication code is sequenced as the principal diagnosis. If the complication is classified to 996 through 999 series and the code lacks the necessary specificity in describing the complication, an additional code for the specific complication may be assigned.

EXAMPLE: Patient was being treated for an iatrogenic postoperative pneumothorax due to recent cardiovascular surgery. The diagnosis codes would include 997.3, Respiratory complications, and 512.1, Iatrogenic pneumothorax.

Guideline II.H. Uncertain diagnosis: If the diagnosis documented at the time of discharge is qualified as "probable," "suspected," "likely," "questionable," "possible," or "still to be ruled out," code the condition as if it existed or was established. The bases for these guidelines are the diagnostic workup, arrangements for further workup or observation, and initial therapeutic approach that correspond most closely with the established diagnosis. Note: This guideline is applicable only to short-term, acute, long-term, and psychiatric hospitals.

Reporting of Additional Diagnoses

The UHDDS item #11-B defines other diagnoses as "all conditions that coexist at the time of admission, that develop subsequently, or that affect the treatment received and/or the length of stay. Diagnoses that relate to an earlier episode which have no bearing on the current hospital stay are to be excluded." Since 1985, when the UHDDS definitions were used by acute care short-term hospitals to report inpatient data elements in a standardized manner, the application of the UHDDS definitions has been expanded. Today, the UHDDS definitions are applicable to all nonoutpatient settings (acute care, short-term, long-term care, and psychiatric hospitals; home health agencies; rehab facilities; nursing homes; and so forth).

For reporting purposes, the general rule is that the definition for other diagnoses is interpreted to include additional conditions affecting patient care in terms of requiring:

- Clinical evaluation

- Therapeutic treatment

- Diagnostic procedures

- Extended length of hospital stay

- Increased nursing care and/or monitoring

The following guidelines are to be applied in designating other diagnoses when neither the Alphabetic Index nor the Tabular List in ICD-9-CM provides direction.

Guideline III.A. Previous conditions: If the provider has included a diagnosis in the final diagnostic statement, such as the discharge summary or the face sheet, the diagnosis should ordinarily be coded. Some providers include in the diagnostic statement resolved conditions or diagnoses and status post procedures from a previous admission that have no bearing on the current stay. Such conditions are not to be reported and are coded only if required by hospital policy.

However, history codes (V10–V19) may be used as secondary codes if the historical condition or family history has an impact on current care or influences treatment.

EXAMPLE: Face sheet states the following diagnoses: acute diverticulitis, congestive heart failure, status post cholecystectomy, status post hysterectomy.

All are coded except the status post cholecystectomy and hysterectomy. The heart failure and the diverticulitis affect the current hospitalization and thus are coded.

Guideline III.B. Abnormal findings: Abnormal findings (laboratory, x-ray, pathologic, and other diagnostic results) are not coded and reported unless the provider indicates their clinical significance. When the findings are outside the normal range and the attending provider has ordered other tests to evaluate the condition or prescribed treatment, the coder should ask the provider whether the abnormal findings should be added. **Note:** This differs from the coding practices in the outpatient setting for coding encounters for diagnostic tests that have been interpreted by a provider.

Guideline III.C. Uncertain diagnosis: If the diagnosis documented at the time of discharge is qualified as "probable," "suspected," "likely," "questionable," "possible," or "still to be ruled out," code the condition as if it existed or was established. The bases for these guidelines are the diagnostic workup, arrangements for further workup or observation, and initial therapeutic approach that correspond most closely with the established diagnosis. **Note:** This guideline is applicable only to short-term, acute, long-term care, and psychiatric hospitals.

Prospective Payment System

The prospective payment system (PPS) is a method of payment undertaken by CMS to control the cost of inpatient hospital services to Medicare recipients. Title VI of the Social Security Amendments of 1983 established the PPS to provide payment to hospitals for each Medicare case at a set reimbursement rate, rather than on a fee-for-service or per-day basis. The payment rates to hospitals, then, are established before services are rendered and are based on diagnosis-related groups (DRGs).

DRGs represent an inpatient classification system designed to categorize patients who are medically related with respect to diagnoses and treatment, and who are statistically similar in their lengths of stay. Each DRG has a preset reimbursement amount that the hospital receives whenever the DRG is assigned.

Payment rates for each DRG are determined from two basic sources. First, each DRG is assigned a relative weight. The relative weight represents the average resources required to care for cases in that particular DRG relative to the national average of resources used to treat all Medicare cases. The average Medicare case is assigned a relative weight of 1.0000. Thus, cases in a DRG with a weight of 2.0000, on average, require twice as many resources as the average Medicare case; on the other hand, cases in a DRG with a weight of 0.5000, on average, require half as many resources as the average Medicare case. Each year, the relative weights of the DRGs are updated to reflect changes in treatment patterns, technology, and any other factors that may change the relative use of hospital resources.

The second source that determines DRG payment rate is the individual hospital's payment rate per case. This payment rate is based on a regional or national adjusted standardized amount that considers the type of hospital; designation of the hospital as large urban, other urban, or rural; and a wage index for the geographic area where the hospital is located.

Thus, the actual amount the hospital is reimbursed for each Medicare inpatient is determined by multiplying the hospital's individual payment rate by the relative weight of the DRG, less any applicable deductible amount. For any given patient in a DRG, the hospital knows, in advance, the amount of reimbursement it will receive from Medicare. It is the responsibility of the hospital to ensure that its resource use is in line with that payment.

In addition to the basic payment rate, Medicare provides for an additional payment per case for outliers. Outliers are cases where patients require considerably more resources than average because of either their length of stay (LOS) or cost of care. After a threshold LOS or cost of care has been reached, an additional payment is made. For example, a patient admitted for a transurethral resection of prostate without any significant complications or comorbidities stays in the hospital, on average, 2.5 days. If the patient requires considerably more care until the LOS is more than 18 days, the hospital, when it presents documentation supporting the necessity of care, will be reimbursed the additional amount.

DRG assignment is based on information that includes:

- Diagnoses (principal and secondary)
- Surgical procedures (principal and secondary)
- Patient's age
- Discharge status
- Presence of complicating/comorbid conditions

CMS evaluates the Medicare PPS annually. CMS's Notice of Proposed Rulemaking is published in the *Federal Register* each May. This notice, on which the public may comment, announces the final decisions on all ICD-9-CM code changes and proposed revisions to the DRG system. CMS's Final Rule announcing final revisions to the PPS, including the DRG system, is published in the *Federal Register* in July or August, and the changes become effective October 1 each year.

Before October 1, 1995, hospitals were required to obtain the physician's signature on each Medicare and Civilian Health and Medical Program of Uniformed Services (CHAMPUS) health record, which attested to the diagnoses and procedures documented on the face sheet. Then, on July 11, 1995, the U.S. Department of Health and Human Services and the White House announced that physician attestation was no longer required for Medicare discharges, effective October 1, 1995. Shortly thereafter, elimination of the physician attestation requirement for CHAMPUS discharges was announced. It was anticipated that these actions would decrease administrative costs and paperwork for hospitals. With the end of physician attestation requirements, all HIM professionals, but especially coders, have faced greater responsibility for ensuring the accurate and ethical coding of health records. AHIMA has developed several documents related to data quality within the past few years as guides toward attaining and maintaining high-quality coding. The Standards of Ethical Coding (updated in January 2000) and an AHIMA practice brief on data quality (2003) are contained in appendices E and F, respectively, of this book.

Quality Improvement Organizations

To ensure that the federal government pays only for medically necessary, appropriate, and high-quality healthcare services, CMS contracts with medical review organizations called quality improvement organizations (QIOs). QIOs conduct outcomes measurement projects to evaluate treatment received by Medicare beneficiaries. At times, during the course of the QIO review, a DRG change or coding change may be identified. The hospital is then notified of the change and may request a QIO re-review in light of the procedure and diagnostic information obtained by the QIO that resulted in a change of DRG assignment. Review decisions made at that time are final and no further review is available.

Coding for Medical Necessity

Accurate ICD-9-CM diagnosis coding is essential to establish the medical necessity of a particular service as required by Medicare's reasonable and necessary medical coverage policies and other third-party payers' desire to know the reason for the service. Medicare fiscal intermediaries and carriers that process Part A and Part B Medicare claims may develop local coverage decisions (LCDs), formerly known as local medical review policies (LMRPs). These policies ensure that claims are submitted only for those services that have been deemed reasonable and necessary for the patient's condition. National coverage determinations (NCDs) also exist for many laboratory tests, for which Medicare payment is contingent on a particular condition being established as the reason the test was ordered. The coder must be certain that documentation contains all of the reasons why the physician ordered a diagnostic or therapeutic service. Then the coder must assign all of the appropriate ICD-9-CM codes for the claim to be reviewed accurately for medical necessity and paid appropriately. The requirements for determining medical necessity have moved the coding personnel outside the traditional health information management department into hospitals' emergency departments, admitting/registration or access departments, central scheduling centers, and a variety of clinical departments performing many outpatient services, such as radiology and laboratory. The need to know if a patient's condition meets the medical necessity requirements of a particular service is essential prior to issuing an advance beneficiary notice (ABN). The purpose of the ABN is to inform patients why Medicare may not pay for the service and to explain to them that they will be financially responsible if they agree to the service being performed. Medical necessity processing has brought the coding function closer to the point of care and, in some institutions, improved the documentation related to the reasons for out-patient testing.

Chapter 4

Infectious and Parasitic Diseases

Chapter 1, Infectious and Parasitic Diseases (001–139)

Chapter 1, Infectious and Parasitic Diseases, in the Tabular List in ICD-9-CM, volume 1, is based on the organism responsible for a disease or condition. Communicable diseases are classified in an inclusion note at the beginning of the chapter. Chapter 1 also includes a few diseases of unknown, but possibly of infectious, origin. Noncommunicable diseases are classified by site in other chapters of ICD-9-CM.

Chapter 1 is subdivided into the following categories and section titles:

Categories	Section Titles
001–009	Intestinal Infectious Diseases
010–018	Tuberculosis
020–027	Zoonotic Bacterial Diseases
030–041	Other Bacterial Diseases
042	Human Immunodeficiency Virus (HIV) Infection
045–049	Poliomyelitis and Other Non-arthropod-borne Viral Diseases of Central Nervous System
050–057	Viral Diseases Accompanied by Exanthem
060–066	Arthropod-borne Viral Diseases
070–079	Other Diseases due to Virus and Chlamydiae
080–088	Rickettsioses and Other Arthropod-borne Diseases
090–099	Syphilis and Other Venereal Diseases
100–104	Other Spirochetal Diseases
110–118	Mycoses
120–129	Helminthiases
130–136	Other Infectious and Parasitic Diseases
137–139	Late Effects of Infectious and Parasitic Diseases

Chapter 4 serves as an introduction to coding instructions specific to tuberculosis, septicemia, late effects of infectious and parasitic diseases, and human immunodeficiency virus

(HIV). Appendix A of *Basic ICD-9-CM Coding* includes a listing of common bacteria and their associated diseases.

In coding infectious and parasitic diseases, the entire health record must be reviewed to identify:

- Body site: Intestine, kidney, or blood

- Severity of the disease: Acute versus chronic

- Specific organism: Candida, bacteria, virus, or parasite

- Etiology of infection: Food poisoning

- Associated signs, symptoms, or manifestations: Gangrene, bleeding, or Kaposi's sarcoma

Combination Codes and Multiple Coding

Chapter 1 of ICD-9-CM includes many combination codes to identify both the condition and the causative organism.

EXAMPLE:	112.0	Candidiasis of mouth
	006.1	Chronic intestinal amebiasis without mention of abscess
	130.1	Conjunctivitis due to toxoplasmosis

Multiple coding is often necessary to completely describe an infectious condition or disease. The coding guidelines discussed in chapter 3 of *Basic ICD-9-CM Coding* also apply here.

Mandatory multiple coding is required when infections and parasitic diseases produce a manifestation within another body system. The Alphabetic Index to Diseases identifies when mandatory multiple coding is required by listing two codes after the main term with the second code listed in brackets. The first code identifies the underlying infectious or parasitic condition. The second code identifies the manifestation that occurs as a result of it.

> **EXAMPLE:** Arthritis due to Lyme disease 088.81 *[711.8]*
>
> The underlying cause and first-listed code is 088.81. The second code describes the arthritis associated with this tick-transmitted illness, 711.8, with a required fifth digit to identify the joint(s) involved.

Categories 041 and 079

Typically, both categories 041 and 079 are assigned as an additional diagnosis to describe the causative organism in diseases that are classified elsewhere in ICD-9-CM. Category code 041, Bacterial infection in conditions classified elsewhere and of unspecified site, is assigned when the organism is a bacteria. Category code 079, Viral and chlamydial infection in conditions classified elsewhere and of unspecified site, is assigned when the organism is a virus or chlamydia. In both categories, the codes may be located using the main term "Infection" in the Alphabetic Index to Diseases.

Category 041 is further subdivided to identify specific bacteria such as streptococcus, staphylococcus, pneumococcus, and so forth.

> **EXAMPLE:** Urinary tract infection due to E. coli
>
> 599.0 Urinary tract infection, site not specified
> 041.4 Escherichia coli (E. coli)

Category 079 is further subdivided to identify specific viruses, such as adenovirus; ECHO virus; Coxsackie virus; retrovirus; human T-cell lymphotrophic virus, types I and II; human immunodeficiency virus, type 2; and so forth.

> **EXAMPLE:** Acute viral osteomyelitis of the hip
>
> 730.05 Acute osteomyelitis, pelvic region and thigh
> 079.99 Unspecified viral infection

Tuberculosis (010–018)

Because tuberculosis can develop anywhere in the body, this disease has category codes that identify the specific anatomical site involved, such as pulmonary, genitourinary, meninges, central nervous system, and so forth.

The fifth-digit subclassification for use with the tuberculosis codes is noted at the beginning of the section, "Tuberculosis." The fifth digit requires identification of the method used to establish the diagnosis of tuberculosis. The fifth digit 0 is assigned when the method of diagnosis is not documented. The fifth digit 2 is assigned when a bacteriological or histological examination is performed, but the results are not available in the health record.

Septicemia (038)

Septicemia results from the entry of pathogens into the bloodstream. Symptoms include spiking fever, chills, and skin eruptions in the form of petechiae or purpura. Blood cultures are usually positive; however, a negative culture does not exclude the diagnosis of septicemia in patients with clinical evidence of the condition. Clinical evidence may include the symptoms just listed, as well as hyperventilation with respiratory alkalosis, changes in the mental status of the patient, and thrombocytopenia.

ICD-9-CM classifies septicemia by the underlying organism involved. Bacterial septicemia is classified to category 038, which is further subdivided to identify the specific bacteria, such as staphylococcus. Without further specification, septicemia is reported with code 038.9. Septicemia due to Candida albicans is reported with code 112.5.

The terms *septic shock, severe sepsis, sepsis,* and *septicemia* may be used interchangeably by physicians, but they are clinically distinct conditions and are no longer considered synonymous terms. In the past several years, ICD-9-CM has been updated to reflect current medical terminology regarding septic shock, sepsis, and septicemia.

Bacteremia is defined as the presence of bacteria in the blood. Septicemia is defined as a systemic disease associated with the presence of pathological organisms or toxins in the blood, which may include bacteria, fungi, viruses, or other organisms. The systemic inflammatory response syndrome (SIRS) is the systemic response to infection or trauma, with symptoms that include fever, tachycardia, tachypnea, and leukocytosis. Sepsis is defined as SIRS due to an infection. This definition of sepsis replaces all previous coding advice that equated sepsis with septicemia. Finally, severe sepsis is defined as sepsis with associated organ dysfunction.

The term *septicemia* is still used in ICD-9-CM in keeping with the international version of ICD-9. In the less acutely ill patient, the term *sepsis* may simply be used to reflect the presence of an infection. However, physicians may describe a more acutely ill patient with the term *sepsis* or *severe sepsis*. The term *septic shock* is the end point for the continuum from sepsis to severe sepsis to septic shock. In order to clarify the terminology in ICD-9-CM, the term *sepsis* has been added as an inclusion term under code 995.91, Systemic inflammatory response due to infectious process without organ dysfunction. The term *sepsis* is indexed to code 995.91. Prior to October 1, 2003, sepsis had been indexed to code 038.9, Septicemia. The term *severe sepsis* is indexed to code 995.92, Systemic inflammatory response syndrome (SIRS) with organ dysfunction. Patients with septic shock have sepsis with hypotension, a failure of the cardiovascular system. Therefore, septic shock meets the definition of severe sepsis.

A note has been added under the code 785.52, Septic shock, instructing coders that code 995.92, SIRS due to infectious process with organ dysfunction, or 995.94, SIRS due to non-infectious process with organ dysfunction, must also be assigned. A note is also present under category 038, Septicemia, to instruct coders to assign an additional code for the corresponding SIRS. Another note appears under code 995.92 instructing the coder to assign the code for septic shock.

By using both an infection or trauma code and a code from subcategory 995.9, the record will accurately reflect the severity of the patient's condition. The "code first" note at subcategory 995.9 provides instruction that the underlying cause of the SIRS (systemic infection or trauma) should be coded first. In the absence of a specified underlying condition, the default first code should be 038.9. If only the term *sepsis* is documented, codes 038.9 and 995.91 would be assigned in that sequence. Either sepsis or SIRS must be documented to assign a code from subcategory 995.9.

If documentation is not clear whether the sepsis was present on admission, the provider should be queried. After provider query, if the sepsis is determined at that point to have met the definition of principal diagnosis, the underlying systemic infection (038.xx, 112.5, and so forth) may be used as principal diagnosis along with code 995.91, Systemic inflammatory response syndrome due to infectious process without organ dysfunction.

When the term *sepsis, severe sepsis,* or *SIRS* is used with an underlying infection other than septicemia, for example, pneumonia, cellulitis, or nonspecific urinary tract infection, a code from category 038 should be assigned first, then code 995.91, followed by a code for the initial infection, such as the pneumonia. The reason for this is that the term *sepsis* or *SIRS* indicates that the patient's infection has advanced to a systemic infection and the systemic infection code should be sequenced before the localized infection code. The instructional note under subcategory 995.9 instructs the coder to assign the underlying condition first.

To code patients with severe sepsis, the code for the systemic infection (038 category, 112.5, or other underlying systemic infection, or a trauma category code) should be sequenced first, followed by either code 995.92, SIRS due to infectious process with organ dysfunction, or 995.94, SIRS due to noninfectious process with organ dysfunction. Codes for the specific organ dysfunction should also be assigned.

When septic shock is documented, the coder should code first the initiating systemic infection or trauma, then either code 995.92 or 995.94, followed by code 785.52 for the septic shock. These instructions refer to coding of sepsis in adult, nongravid patients because separate codes exist for sepsis complicating a pregnancy and in newborns.

Coding Guidelines for Septicemia, Systemic Inflammatory Response Syndrome (SIRS), Sepsis, Severe Sepsis, and Septic Shock

The ICD-9-CM Official Guidelines for Coding and Reporting, effective April 1, 2005, contain updated guidelines for coding septicemia, SIRS, sepsis, severe sepsis, and septic shock. Please refer to appendix I in this text for a complete review. Long-standing coding guidelines also state:

> Negative or inconclusive blood cultures do not preclude a diagnosis of septicemia or sepsis in patients with clinical evidence of the condition, however, the provider should be queried.

New information has been added regarding sepsis as principal or secondary diagnosis and the process to be followed when documentation is unclear as to whether sepsis was present on admission. Additional information was added concerning the sequencing of septic shock, septic shock without documentation of severe sepsis, newborn sepsis, sepsis due to a procedural infection, and external cause of injury codes with SIRS.

Late Effects of Infectious and Parasitic Diseases (137–139)

Three categories are identified for use in describing late effects of infectious and parasitic diseases:

Category 137   Late effects of tuberculosis
Category 138   Late effects of acute poliomyelitis
Category 139   Late effects of other infectious and parasitic diseases

Late effects are located under the main term "Late" with the subterm "effect." In sequencing, the first code listed is the residual condition that is present in the patient today (retardation, hemiplegia, and so forth) followed by the late effect code (137.0, 137.2, 138, and so forth) identifying the underlying cause, unless the Alphabetic Index directs otherwise.

> **EXAMPLE:**   Mental retardation due to old viral encephalitis
>
> 319   Unspecified mental retardation
> 139.0   Late effects of viral encephalitis

Human Immunodeficiency Virus (HIV) Disease

The human immunodeficiency virus attacks the body's immune system and leads to associated infections and malignant tumors. HIV is the virus that leads to acquired immunodeficiency syndrome, which is known as AIDS. HIV destroys the body's ability to fight off disease, so that common infections from which healthy people generally recover can prove fatal to people who have contracted the virus.

HIV infection is caused by one of two related retroviruses, HIV-1 and HIV-2, that produce a wide range of conditions varying from the presence of contagious infections with no apparent symptoms to disorders that are severely disabling and eventually fatal. HIV-1 is widespread throughout the world and causes acquired immunodeficiency syndrome (AIDS). Found primarily in West Africa, HIV-2 seems to be less virulent and causes a different type of illness.

Essentially, the total HIV-1 infection process involves five phases:

1. The first phase, a window period, occurs four weeks to six months after infection with HIV-1 and is asymptomatic.

2. The second phase manifests itself as a short period of flu-like symptoms that include fever, lymphadenopathy, skin rash, and malaise. This phase is called acute primary infection and lasts for approximately one to two weeks.

3. A third phase follows the brief flu-like illness and consists of a prolonged asymptomatic period that can last from one to fifteen or more years.

4. Eventually, the person infected with HIV-1 experiences the fourth phase of HIV-1 infection: symptoms of immune suppression, such as persistent low-grade fever, night sweats, continuous or intermittent diarrhea, lymphadenopathy, unintended weight loss, oral lesions, fatigue, rashes, cognitive slowing, and peripheral neuropathy.

5. Any of the preceding symptoms indicate that the disease could shift into the fifth phase, AIDS, within the next two to three years. The symptoms of AIDS include severe opportunistic infections, tumors in any body system, and neurologic manifestations.

There is no cure for HIV infection, and HIV treatment is complex. One major emphasis of treatment is to find effective combinations of antiviral medications that a person can tolerate over an indefinite period. Another is to prevent opportunistic infections that can prove fatal. Anti-HIV therapy is generally initiated when the T-cell count of an infected person goes below 200, indicating a severely weakened immune system.

To ensure uniform reporting of AIDS cases, the Centers for Disease Control (CDC) has developed specific definition criteria that must be met prior to establishing a diagnosis of AIDS.

HIV Classification

When first created, the classification of HIV was complex. It included three category codes to identify the phases of the HIV infection. Unfortunately, the terminology often found in the health record did not correspond to what was available in ICD-9-CM and, as such, created much confusion.

Effective October 1, 1994, the HIV classification was simplified to include the following categories and codes:

- 042, Human immunodeficiency virus (HIV) disease: Patients with HIV-related illness should be coded to 042. Category 042 includes AIDS, AIDS-like syndrome, AIDS-related complex, and symptomatic HIV infection.

- V08, Asymptomatic human immunodeficiency virus (HIV) infection: Patients with physician-documented asymptomatic HIV infection who have never had an HIV-related illness should be coded to V08.

- 795.71, Nonspecific serologic evidence of human immunodeficiency virus (HIV): Code 795.71 should be used for patients (including infants) with inconclusive HIV test results.

Code only confirmed cases of HIV infection/illness. Health records with diagnostic statements of "suspected," "likely," "possible," or "questionable" HIV infection are to be returned to the physician for clarification. The instructions to code only confirmed cases of HIV infection/illness represent an exception to the general ICD-9-CM inpatient coding guidelines that state that diagnoses identified as "suspected" or "possible" should be coded as if they have been established. In this context, "confirmation" does not require documentation of positive serology or culture for HIV. The physician's diagnostic statement that the patient is HIV positive or has an HIV-related illness is sufficient.

Coding Guidelines for HIV Disease

Official coding guidelines exist for the coding of HIV infections. See Part I, C. Chapter-Specific Coding Guidelines, 1. Chapter 1: Infectious and Parasitic Diseases (001–139) for the complete set of HIV coding guidelines.

The circumstances of admission for patients with HIV-related illness govern the selection of principal diagnosis in keeping with its UHDDS definition of that "condition established after study to be chiefly responsible for occasioning the admission of the patient to the hospital for care."

Patients who are admitted for an HIV-related illness should be assigned a minimum of two codes in the following order:

1. Code 042 to identify the HIV disease

2. Additional codes to identify other diagnoses, such as Kaposi's sarcoma

> **EXAMPLE:** Disseminated candidiasis secondary to AIDS
>
> 042   Human immunodeficiency virus [HIV] disease
> 112.5   Disseminated candidiasis

> **EXAMPLE:** Acute lymphadenitis with HIV infection
>
> 042   Human immunodeficiency virus [HIV] disease
> 683   Acute lymphadenitis

During pregnancy, childbirth, or the puerperium, a patient admitted because of an HIV-related illness should receive a principal diagnosis of 647.6x, Other specified infectious and parasitic diseases in the mother classifiable elsewhere, but complicating the pregnancy, childbirth, or the puerperium, followed by 042 and the code(s) for the HIV-related illness(es). This is an exception to the sequencing rule discussed above.

> **EXAMPLE:** Delivery of a liveborn male in mother with AIDS
>
> 647.61   Other specified infectious and parasitic diseases in the mother classifiable elsewhere, but complicating the pregnancy, childbirth, or the puerperium
> 042   Human immunodeficiency virus (HIV) disease
> V27.0   Outcome of delivery, single liveborn

> **EXAMPLE:** Patient is admitted for evaluation and treatment of pneumonia; workup reveals Pneumocystis carinii pneumonia. Patient is also 25 weeks pregnant and has AIDS.
>
> 647.63   Other specified infectious and parasitic diseases in the mother classifiable elsewhere, but complicating the pregnancy, childbirth, or the puerperium
> 042   Human immunodeficiency virus [HIV] disease
> 136.3   Pneumocystosis

If a patient with symptomatic HIV disease or AIDS is admitted for an unrelated condition, such as a traumatic injury, the code for the unrelated condition should be the principal diagnosis. An additional diagnosis would include code 042, as well as all other manifestations or conditions associated with the HIV disease.

> **EXAMPLE:** Patient was admitted with a diagnosis of acute appendicitis and an appendectomy was performed. Patient also has AIDS.
>
> 540.9   Acute appendicitis
> 042   Human immunodeficiency virus [HIV] disease
> 47.09   Other appendectomy

Code V08, Asymptomatic HIV infection status, is applied when the patient without any documentation of symptoms is reported as being HIV positive, known HIV, HIV test positive, or similar terminology. Do not use this code if the term *AIDS* is used or if the patient is treated for any HIV-related illness or is described as having any condition(s) resulting from his or her HIV positive status. Use code 042 in these cases.

During pregnancy, childbirth, or the puerperium, a patient admitted with a diagnosis of asymptomatic HIV infection (or similar terminology as described above) should receive a principal diagnosis of 647.6x, Other specified infectious and parasitic diseases in the mother classifiable elsewhere, but complicating the pregnancy, childbirth, or the puerperium, followed by code V08, Asymptomatic human immunodeficiency virus (HIV) infection. In addition, codes should be assigned to describe other complications of pregnancy, childbirth, or the puerperium, as appropriate. Codes from chapter 15, Pregnancy, always take sequencing priority.

> **EXAMPLE:** Normal delivery of liveborn female; patient has a diagnosis of HIV infection with no related symptoms.
>
> 647.61   Other specified infectious and parasitic diseases in the mother
> V27.0   Outcome of delivery, single liveborn
> V08   Asymptomatic human immunodeficiency virus (HIV) infection

Code 795.71, Inconclusive serologic test for human immunodeficiency virus [HIV], is reported for patients with inconclusive HIV serology, but with no definitive diagnosis or manifestations of the illness.

A point to remember: Patients with any known prior diagnosis of an HIV-related illness should be assigned code 042. After a patient has developed an HIV-related illness, the patient should always be assigned code 042 on every subsequent admission. Patients previously diagnosed with any HIV illness (042) should never be assigned code 795.71 or V08.

Testing for HIV

Patients requesting testing for HIV should be assigned code V73.89, Screening for other specified viral disease. In addition, code V69.8, Other problems related to lifestyle, may be assigned to identify patients who are in a known high-risk group for HIV. Code V65.44, HIV counseling, also may be assigned if these services are provided during the encounter.

If the results of the test are positive and the patient is asymptomatic, code V08, Asymptomatic HIV infection, should be assigned. If the results are positive and the patient is symptomatic with an HIV-related illness, such as Kaposi's sarcoma, code 042, HIV disease, should be assigned.

Review Exercise: Chapter 4

Assign ICD-9-CM codes to the following:

1. Aseptic meningitis due to AIDS

   _____ 042   047.8 _____

2. Asymptomatic HIV infection

   _____ V08 _____

3. Staphylococcal aureus septicemia with SIRS

   _____ 038.11   995.91 _____

4. Dermatophytosis of the foot

   _____ 110.4 _____

Review Exercise: Chapter 4 (Continued)

5. Fracture, right radius, shaft; AIDS

   813.21, 042

6. Nodular pulmonary tuberculosis; confirmed histologically

   011.15

7. Acute poliomyelitis

   045.90

8. Left lower extremity paralysis; late effect of poliomyelitis

   344.30   138

9. Viral hepatitis A

   070.1

10. Staphylococcal food poisoning

    005.0

11. AIDS with encephalopathy, and esophageal candidiasis

    042 348.39 112.84

12. Acute gonococcal cervicitis and gonococcal endometritis

    098.15   098.16

13. Syphilitic endocarditis involving the aortic valve

    093.22

14. Septic nasopharyngitis

    034.0

15. Filarial orchitis

    125.9 [604.91]   ?

16. Osteitis due to yaws

    102.6

17. Acute cystitis due to E. coli

    595.0   041.4

18. Vaginitis due to Candida albicans

    112.1

19. Tuberculous osteomyelitis of knee; confirmed by histology

    015.25   730.86

20. Toxic shock syndrome due to Group A Streptococcus

    040.82   041.01

Chapter 5

Neoplasms

Chapter 2, Neoplasms (140–239)

The term *neoplasm* refers to any new or abnormal growth. Chapter 2 in the Tabular List in ICD-9-CM, volume 1, classifies *all* neoplasms. The following categories and section titles are included:

Categories	Section Titles
140–195	Malignant Neoplasms, Stated or Presumed to Be Primary, of Specified Sites, Except of Lymphatic and Hematopoietic Tissue
196–198	Malignant Neoplasms, Stated or Presumed to Be Secondary, of Specified Sites
199	Malignant Neoplasms, without Specification of Site
200–208	Malignant Neoplasms, Stated or Presumed to Be Primary, of Lymphatic and Hematopoietic Tissue
210–229	Benign Neoplasms
230–234	Carcinoma in Situ
235–238	Neoplasms of Uncertain Behavior
239	Neoplasms of Unspecified Nature

In ICD-9-CM coding, neoplasms are classified according to three criteria:

1. Behavior of the neoplasm, such as malignant or benign

2. Anatomical site involved, such as lung, brain, or stomach

3. Morphology type, such as leukemia, melanoma, or adenocarcinoma

Common morphology types can be found in appendix C at the back of this book.

Coding Guidelines

The ICD-9-CM Official Guidelines for Coding and Reporting contain a chapter-specific set of rules concerning the coding of neoplasms. See Section I. C. Chapter-Specific Coding Guidelines, 2. Chapter 2 Neoplasms (140–239) for a complete review of the specific guidelines that address coding and sequencing of primary and secondary sites, complications, V10 codes for personal history, admissions for chemotherapy or radiation therapy, admissions to determine extent of malignancy, and sign and symptom codes. The newest addition to these guidelines addresses encounters for prophylactic organ removal due to genetic susceptibility to cancer or a family history of cancer.

Neoplasm Behavior

Definitions describing the behavior of seven specific neoplasms include:

- **Malignant:** Malignant neoplasms are collectively referred to as cancers. A malignant neoplasm can invade and destroy adjacent structures, as well as spread to distant sites to cause death.

- **Primary:** A primary neoplasm is the site where a neoplasm originated.

- **Secondary:** A secondary neoplasm is the site(s) to which the neoplasm has spread via:

  —Direct extension, in which the primary neoplasm infiltrates and invades adjacent structures

  —Metastasis to local lymph vessels by tumor cell infiltration

  —Invasion of local blood vessels

  —Implantation in which tumor cells shed into body cavities

- **In situ:** In an in situ neoplasm, the tumor cells undergo malignant changes but are still confined to the point of origin without invasion of surrounding normal tissue. The following terms also describe in situ malignancies: noninfiltrating, noninvasive, intra-epithelial, or preinvasive carcinoma.

- **Benign:** In benign neoplasms, growth does not invade adjacent structures or spread to distant sites but may displace or exert pressure on adjacent structures.

- **Uncertain behavior:** Neoplasms of uncertain behavior are tumors that a pathologist cannot determine as being either benign or malignant because some features of each are present.

- **Unspecified nature:** Neoplasms of unspecified nature include tumors in which neither the behavior nor the histological type is specified in the diagnosis.

Neoplasm Table

As mentioned in chapter 1, the Alphabetic Index to Diseases contains two tables. One of them is known as the neoplasm table. This table is indexed under the main term "Neoplasm."

The neoplasm table contains seven columns. The first column lists the anatomical sites in alphabetical order. The next six columns identify the behavior of the neoplasm. The first three of these six columns include codes for malignant neoplasms and are further classified as primary, secondary, and carcinoma (ca) in situ. The fourth column identifies codes for benign neoplasms. The last two columns include codes for neoplasms of uncertain behavior and of unspecified type.

A point to remember: When many sites are indented under a main term, the listing for that term may run several pages long. Remember to search through all of the subterms under the main heading.

Exercise 5.1

Using only the neoplasm table, assign codes to the following:

100%

1. Malignant neoplasm originating in the lingual tonsil

   _141.6_

2. Neoplasm of cerebrum, behavior uncertain

   _237.5_

3. Benign neoplasm of liver

   _211.5_

4. Carcinoma in situ of cervix

   _233.1_

5. Neoplasm of abdomen (behavior unspecified)

   _239.8_

6. Secondary malignant neoplasm involving the lower lobe of lung

   _197.0_

Morphology Codes

Morphology codes (M codes) consist of five digits: the first four digits identify the histological type of the neoplasm; the fifth digit indicates the behavior. A complete listing of morphology codes can be found in appendix A of ICD-9-CM, volume 1. The M codes are used primarily by cancer or tumor registries in hospitals to identify the specific histology and behavior of the neoplasm.

The one-digit behavior codes that follow the morphology code are:

/0 Benign

/1 Uncertain whether benign or malignant
    Borderline malignancy

/2 Carcinoma in situ
    Intraepithelial
    Noninfiltrating
    Noninvasive

/3 Malignant, primary site

/6 Malignant, metastatic site
    Secondary site

/9 Malignant, uncertain whether primary or metastatic site

Morphology codes appear next to each neoplastic term in the Alphabetic Index.

EXAMPLE: Adenocarcinoma (M8140/3)—*see also* Neoplasm, by site, malignant

In the preceding example, M8140 identifies the histological type as adenocarcinoma and the digit /3 indicates the malignant behavior as a primary site.

Although the behavior code listed in ICD-9-CM is appropriate to the histological type of neoplasm, the behavior type should be changed to fit the diagnostic statement.

EXAMPLE: Patient was admitted to the hospital with a diagnosis of adenocarcinoma of the lung with metastasis to the bone.

M8140/3   Adenocarcinoma (lung)
M8140/6   Metastatic adenocarcinoma (bone)

ICD-9-CM codes do not use the behavior digit /9 because all malignant neoplasms are coded as primary or secondary, based on the documentation in the health record.

Occasionally, a difficulty arises in assigning a morphologic number when a diagnosis contains two qualifying adjectives with different morphology codes. In such cases, the higher number should be selected.

EXAMPLE: Patient was admitted to the hospital with a diagnosis of papillary serous carcinoma of the ovary.

The following two morphology codes are available:

M8050/3   Papillary carcinoma (ovary)
M8460/3   Serous carcinoma (ovary)

Because the higher number is M8460/3, this code is assigned.

V Codes

V codes provide a method for reporting encounters for chemotherapy, radiation therapy, and follow-up visits, as well as a way to indicate a history of primary malignancy or a family history of cancer.

Coding Guidelines for V Codes

Following is a set of guidelines for using V codes:

- If the treatment is directed at the malignancy, designate the malignancy as the principal diagnosis. When the purpose of the encounter or hospital admission is for radiation therapy or radiotherapy (V58.0) or for chemotherapy (V58.1), use the V code as the principal diagnosis and sequence the malignancy as an additional diagnosis. Do not use V58.0 or V58.1 as the only code reported. The need for the therapy should be explained with the use of a code from the 140–208 categories. Also, it is inappropriate to report V58.0 or V58.1 with only a V10 category code as a secondary code. Chemotherapy is not likely to be given to a patient who has a history of cancer and not the active disease process. V58.0 or V58.1 can be used with the V10 category code when an additional code for a malignancy of a secondary site, for example, categories 196–198, is included. This indicates that the cancer treatment is being directed to the secondary site with the V10 category code indicating the primary site.

  EXAMPLE: Patient with right upper outer quadrant (UOQ) breast carcinoma was admitted for chemotherapy.

  The following codes are reported:

  V58.1   Encounter for chemotherapy
  174.4   Malignant neoplasm of upper outer quadrant of breast

- When a patient is admitted for the purpose of radiotherapy or chemotherapy and develops a complication, such as uncontrolled nausea and vomiting or dehydration, the principal diagnosis is the admission for radiotherapy (V58.0) or the admission for the chemotherapy (V58.1). Additional codes would include the cancer and the complication(s).

> **EXAMPLE:** Patient was admitted for chemotherapy for acute lymphocytic leukemia. During the hospitalization, the patient developed severe nausea and vomiting treated with medications.
>
> The following codes are reported:
>
> V58.1   Encounter for chemotherapy
> 204.00 Acute lymphocytic leukemia
> 787.01 Nausea with vomiting
> 99.25   Chemotherapy

- When the primary malignancy has been previously excised or eradicated from its site, and there is no adjunct treatment directed to that site and no evidence of any remaining malignancy at the primary site, use the appropriate code from category V10 to indicate the former site of the primary malignancy. Any mention of extension, invasion, or metastasis to a nearby structure or organ or to a distant site is coded as a secondary malignant neoplasm to that site and may be the principal diagnosis in the absence of the primary site. The V10 category essentially describes the patient who is "cured" of the malignancy.

A point to remember: The instructional notes listed under each subcategory in category V10 refer to specific code ranges for primary malignancy categories (140–195 and 200–208) and carcinoma in situ categories (230–234). The history of secondary malignancies (196–198) is not reported with the V10 codes (*Coding Clinic* 1990; *Coding Clinic* 1998; *Official Coding Guidelines*).

Exercise 5.2

Use the Alphabetic Index to assign diagnosis and morphology codes (M codes) to questions 1 through 6; then assign the appropriate disease, procedure, and morphology codes to questions 7 and 8.

1. C cell carcinoma

   _M8510/3 , 193_

2. Theca cell carcinoma

   _M8600/3 , 183.0_

3. Acute monocytic leukemia

   _M9891/3 , 206.00_

4. Multiple myeloma

   _M9730/3 , 203.00_

5. Wilms' tumor

   _M8960/3 , 189.0_

6. Choriocarcinoma (male patient, age 31)

   _M9100/3 , 186.9_

7. Patient was admitted with a diagnosis of bone metastasis originating from the right upper lobe (RUL) of the lung. Pathology was consistent with oat cell carcinoma. This admission was for chemotherapy that was administered.

   _V58.11, 162.3 , 198.5 , 99.25_

8. Patient was admitted with a history of right breast carcinoma with mastectomy performed two years ago and no treatment currently given for breast carcinoma. Patient presents with complaints of vision disturbances. Workup revealed metastasis to the brain.

   _V10.3, 368.9, 198.3_

[handwritten margin notes: 6. M8000/3, M8042/2 oat cell]

Alphabetic Index Instructions

The main terms and subentries in the Alphabetic Index to Diseases and Injuries assist the coder in locating the morphological type of neoplasms. When a specific code or site is not listed in the index, cross-references direct the coder to the neoplasm table. The following steps should be followed in coding neoplasms:

1. **Locate the morphology of the tumor in the Alphabetic Index.** ICD-9-CM classifies neoplasms by system, organ, or site. Exceptions to this rule are:

   • Neoplasms of the lymphatic and hematopoietic system

   • Malignant melanomas of the skin

- Lipomas

- Common tumors of the bone, uterus, and ovary

Because of these exceptions, the Alphabetic Index must first be checked to determine if a code has been assigned for that specific histology type.

Leiomyoma (M8890/0)—*see also . . .*
    uterus (cervix) (corpus) 218.9
        interstitial 218.1
        intramural 218.1
        submucous 218.0
        subperitoneal 218.2
        subserous 218.2
    vascular (M8894/0)—*see* Neoplasm,
        connective tissue, benign

As the preceding example shows, the Alphabetic Index offers direction to the neoplasm table for selection of codes, but occasionally the index itself will provide the codes more directly.

2. **Follow instructions under the main term in the Alphabetic Index.** Instructions in the Alphabetic Index should be followed when determining which column to use in the neoplasm table.

Adenomyoma (M8932/0)—*see also*
    Neoplasm, by site, benign
  prostate 600.2

The directions in the Alphabetic Index can be overridden if the documentation in the health record specifies a different behavior.

    EXAMPLE: Malignant adenoma of colon

                153.9   Malignant neoplasm of colon, unspecified

Although the Alphabetic Index says to "*see also* Neoplasm, by site, benign," the coder should assign code 153.9, Malignant neoplasm of colon, unspecified, rather than code 211.3, Benign neoplasm of the colon.

When a diagnostic statement indicates which column of the neoplasm table to reference but does not identify the specific type of tumor, the neoplasm table should be consulted directly.

    EXAMPLE: Carcinoma in situ of cervix

                233.1   Carcinoma in situ of cervix uteri

After consulting the neoplasm table, code 233.1 from the in situ column is selected.

Tabular List Instructions

Specific instructions for coding neoplasms appear in the Tabular List as well as in the Alphabetic Index. The following information applies to the coding of neoplasms:

1. **Code functional activity associated with a neoplasm.** Some categories in the neoplasm chapter in the Tabular List offer the instructional notation "Use additional code" as advice to also code any functional activity associated with a particular neoplasm, such as increased or decreased hormone production due to the presence of a tumor.

---

183   Malignant neoplasm of ovary and other uterine adnexa

> Excludes: Douglas' cul-de-sac (158.8)

183.0   Ovary
Use additional code to identify any functional activity

> **EXAMPLE:**   Patient was admitted to the hospital with carcinoma of the ovary and menometrorrhagia due to hyperestrogenism.
>
> 183.0   Malignant neoplasm of ovary
> 256.0   Hyperestrogenism
> 626.2   Excessive or frequent menstruation

2. **Note variations in categories 150 and 201.** Two categories in the malignant section depart from the usual principles of classification. In each case, the fourth-digit subdivisions are not mutually exclusive. The two categories are:

- Malignant neoplasms of the esophagus (150)

- Hodgkin's disease (201)

> **EXAMPLE:**   150.0   Cervical esophagus
> 150.1   Thoracic esophagus
> 150.2   Abdominal esophagus
> 150.3   Upper third of esophagus
> 150.4   Middle third of esophagus
> 150.5   Lower third of esophagus

In the preceding example, the anatomy of the esophagus is classified in two ways because no uniform agreement exists on the use of these terms. Some physicians prefer the terms *upper, middle,* and *lower* to describe the site of the esophagus; others prefer *cervical, thoracic,* and *abdominal.* The code that correlates with documentation in the health record should be assigned.

> **EXAMPLE:**   201.0x   Hodgkin's paragranuloma
> 201.1x   Hodgkin's granuloma
> 201.2x   Hodgkin's sarcoma
> 201.4x   Lymphocytic-histiocytic predominance
> 201.5x   Nodular sclerosis
> 201.6x   Mixed cellularity
> 201.7x   Lymphocytic depletion
> 201.9x   Hodgkin's disease, unspecified

In the preceding example, a dual axis reflects the different terminology used by pathologists. One pathologist may use Hodgkin's paragranuloma; another may indicate the type of involvement as Hodgkin's lymphoma of mixed cellularity. Again, no uniform agreement exists on the use of these terms, so the terminology in the health record should be the guide in assigning a code.

Exercise 5.3

Using volumes 1 and 2 of ICD-9-CM (referring to the Alphabetic Index to Diseases and the neoplasm table), assign codes to the following. Do not assign morphology codes.

1. Malignant melanoma of skin of scalp

   172.4

2. Lipoma of face

   214.0

3. Glioma of the parietal lobe of brain

   239.6 , ✓ 191.3

4. Adenocarcinoma of prostate

   185 ,

5. Carcinoma in situ of vocal cord

   231.0 ,

6. Hypoglycemia due to islet cell adenoma of pancreas

   211.7, 251.1 ,

7. Epidermoid carcinoma of the middle third of the esophagus

   150.4 ,

8. Galactorrhea due to pituitary adenoma

   239.7, 676.60   ✓ 227.3, 611.6

9. Benign melanoma of skin of shoulder

   216.6

10. Adenoma of adrenal cortex with Conn's syndrome

   227.0 255.12 .

Coding of the Anatomical Site

ICD-9-CM provides guidelines for coding the anatomical site of a neoplasm to the highest degree of specificity. These guidelines are discussed in the following sections.

Classification of Malignant Neoplasms

Malignant neoplasms are separated into primary sites (140–195) and secondary or metastatic sites (196–198), with further subdivisions by anatomic sites.

Neoplasms of the lymphatic and hematopoietic system are always coded to categories 200 through 208, regardless of whether the neoplasm is stated as primary or secondary. Neoplasms of the lymphatic and hematopoietic system, such as leukemias and lymphomas, are considered widespread and systemic in nature and, as such, do not metastasize. Therefore, they are not coded to category 196, Secondary and unspecified malignant neoplasms of lymph nodes, which includes codes identifying secondary or metastatic neoplasms of the lymphatic system.

Determination of the Primary Site

The primary site is defined as the origin of the tumor. Physicians usually identify the origin of the tumor in the diagnostic statement. In some cases, however, the physician cannot identify the primary site. For these situations, ICD-9-CM provides an entry in the neoplasm table titled "unknown site or unspecified" assigned to code 199.1. Code 199.1 can be assigned whether or not the site is primary or secondary (metastatic) in nature.

Category 195

Category 195, Malignant neoplasms of other and ill-defined sites, is available for use only when a more specific site cannot be identified. This category includes malignant neoplasms of contiguous sites, not elsewhere classified, whose point of origin cannot be determined.

> **EXAMPLE:** Carcinoma of the neck
>
> 195.0   Malignant neoplasm of head, face, and neck

Definition of the Asterisk *

At the beginning of the neoplasm table, a boxed note defines the use of the asterisk (*). When the asterisk follows a specific site in the neoplasm table, the following rules apply:

- When the neoplasm is identified as a squamous cell carcinoma or an epidermoid carcinoma, that condition should be classified as a malignant neoplasm of the skin.

> **EXAMPLE:** Squamous cell carcinoma of the ankle
>
> 173.7   Malignant neoplasm of skin of lower limb, including hip (ankle)

The asterisk following the term *ankle* in the neoplasm table indicates that it would be incorrect in this case to assign code 195.5, Malignant neoplasm of lower limb, because the neoplasm is a squamous cell carcinoma. Instead, the malignant column for the entry "skin . . . ankle" in the neoplasm table should be referenced to assign the correct code: 173.7.

- When the neoplasm is identified as a papilloma of any type, that condition should be classified as a benign neoplasm of the skin.

> **EXAMPLE:** Papilloma of the arm
>
> 216.6   Benign neoplasm of skin of upper limb, including shoulder (arm)

The asterisk following the term *arm* in the neoplasm table indicates that it would be incorrect to assign code 229.8, Benign neoplasm of other specified sites, if the neoplasm is a papilloma. The benign column for the entry "skin, . . . arm" in the neoplasm table should be referenced to assign the correct code: 216.6.

Coding of Contiguous Sites

In some cases, the origin of the tumor (primary site) may involve two adjacent sites. Therefore, neoplasms with overlapping site boundaries are classified to the fourth-digit subcategory 8, titled "Other."

EXAMPLE: A malignant lesion of the jejunum and ileum

152.8   Malignant neoplasm of other specified sites of small intestine

---

152   Malignant neoplasm of small intestine, including duodenum
152.8   Other specified sites of small intestine
Duodenojejunal junction
Malignant neoplasm of contiguous or overlapping
   sites of small intestine whose point
   of origin cannot be determined

Code 152.8 is obtained by referencing the entry "intestine, . . . small . . . contiguous sites" in the neoplasm table.

Exercise 5.4

Assign ICD-9-CM codes to the following:

1. Subacute leukemia

2. Basal cell carcinoma of buttock

3. Papilloma of back

4. Adenocarcinoma of head of pancreas

5. Epidermoid carcinoma in situ of tongue, dorsal surface

6. Hemangioma of skin of lower leg

7. Acute myeloid leukemia in remission

8. Squamous cell carcinoma of leg

9. Hodgkin's granuloma of intra-abdominal lymph nodes and spleen

10. Paget's disease with infiltrating duct carcinoma of breast involving central portion, nipple, and areola

Classification of Primary Sites

As defined earlier in this chapter, a primary site refers to the site where the tumor originated. This subsection discusses some of the complexities involved in determining whether a neoplasm should be coded as a primary or a secondary site.

Surgical Removal Followed by Adjunct Therapy

When surgical removal of a primary site malignancy is followed by adjunct chemotherapy or radiotherapy, the malignancy code (from categories 140 through 198 or 200 through 208) is assigned as long as chemotherapy or radiotherapy is actively administered. Even though the neoplasm has been removed surgically, the patient is still receiving therapy for that condition and the active code for the malignant neoplasm must be assigned, rather than a V10 category code describing "history of carcinoma."

Surgical Removal Followed by Recurrence

If a primary malignant neoplasm previously removed by surgery or eradicated by radiotherapy or chemotherapy recurs, the primary malignant code for that site is assigned, unless the Alphabetic Index directs otherwise.

> **EXAMPLE:** Recurrence of carcinoma of inner aspect of lower lip
>
> 140.4   Malignant neoplasm of lower lip, inner aspect

The Alphabetic Index refers to the neoplasm table, where code 140.4 is found for neoplasm of the inner aspect of the lower lip.

> **EXAMPLE:** Recurrence of breast carcinoma in a mastectomy site
>
> 198.2   Secondary malignant neoplasm of skin

The Alphabetic Index refers to the neoplasm table where an entry of "mastectomy site" is found and code 198.2 is assigned. It should be noted that even though this is a recurrence in the same area, ICD-9-CM directs the use of a secondary malignancy code because the breast has been removed.

"Metastatic from" in Diagnostic Statements

When cancer is described as "metastatic from a specific site," it is interpreted as a primary neoplasm of that site.

> **EXAMPLE:** Carcinoma in cervical lymph nodes metastatic from lower esophagus
>
> 150.5   Malignant neoplasm of lower third of esophagus
> 196.0   Secondary malignant neoplasm of lymph nodes of head, face, and neck

The lower esophagus is the primary site (150.5). The secondary site is the cervical lymph nodes (196.0).

Exercise 5.5

Assign ICD-9-CM codes to the following. Do not assign M codes to these exercises.

1. Recurrent choriocarcinoma in female patient

   _____

2. Carcinoma of cervical lymph nodes from epidermoid carcinoma of larynx cartilage

   _____

3. Recurrence of papillary carcinoma of bladder dome, low-grade transitional cell

   _____

4. Burkitt's lymphoma in multiple lymph nodes and spleen

   _____

5. Carcinoma of the brain from the lower lobe of the lungs

   _____

Classification of Secondary Sites

The patient's health record is the best source of information for differentiating between a primary and a secondary site. A secondary site may be referred to as a metastatic site in the record documentation. The following subsection describes some of the principal terms used in diagnostic statements that refer to secondary malignant neoplasms.

"Metastatic To" and "Direct Extension To"

The terms "metastatic to" and "direct extension to" are both used in classifying secondary malignant neoplasms in ICD-9-CM. For example, cancer described as "metastatic to a specific site" is interpreted as a secondary neoplasm of that site.

EXAMPLE: Metastatic carcinoma of the colon to the lung

153.9   Malignant neoplasm of colon, unspecified
197.0   Secondary malignant neoplasm of lung

The colon (153.9) is the primary site, and the lung (197.0) is the secondary site.

"Spread To" and "Extension To"

When expressed in terms of malignant neoplasm with "spread to" or "extension to," diagnoses should be coded as primary sites with metastases.

EXAMPLE: Adenocarcinoma of the stomach with spread to the peritoneum

151.9   Malignant neoplasm of stomach, unspecified
197.6   Secondary malignant neoplasm of retroperitoneum and
        peritoneum

The stomach (151.9) is the primary site, and the peritoneum (197.6) is the secondary site.

Metastatic of One Site

If only one site is stated in the diagnostic statement and it is identified as metastatic, the coder determines whether the site should be coded as primary or secondary (assuming the health record does not provide additional information to assist in assigning a code).

> **EXAMPLE:** Metastatic serous papillary ovarian carcinoma

In the preceding example, the diagnostic statement identifies the carcinoma as metastatic. Before the code can be assigned, however, the following two steps must be taken:

1. In the Alphabetic Index, locate the morphology type of the neoplasm as described in the diagnostic statement.

   > **EXAMPLE:** In the preceding example, the morphology type is carcinoma with subterms "serous" and "papillary."

2. Review subterms for the specific site as identified in the diagnostic statement. If the specific site is identified, assign that code. If the specific site is not included as a subterm, assign the code for primary of an unspecified site.

   > **EXAMPLE:** In the preceding example, the specific site, ovary, is not identified; however, a code is provided for primary of unspecified site.
   > The following is displayed in the Alphabetic Index:
   >
   > **Carcinoma** (M8010/3) . . .
   >
   > serous (M8441/3)
   > papillary (M8460/3)
   > specified site—*see* Neoplasm, by site, malignant
   > unspecified site 183.0

   Code 183.0, Malignant neoplasm of ovary, is assigned as the principal diagnosis to indicate the primary malignant site.

3. When the code obtained in step 2 is 199.0 or 199.1, the directions in step 5 must be followed.

4. Now that the primary site of the carcinoma has been identified, a code must be assigned to describe the metastatic or secondary site. A review of the diagnostic statement finds no other site identified. Therefore, the neoplasm table must be used to determine the metastatic code. Because the metastatic site is unspecified, review the neoplasm table for a subterm of "unknown site or unspecified." From the second column, "Malignant, Secondary," select the code 199.1.

5. When the morphology is not stated, or the code obtained in step 2 is 199.0 or 199.1, the site described as metastatic in the diagnostic statement should be coded as a primary malignant neoplasm, unless it is included in the following list of exceptions.

   The following sites are exceptions to this rule and must be coded as secondary neoplasms of that site:

Bone	Brain
Diaphragm	Heart
Liver	Lymph nodes
Mediastinum	Meninges
Peritoneum	Pleura
Retroperitoneum	Spinal cord
Sites classifiable to 195.0–8	

EXAMPLE: Metastatic carcinoma of the bronchus. The morphology is carcinoma. Upon indexing "Carcinoma," the first step is to look for a subterm of unspecified site. In reviewing the entries, no subterm is found for unspecified site. However, "see also Neoplasm, by site, malignant" appears after the main term "Carcinoma."

6. The next step is to turn to the neoplasm table and look for a subterm of unspecified site. A code is selected from the "Malignant, Primary" column—199.1. However, step 5 informs coders to assign the site listed in the diagnostic statement as the primary site if code 199.1 is identified. The next step is to review the exception list to determine if bronchus is included in the list. Because bronchus is not included in the list, it is assigned as the primary site and identified by code 162.9, Malignant neoplasm of bronchus and lung, unspecified. To assign a code for the secondary site, unknown in this example, use the "Malignant, Secondary" column of the neoplasm table to locate the subterm of "unknown site or unspecified"—199.1.

Exercise 5.6

Assign ICD-9-CM codes to the following diagnoses:

1. Metastatic carcinoma of bone

   a. What is the morphology type of this neoplasm? _____

   b. What is the code for primary carcinoma of unspecified site? _____

   c. Is bone included in the exception list? _____

   d. What is the primary site? _____

   e. What is the secondary site? _____

2. Adenocarcinoma of sigmoid colon with extension to peritoneum

   _____

3. Metastatic carcinoma of mediastinum

   _____

4. Metastatic carcinoma of bile duct to local lymph nodes

   _____

5. Adenocarcinoma of prostate with metastasis to pelvic bones

   _____

Review Exercise: Chapter 5

Assign the appropriate ICD-9-CM codes (including morphology codes) for the following diagnoses and procedures:

1. Malignant carcinoid of appendix with appendectomy and resection of cecum

   153.5, M8240/3, 47.09, 45.72

2. Lipoma of kidney

   214.3

3. Metastatic carcinoma to liver from rectum

   197.7, M8000/6, 154.1

4. Hepatocellular carcinoma

   155.0 M8170/3

5. Carcinoma in situ of cervix

   233.1

6. Acute exacerbation of chronic leukemia

   208.10

7. Hodgkin's disease (mixed cellularity), head and neck with cervical lymph node biopsy

   201.61, M9652/3, 40.11

8. Epidermoid carcinoma of the upper lip; wide resection of lesion; chemotherapy

   M8070/3 27.42 V58.11

9. Subacute monocytic leukemia in remission

   206.21

10. Generalized carcinomatosis, primary site undetermined with abdominal paracentesis

    199.0, M8010/6, 54.91

11. Small cell carcinoma of the right lower lobe of the lung with metastasis to the mediastinum; partial right lower lobectomy

    162.5, M8041/3, 197.1, M8000/6, 01.53

12. Poorly differentiated lymphocytic lymphoma of the brain; admission for photon radiation therapy; radiation administered without complications

    200.11, V58.0, 92.24

13. Adenocarcinoma of the right breast, upper outer quadrant, with metastasis to the axillary lymph nodes; modified radical mastectomy

    174.4, M8000/6, 196.3, 85.43

14. Malignant melanoma of the lower arm with radical excision

    M8720/3, 172.6, 86.4

M8000/6

2 order

M8000/3
M8000/6

Review Exercise: Chapter 5 (Continued)

15. Admission for chemotherapy; 25-year-old male with inoperable giant cell glioblastoma; chemotherapy

    191.9, V58.11, 99.25

16. Cavernous angioma of the trunk (skin) with excision of skin lesion

    228.01, 86.3

17. Acute lymphocytic leukemia; admission for chemotherapy; chemotherapy

    204.00, V58.11 99.25

18. Ewing's sarcoma of the left femur with excision of lesion of bone

    195.5, M9260/3, 77.60

19. Squamous cell carcinoma of the leg with excision of skin lesion

    195.5 M8070/3 86.3

20. Tumor of abdomen

    239.2

Chapter 6

Endocrine, Nutritional and Metabolic Diseases, and Immunity Disorders

Chapter 3, Endocrine, Nutritional and Metabolic Diseases, and Immunity Disorders (240–279)

Chapter 3, Endocrine, Nutritional and Metabolic Diseases, and Immunity Disorders, in the Tabular List in volume 1 of ICD-9-CM includes conditions such as diabetes, cystic fibrosis, electrolyte imbalances, and disorders of the thyroid, parathyroid, and adrenal glands. In addition, chapter 3 provides codes for nutritional deficiencies, vitamin deficiencies, and other disorders of metabolism, as well as immune disorders.

Chapter 3 is subdivided into the following categories and section titles:

Categories	Section Titles
240–246	Disorders of Thyroid Gland
250–259	Diseases of Other Endocrine Glands
260–269	Nutritional Deficiencies
270–279	Other Metabolic and Immunity Disorders

Chapter 6 introduces coding instruction as it specifically relates to diabetes and to fluid, electrolyte, and acid-base imbalances.

Diabetes Mellitus

Diabetes mellitus is a metabolic disease in which the pancreas does not produce insulin normally. The cause of diabetes mellitus can be attributed to both hereditary and nonhereditary factors, such as obesity, surgical removal of the pancreas, or the action of certain drugs. When the pancreas fails to produce insulin, glucose (sugar) is not broken down to be used and stored by the body's cells. As a result, too much sugar accumulates in the blood, causing hyperglycemia, which, in turn, spills over into the urine, causing glycosuria. Saturating the blood and urine with glucose draws water out of the body, causing dehydration and thirst. Other symptoms include excessive hunger, marked weakness, and weight loss.

Laboratory findings indicating diabetes mellitus include:

- Elevated blood sugar after a glucose tolerance test: 160 mg/100 ml blood, one hour after a meal; 120 mg/100 ml blood, two hours after a meal (normal = 115–130 mg/100 ml blood, one hour after a meal)

- Evidence of glycosuria in a urine specimen

Treatment consists of insulin regulation by either insulin injection or oral antidiabetic agents, and/or a controlled diet.

Improper metabolism of fat produces a toxic condition called acidosis or ketoacidosis. This condition is recognized by an "alcoholic" odor on the patient's breath. Manifestations of ketoacidosis are anorexia, air hunger, and, eventually, coma and death. Complications include hypercholesterolemia, premature atherosclerosis, neuropathy, retinopathy, increased susceptibility to infection leading to skin rashes, and/or gangrene.

Category 250

Category 250, Diabetes mellitus, is subdivided to fourth-digit subcategories to identify the presence or absence of complications and/or manifestations.

250   Diabetes Mellitus
   250.0   Diabetes mellitus, without mention of complications
   250.1   Diabetes with ketoacidosis
   250.2   Diabetes with hyperosmolarity
   250.3   Diabetes with other coma
   250.4   Diabetes with renal manifestations
   250.5   Diabetes with ophthalmic manifestations
   250.6   Diabetes with neurological manifestations
   250.7   Diabetes with peripheral circulatory disorders
   250.8   Diabetes with other specified manifestations
   250.9   Diabetes with unspecified complication

Fifth-Digit Subclassification

Two forms of diabetes mellitus exist: type I and type II. If the type of diabetes is not documented in the medical records, the ICD-9-CM code assignment default is type II. These two types of diabetes mellitus were previously known as insulin dependent and non-insulin dependent. The distinction today is on the functioning of the pancreatic beta cells.

Type I diabetes was previously referred to as insulin-dependent type (IDDM). Most type I diabetics develop the condition before reaching puberty. For this reason, type I diabetes mellitus is also referred to as juvenile diabetes. Type I diabetes occurs when there is an absolute lack of insulin production. The diabetes begins most often in children and young adults, although type I diabetes can develop at any age. The cause is unknown.

Type II diabetes was previously referred to as non-insulin-dependent diabetes (NIDDM) or adult-onset diabetes. Type II diabetes is the more common form of diabetes mellitus, affecting 90 percent of the diabetic population. It is common in older adults but also can occur in teenagers and young adults. Risk factors include obesity and heredity. The cause is unknown.

Type I diabetes mellitus refers to the absence of pancreatic beta cells. Type II diabetes mellitus refers to the lack of proper functioning of pancreatic beta cells. The use of insulin is not a determining factor in the type of diabetes present in a patient. Type I diabetic patients must use insulin. Type II diabetic patients may or may not use insulin depending on their diabetic condition and the other health conditions they may have. Pregnant women who develop gestational diabetes may also require insulin to maintain proper blood glucose levels during the pregnancy.

The following fifth digits with category 250 have been revised to conform to the accepted terminology for diabetes mellitus. In addition to the fifth-digit title changes, a second code to indicate the long-term (current) use of insulin is assigned with the fifth digits of 0 and 2. The use of insulin by patients with type II diabetes mellitus and women with gestational diabetes will be identified by the V58.67 code. The following fifth digits are available for use with category 250:

- 0 type II or unspecified type, not stated as uncontrolled

  Fifth digit 0 is for use for type II patients, even if the patient requires insulin.

  Use additional code, if applicable, for associated long-term (current) insulin use, V58.67

- 1 type I [juvenile type], not stated as uncontrolled

- 2 type II or unspecified type, uncontrolled

  Fifth digit 2 is used for type II patients, even if the patient requires insulin.

  Use additional code, if applicable, for associated long-term (current) insulin use, V58.67

- 3 type I [juvenile type], uncontrolled

When coding the case of a patient who receives insulin during a hospitalization, it should not be assumed that the patient is a type I diabetic. Type II diabetics often may require the administration of insulin for a short time to regulate their diabetes; however, this does not imply that the patient is now a type I diabetic.

If the documentation in a medical record does not indicate the type of diabetes but does indicate that the patient uses insulin, the appropriate fifth digit for type II must be used. For type II patients who routinely use insulin, code V58.67, Long-term (current) use of insulin, should also be assigned to indicate the patient uses insulin. Code V58.67 should not be assigned if insulin is given temporarily to bring a type II patient's blood sugar under control during an encounter.

Documentation in the health record must support assignment of a type I diabetes. Furthermore, use of fifth digits 2 or 3 also must be confirmed by appropriate documentation. The physician must document the diabetes as "out of control" or "uncontrolled."

Complications and Manifestations

Some diabetics develop other conditions (for example, retinopathy, neuropathy, and others) that may or may not be due to diabetes mellitus. ICD-9-CM provides codes when a causal relationship exists between a condition and the diabetes:

250.4   **Diabetes with renal manifestations**
250.5   **Diabetes with ophthalmic manifestations**
250.6   **Diabetes with neurological manifestations**
250.7   **Diabetes with peripheral circulatory disorders**
250.8   **Diabetes with other specified manifestations**

To assign these codes, documentation in the health record must support this causal relationship. When a causal relationship exists, the principal diagnosis code assigned is a diabetic code from category 250, followed by the code for the manifestation or complication. The diabetes codes and the secondary codes that correspond to them are paired codes that follow the etiology/manifestation convention of the classification.

> **EXAMPLE:**   Proliferative diabetic retinopathy due to type I diabetes mellitus
>
> 250.51   Diabetes with ophthalmic manifestations
> 362.02   Proliferative diabetic retinopathy

The principal diagnosis is diabetes with ophthalmic manifestations (250.51), followed by proliferative diabetic retinopathy (362.02).

When a patient develops several complications due to diabetes, more than one code from subcategories 250.4 through 250.8 may be assigned to describe the patient's condition completely. Assign as many codes from category 250 as needed to identify all of the associated conditions that the patient has.

> **EXAMPLE:**   Diabetic polyneuropathy and peripheral angiopathy due to insulin-dependent diabetes mellitus
>
> 250.61   Diabetes with neurological manifestations, type I
> *357.2   Polyneuropathy in diabetes*
> 250.71   Diabetes with peripheral circulatory disorders, type I
> *443.81   Peripheral angiopathy in diseases classified elsewhere*

As in the preceding example of diabetic polyneuropathy, the Tabular List often displays a manifestation in italic type as a reminder that the manifestation (for example, polyneuropathy) should not be used as a principal diagnosis.

Official coding guidelines exist for the coding of diabetes mellitus. See Section I. C. Chapter Specific Guidelines, Chapter 3: Endocrine, Nutritional, and Metabolic Diseases and Immunity Disorders (240–279).

Metabolic Disorders

Category 276 includes the following conditions:

276   **Disorders of fluid, electrolyte and acid-base imbalance**
   276.0   **Hyperosmolality and/or hypernatremia**
   276.1   **Hyposmolality and/or hyponatremia**
   276.2   **Acidosis**
   276.3   **Alkalosis**
   276.4   **Mixed acid-base balance disorder**
   276.5   **Volume depletion**
   276.6   **Fluid overload**
   276.7   **Hyperpotassemia**
   276.8   **Hypopotassemia**
   276.9   **Electrolyte and fluid disorders, not elsewhere classified**

The preceding conditions are usually symptoms of a larger disease process and, as such, should be coded as additional diagnoses when documented in the health record. In some cases, however, the patient may be admitted for treatment of one of these symptoms, with the underlying condition not requiring much care. In such cases, the symptom or metabolic disorder may be assigned as the principal diagnosis.

Volume depletion may refer to depletion of total body water (dehydration) or depletion of the blood volume (hypovolemia). Dehydration, a lack of adequate water in the body, can be a medical emergency. Common in infants and elderly people, severe dehydration can occur with vomiting, excessive heat and sweating, diarrhea, or lack of food or fluid intake. Symptoms include extreme thirst, tiredness, light-headedness, abdominal or muscle cramping, dry mouth, or restlessness. Blood volume may be maintained despite dehydration, with fluid being pulled from other tissues. Conversely, hypovolemia may occur without dehydration when "third-spacing" of fluids occurs, for example, with significant edema or ascites. Hypovolemia is an abnormally low circulating blood volume. Blood loss may be due to internal bleeding from the intestine or stomach, external bleeding from an injury, or loss of blood volume and body fluid associated with diarrhea, vomiting, dehydration, or burns. If hypovolemia is severe, hypovolemic shock can occur with symptoms such as rapid or weak pulse, feeling faint, pale skin, cool or moist skin, rapid breathing, anxiety, overall weakness, and low blood pressure. Emergency medical attention must be sought. Given that the nature of these two conditions and their respective treatments are different, coding of hypovolemia is different from dehydration.

> **EXAMPLE:** Patient admitted with severe dehydration and gastroenteritis. Treatment was directed toward resolving the dehydration.
>
> 276.51 Dehydration
> 558.9 Other and unspecified noninfectious gastroenteritis and colitis

In the preceding example, dehydration (276.51) is assigned as the principal diagnosis, followed by the underlying cause, gastroenteritis (558.9).

Codes for cystic fibrosis (277.0) have expansions to the fifth-digit level to describe the different manifestations that often occur. Cystic fibrosis is an inherited disease of the exocrine glands and affects the GI and respiratory systems. It is characterized by COPD, pancreatic insufficiency, and abnormally high sweat electrolytes. The degree of pulmonary involvement usually determines the course of the disease. The patient's demise is often the result of respiratory failure and cor pulmonale. Recently, new codes were added to describe cystic fibrosis with pulmonary manifestations, with complications of pancreatic enzyme replacement therapy, and with other manifestations.

Review Exercise: Chapter 6

Assign ICD-9-CM codes to the following:

1. Type II diabetic with nephrosis due to the diabetes

   250.40 581.81

2. Toxic diffuse goiter with thyrotoxic crisis

   242.01

3. Cushing's syndrome

   255.0

4. Hypokalemia

   276.8

5. Cystic fibrosis with pulmonary manifestations

   277.02

6. Uncontrolled type II diabetes mellitus; mild malnutrition

   250.02 263.1

7. Panhypopituitarism

   253.2

8. Sporadic hypogammaglobulinemia

   279.06

(Continued on next page)

Review Exercise: Chapter 6 (Continued)

9. Tyrosinemia

   _270.2_

10. Acute infantile rickets

    _268.0_

11. Lower extremity ulcer on heel of foot secondary to brittle diabetes mellitus, type I, uncontrolled

    _250.83 707.14_

12. Diabetic proliferative retinopathy in a patient with controlled type I diabetes

    _250.51 362.02_

13. Arteriosclerotic heart disease involving native arteries with familial hypercholesterolemia

    _414.01 272.0_

14. Overweight adult with a body mass index (BMI) of 26.5

    _278.02 V85.22_

15. Syndrome of inappropriate secretion of antidiuretic hormone (SIADH)

    _253.6_

16. Marasmus secondary to AIDS

    _042 261_

17. Gouty arthritis

    _274.0_

18. Hypoglycemia in type I diabetic

    _250.81_

19. Hyperthyroidism with nodular goiter; partial thyroidectomy

    _242.30 06.39_

20. Waldenström's hypergammaglobulinemia

    _273.0_

Chapter 7

Diseases of the Blood and Blood-Forming Organs

Chapter 4, Diseases of the Blood and Blood-Forming Organs (280–289)

Chapter 4, Diseases of the Blood and Blood-Forming Organs, in the Tabular List in volume 1 of ICD-9-CM includes anemias, coagulation defects, purpura, and other hemorrhagic conditions and diseases of the white blood cells.

Anemias

Anemia is defined as a decrease in the number of erythrocytes (red blood cells), the quantity of hemoglobin, or the volume of packed red cells in the blood. Laboratory data reflect a decrease in red blood cells (RBCs), hemoglobin (Hgb), or hematocrit (Hct). Anemia is manifested by pallor of skin and mucous membranes, shortness of breath, palpitations of the heart, soft systolic murmurs, lethargy, and fatigability.

Deficiency Anemias

Categories 280–281 include codes for deficiency anemias. The most common type of anemia, iron deficiency anemia (category 280), is caused by an inadequate absorption of or excessive loss of iron. Iron deficiency anemia due to chronic blood loss is reported with code 280.0. The underlying cause of the bleeding—such as an ulcer, menorrhagia, or cancer—also should be coded when documented in the health record. Without further specification, iron deficiency anemia is reported with code 280.9.

Acute posthemorrhagic anemia is anemia due to acute blood loss and is reported with code 285.1. It is defined as a normocytic, normochromic anemia developing as a result of rapid loss of large quantities of RBCs during bleeding. It may occur as a result of a massive hemorrhage that may be due to spontaneous or traumatic rupture of a large blood vessel, rupture of an aneurysm, arterial erosion from a peptic ulcer or neoplastic process, or complications of surgery from excessive blood loss.

Category 281 describes other deficiency anemias that may be referred to as megaloblastic anemias. The etiology of megaloblastic anemias includes a deficiency or defective utilization of vitamin B_{12} or folic acid. The condition can also be caused by the presence of cytotoxic agents (usually antineoplastic or immunosuppressive drugs) that interfere with DNA synthesis. Megaloblastic anemias include:

281.0   Pernicious anemia
281.1   Other vitamin B$_{12}$ anemias
281.2   Folate deficiency
281.3   Other specific megaloblastic anemias, NEC
281.4   Protein deficiency anemias
281.8   Anemia associated with other specific nutritional deficiencies

Hemolytic Anemias

Hemolytic anemia refers to an abnormal reduction of red blood cells caused by an increased rate of red blood cell destruction and the inability of the bone marrow to compensate. Hemolytic anemias may be acquired (category 283) or hereditary (category 282). Hereditary anemias are caused by intrinsic abnormalities involving structural defects of red blood cells or defects of globin synthesis or structure. ICD-9-CM classifies hereditary hemolytic anemias to category 282, which includes the following common hematologic disorders:

282.41–282.49   Thalassemias
282.5   Sickle-cell trait
282.60–282.62   Sickle-cell disease

Typically, acquired hemolytic anemias are caused by extrinsic factors such as trauma (surgery or burns), infection, systemic diseases (Hodgkin's lymphoma, leukemia, or systemic lupus erythematosus), drugs or toxins, liver or renal disease, or abnormal immune responses. ICD-9-CM classifies acquired hemolytic anemia to category 283, with the fourth and fifth digits (when applicable) describing the specific type or cause of disorder; for example,

283.0   Autoimmune hemolytic anemias
283.10–283.19   Non-immune hemolytic anemias

Aplastic anemia is caused by an abnormal reduction of red blood cells due to a lack of bone marrow blood production. Usually, this type of anemia is accompanied by agranulocytosis and thrombocytopenia, in which case it is called pancytopenia. Half of aplastic anemia cases are attributed to exposure to a toxin, and half are determined to be of unknown causes. Toxins that can result in aplastic anemia include radiation, chemotherapy, chloramphenicol, sulfonamides, and phenytoin. ICD-9-CM classifies aplastic anemias to category 284, with the fourth digits indicating the specific type. Congenital, constitutional, or primary aplastic anemia is reported with code 284.8. An additional E code should be assigned to identify the specific toxin or substance. Aplastic anemia without further specification is reported with code 284.9.

Other and Unspecified Anemias

Category 285 classifies other and unspecified anemias, including acute blood loss anemia (285.1) and sideroblastic anemia (285.0). Code 285.9 is used to report anemia, unspecified. Recently, subcategory 285.2 was added to allow three new codes to be reported: 285.21, Anemia of end-stage renal disease; 285.22, Anemia in neoplastic disease; and 285.29, Anemia of other chronic illness.

Coagulation Defects

Coagulation defects are disorders of the platelets that result in serious bleeding due to a deficiency of one or more clotting factors. ICD-9-CM classifies coagulation defects to category 286, with the fourth digit identifying the specific type of defect. Three types of coagulation defects that are recognized are:

1. Classic hemophilia (hemophilia A), which is the most common, occurs as a result of factor VIII deficiency. It is inherited as an X-linked recessive disorder affecting males and transmitted by females. ICD-9-CM classifies classic hemophilia to code 286.0.

2. Hemophilia B (Christmas disease) results from a deficiency of factor IX. As with hemophilia A, this type is transmitted as an X-linked recessive trait. ICD-9-CM classifies hemophilia B to code 286.1.

3. Hemophilia C is an autosomal recessive disease caused by a deficiency in factor XI. ICD-9-CM classifies this condition to code 286.2.

Other conditions are often confused with coagulation defects. For example, a patient being treated with Coumadin, heparin, or another anticoagulant may develop bleeding or hemorrhage. Bleeding that occurs in a patient taking the drug Coumadin or heparin is an adverse effect of the anticoagulant therapy. When this occurs, a code for the condition and associated hemorrhage is assigned, with an additional code of E934.2 to indicate the drug documented by the physician and responsible for the bleeding. Code 286.5, Hemorrhagic disorder due to intrinsic circulating anticoagulants, is not assigned for bleeding in a patient taking an anticoagulant drug.

Another condition confused with coagulation defects is prolonged prothrombin time or other abnormal coagulation profiles. This condition is not coded as a coagulation defect. Code 790.92 is assigned to report an abnormal laboratory finding. However, when a patient is receiving Coumadin therapy, it is expected that the patient will have a prolonged bleeding time, and in such a case, code 790.92 is not assigned.

Purpura and Other Hemorrhagic Conditions

Category 287 includes codes that describe purpura, thrombocytopenia, and other hemorrhagic disorders. Thrombocytopenia is diagnosed when the platelets fall below 100,000/mm. Two types of thrombocytopenia are recognized: primary or idiopathic and secondary. Idiopathic thrombocytopenic purpura (ITP) is an autoimmune disorder with development of antibodies to one's own platelets. In children, the condition often resolves without treatment. In adults, medication such as corticosteroids or thrombopoietins are given. In severe cases, the spleen may be removed to eliminate the platelet destruction by phagocytosis. Primary thrombocytopenia may also be congenital or hereditary. Primary thrombocytopenia is classified in ICD-9-CM to 287.30–287.39 depending on the type. Secondary thrombocytopenia is a complication of another disease. Causes may include viral or bacterial infections, systemic lupus erythematosus, chronic lymphocytic leukemia, sarcoidosis, or carcinoma of the ovary. Drugs such as chemotherapy, heparin, and rifampin can cause the condition. It is also a common, temporary complication of bone marrow transplant. The treatment of the secondary form of this conditions centers on treating the underlying disease or changing medication. If bleeding is severe, a person is given transfusions of platelets to replace those destroyed. ICD-9-CM classifies secondary thrombocytopenia to code 287.4. An additional code should be assigned to identify the drug or external cause (E code).

Diseases of the White Blood Cells

Category 288 classifies diseases of the white blood cells (WBCs), with the fourth digit identifying the specific type of disorder. Two types of WBCs circulate in the body: granular and nongranular (agranular) leukocytes. Granular leukocytes include neutrophils, eosinophils, and basophils. Nongranular leukocytes include lymphocytes and monocytes. Agranulocytosis (also known as neutropenia) is an acute condition characterized by the absence of neutrophils and an extremely low granulocyte count. The most common cause is drug toxicity or hypersensitivity caused by large doses of drugs and/or drugs taken over a long period of time. Neutropenia commonly occurs in patients receiving chemotherapy. ICD-9-CM classifies neutropenia to code 288.0.

Other Blood and Blood-Forming Organ Diseases

The last category in chapter 4 of ICD-9-CM (category 289) includes conditions not classified elsewhere, including familial and secondary polycythemia, chronic lymphadenitis, hypersplenism, chronic congestive splenomegaly, and methemoglobinemia.

Secondary polycythemia occurs as a result of tissue hypoxia and is associated with chronic obstructive pulmonary disease, congenital heart disease, and prolonged exposures to high altitudes (higher than 10,000 feet). ICD-9-CM classifies secondary polycythemia to code 289.0.

Review Exercise: Chapter 7

Assign ICD-9-CM codes to the following (morphology codes are not necessary):

1. Sickle-cell (Hb-SS) disease with crisis

   282.62

2. Iron deficiency anemia secondary to blood loss

   280.0

3. Von Willebrand's disease

   286.4

4. Chronic congestive splenomegaly

   289.51

5. Congenital nonspherocytic hemolytic anemia

   282.3

6. Idiopathic thrombocytopenic purpura

   287.31

7. Malignant neutropenia

   288.0

8. Fanconi's anemia

   284.0

Review Exercise: Chapter 7 (Continued)

9. Microangiopathic hemolytic anemia

   283.19

10. Aplastic anemia secondary to antineoplastic medication for breast cancer ?

   284.8, (174.9), E933.1

11. Disseminated intravascular coagulation

   286.6

12. Acute hemorrhaging duodenal ulcer with acute blood loss anemia ?

   532.00, (285.1)

13. Acquired hemolytic anemia due to AIDS

   042, 283.9

14. Chronic mesenteric lymphadenitis with biopsy of lymphatic structure

   289.2, 40.11

15. Cooley's anemia; splenectomy   Total

   282.49,   41.5

16. Polycythemia secondary to living in a high-altitude region

   289.0, (E902.0)

17. Glucose-6-phosphate dehydrogenase (G-6-PD) anemia

   282.2

18. Goat's milk anemia

   281.2

19. Deficiency of factor I

   286.3

20. Hematuria, identified as a result of the patient's Coumadin therapy, properly administered

   599.7, (E934.2)

Chapter 8

Mental Disorders

Chapter 5, Mental Disorders (290–319)

Chapter 5, Mental Disorders, in the Tabular List in volume 1 of ICD-9-CM classifies mental disorders into the following categories and section titles:

Categories	Section Titles
290–299	Psychoses
300–316	Neurotic Disorders, Personality Disorders, and Other Nonpsychotic Mental Disorders
317–319	Mental Retardation

The codes in chapter 5 are compatible with those included in the *Diagnostic and Statistical Manual of Mental Disorders, Fourth Edition, Text Revision (DSM-IV-TR)*, published by the American Psychiatric Association.

DSM-IV-TR

The *Diagnostic and Statistical Manual of Mental Disorders, Fourth Edition, Text Revision (DSM-IV-TR),* provides clear descriptions of diagnostic categories that allow clinicians and investigators to diagnose, communicate about, study, and treat people with various mental disorders. All DSM-IV-TR categories are listed in chapter 5 of ICD-9-CM; however, there are some variations, especially in the narrative text of the codes.

DSM-IV uses a multiaxial system involving an assessment on five different axes:

- Axis I (Clinical Disorders and Other Conditions That May Be a Focus of Attention) includes all psychiatric disorders except personality disorders and mental retardation.

- Axis II includes personality disorders and mental retardation.

- Axis III identifies the presence of general medical conditions.

- Axis IV is used to note clinically relevant psychosocial and environmental problems.

- Axis V is used to indicate the individual's overall psychological, social, and occupational functioning.

In addition, axes I, II, and III provide diagnostic information.

Glossary of Mental Disorders and Chapter Introduction

A glossary of mental disorders has been removed from the official government ICD-9-CM (CD-ROM version) effective October 1, 2004. It previously was located in appendix B of volume 1. The appendix had not been maintained for many years and was no longer completely accurate. Although the appropriate code assignment should be determined on the basis of documentation in the health record, the glossary served as a reference tool for a basic understanding of psychiatric terms. Coders may refer to DSM-IV-TR for definitions of the mental disorders classified in chapter 5 of ICD-9-CM.

Previously, chapter 5 of ICD-9-CM contained an introduction that gave credit to the American Psychiatric Association (APA) in modifying ICD-9 to provide detail useful to American clinicians and coders in using the chapter. APA continues to work to improve ICD-9-CM, but the introduction was dated and no longer useful.

Updating of Code Descriptions

Effective October 1, 2004, numerous substantial changes were made to the titles of category and subcategory codes within chapter 5 of ICD-9-CM. Although the diagnostic codes used in the DSM-IV-TR classification system have been taken from ICD-9-CM, the diagnostic terminology has evolved over several revisions of the DSM in order to keep up with current clinical usage. In contrast, the terminology used in ICD-9-CM has not changed much since the introduction of ICD-9 in the late 1970s. The APA has worked closely with the National Center for Health Statistics over the years to ensure a seamless crosswalk between the two systems so that coders can easily determine the ICD-9-CM diagnosis codes that correspond to the DSM diagnoses. The adoption of ICD-10-CM in the future will have a near-perfect compatibility between the two systems as the diagnostic terms are virtually identical. Due to the delay in adopting ICD-10-CM and the HIPAA designation that ICD-9-CM be the only diagnosis code set to be used, code title changes have been made to replace as much as possible the obsolete ICD-9-CM diagnostic terminology of mental disorders with DSM-IV-TR (and ICD-10-CM) terminology. For example, category 290, formerly titled "Senile and presenile organic psychotic conditions," is currently titled "Dementias."

Multiple Coding

When coding mental disorders, instructional notations to assign additional codes to fully describe the patient's condition are frequently encountered. Examples of three such instructional notations follow:

- Instructional note to assign an additional code to identify any associated neurological disorder.

  EXAMPLE: **299.1 Childhood disintegrative disorder**
  Heller's syndrome

  Use additional code to identify any associated neurological disorder.

- Instructional note to assign an additional code to identify any associated mental disorder, as well as physical condition.

> **EXAMPLE:** **301   Personality disorders**
> Includes: character neurosis
>
> Use additional code to identify any associated neurosis or psychosis, or physical condition.

- Instructional note to assign a specific code for the presence of another condition (for example, cerebral atherosclerosis).

> **EXAMPLE:** **290.4   Vascular dementia**
> Multi-infarct dementia or psychosis
>
> Use additional code to identify cerebral atherosclerosis (437.0).

Fifth-Digit Subclassification

The use of fifth digits occurs quite frequently in the chapter on mental disorders of ICD-9-CM. Although this specificity exists in the classification system, documentation in the health record often does not provide the information required to assign a specific fifth digit. The fifth digit for unspecified course of illness is assigned when further information is unavailable. Never assume the course of illness from general statements made in the health record.

Exercise 8.1

Assign ICD-9-CM codes to the following:

1. Autistic disorder, active

   299.00

2. Continuous cocaine dependence

   304.21

3. Latent schizophrenia, chronic

   295.52

4. Acute senile dementia in Alzheimer's disease

   331.0   294.10

5. Epileptic psychosis with generalized grand mal epilepsy

   294.8   345.90   345.10

Inclusion and Exclusion Notes

Chapter 5 of ICD-9-CM contains many special inclusion notes, such as those in the following two examples:

> **EXAMPLE:** **295   Schizophrenic disorders**
> Includes: schizophrenia of the types described in 295.0–295.9 occurring in children

The preceding inclusion note says that codes 295.0–295.9 may be assigned in the pediatric population, if applicable.

EXAMPLE: **298**   **Other nonorganic psychoses**

Includes: psychotic conditions due to or provoked by:
     emotional stress
     environmental factors as major part of etiology

The preceding inclusion note serves to advise that psychotic conditions due to or provoked by emotional stress (for example, divorce) or environmental factors (for example, a forest fire) are assigned to category 298.

Exclusion notes also are used frequently in chapter 5 to warn that specified forms of a condition are classified elsewhere, such as:

290.0   **Senile dementia, uncomplicated**

Senile dementia:

NOS

simple type

Excludes: *mild memory disturbances, not amounting to dementia,*
     associated with senile brain disease (310.1)
senile dementia with:
     delirium or confusion (290.3)
     delusional [paranoid] features (290.20)
     depressive features (290.21)

The preceding exclusion note advises that mild memory disturbances associated with senile brain disease and senile dementia with specific features—such as confusion, paranoia, or depression—are classified elsewhere.

294.10   **Dementia in conditions classified elsewhere without behavioral disturbance**

Dementia in conditions classified elsewhere NOS

294.11   **Dementia in conditions classified elsewhere with behavioral disturbance**

Aggressive behavior

Combative behavior

Violent behavior

Wandering off

Coders should pay special attention to inclusion and exclusion notes in the previous example regarding the treatment and long-term care of patients with dementia affected by the behavioral aspect of the dementia. Patients who are aggressive and combative or who wander off pose a greater treatment dilemma. Subcategory code 294.1 was expanded to distinguish with and without behavioral disturbance. An inclusion note was added to 294.11 to list those conditions considered to be behavioral disturbances.

Similarly, an excludes note was added to code 294.11 to describe those conditions not considered to be behavioral disturbances.

Alcoholism and Alcohol Abuse

Alcoholism (alcohol dependence) is a chronic condition in which a patient has become dependent on alcohol with increased tolerance and is unable to stop using it, even while facing strong incentives such as impairment of health, deteriorated social interactions, and interference with job performance. Such patients often experience physical signs of withdrawal during any sudden cessation of drinking.

Alcoholism is classified to category 303, Alcohol dependence syndrome. The fourth digits identify a state of acute intoxication (303.0) or other and unspecified forms, including chronic forms (303.9). The fifth digits identify the stage of the alcoholism—unspecified, continuous, episodic, or in remission. An additional code should be assigned to identify any of the following associated conditions:

Alcohol-induced mental disorders (291.0–291.9)
Drug dependence (304.0–304.9)
Physical complication of alcohol, such as:
    Cerebral degeneration (331.7)
    Cirrhosis of the liver (571.2)
    Epilepsy (345.00–345.90)
    Gastritis (535.3)
    Hepatitis (571.1)
    Liver damage (571.3)

Reported with code 305.0x, acute alcohol abuse is described as problem drinking and includes those patients who drink to excess but have not reached a stage of physical dependency. The fifth digit (shown as x in the previous sentence) again identifies the stage of the condition (unspecified, continuous, episodic, or in remission); for example: 305.01, Alcohol abuse, continuous.

A point to remember: The excludes note appearing below code 305.0 indicates that a diagnosis of acute alcohol intoxication in a patient with alcoholism is reported with code 303.0x *(Coding Clinic 1991)*.

Drug Dependence and Abuse

Drug dependence or drug addiction is a chronic mental and physical condition related to the patient's pattern of taking a drug or a combination of drugs. It is characterized by behavioral and physiological responses such as a compulsion to take the drug, to experience its psychic effects, or to avoid the discomfort of its absence. There is increased tolerance and an inability to stop the use of the drug, even with strong incentives.

Category 304 of ICD-9-CM classifies drug addiction. The fourth digit identifies the specific drug or class of drug involved. The fifth digit identifies the stage of the dependence—unspecified, continuous, episodic, or in remission. When several drugs are involved in the drug addiction, ICD-9-CM provides the following codes for use: 304.7x, Combination drugs including an opioid drug, and 304.8x, Combination drugs not including an opioid drug.

Nondependent drug abuse represents problem drug taking and includes those patients who take drugs to excess but have not yet reached a state of dependence. ICD-9-CM classifies nondependent drug abuse to codes 305.2x through 305.9x. The fourth digit identifies the specific class of drug, and the fifth digit indicates the stage of the addiction *(Coding Clinic 1991)*.

Fifth Digits for Alcohol/Drug Dependence and Abuse

The following information can serve as a guide to selecting the appropriate fifth digit for categories 303 and 304 and for code 305.0x. As always, the documentation in the health record should serve as the final determination for the code selected.

0	Unspecified	Inadequate documentation in the health record
1	Continuous	Alcohol: Refers to daily intake of large amounts of alcohol or regular heavy drinking on weekends or days off from work
		Drugs: Daily or almost daily use of drug(s)
2	Episodic	Alcohol: Refers to alcoholic binges lasting weeks or months, followed by long periods of sobriety
		Drugs: Indicates short periods between drug use or use on the weekends
3	Remission	Refers to either a complete cessation of alcohol or drug intake or the period during which a decrease toward cessation is taking place (*Coding Clinic* 1991)

Principal Diagnosis Selection for Patients Admitted for Alcohol or Drug Dependence Treatment

The circumstances of admission for patients with alcohol and/or drug dependence and associated mental disorders govern the selection of principal diagnosis. This is in keeping with the UHDDS definition of principal diagnosis as "the condition established after study to be chiefly responsible for occasioning the admission of the patient to the hospital for care." The following guidelines will help coders determine the appropriate principal diagnosis:

- If the patient is admitted in withdrawal or if withdrawal develops after admission, the withdrawal code is designated as the principal diagnosis. Categories 291 and 292 include codes that describe withdrawal symptoms. The code for the substance abuse/ dependence is listed second; for example, 292.0, Drug withdrawal, and 304.01, Opioid-type dependence, continuous.

- If the patient is admitted with a diagnosis of a substance-related mental condition, such as alcoholic dementia, the principal diagnosis is the mental condition, followed by a code for alcohol/drug dependence or abuse; for example, 291.2, Alcohol-induced persisting dementia, and 303.91, Chronic alcoholism, continuous.

- If the patient is admitted for detoxification or rehabilitation or both, and no related mental condition is documented, the principal diagnosis is the code describing the alcohol and/or drug abuse/dependence; for example, 304.22, Cocaine dependence, episodic.

- If the patient is admitted with an unrelated condition and has a diagnosis of alcohol and/or drug dependence/abuse, the unrelated condition is the principal diagnosis. The code for substance abuse/dependence is listed second; for example, 038.0, Streptococcal septicemia, and 303.90, Chronic alcoholism, unspecified.

- If the patient is admitted for treatment or evaluation of a physical complaint related to alcohol and/or drug abuse/dependence, the physical condition is the principal diagnosis, followed by the code for the alcohol and/or drug abuse/dependence (*Coding Clinic* 1991); for example, 535.30, Alcoholic gastritis, without mention of hemorrhage, and 303.91, Chronic alcoholism, continuous.

Therapy for Alcohol or Drug Dependence

Therapies for patients with diagnoses of substance abuse or dependence consist of detoxification, rehabilitation, or both.

Detoxification

Detoxification is the active management of withdrawal symptoms in a patient who is physically dependent on alcohol and/or drugs. Treatment includes evaluation, observation, and monitoring, as well as administration of thiamine and multivitamins for nutrition and other medications, such as methadone, clonidine, long-acting barbiturates, benzodiazepines, and carbamazepine.

Rehabilitation

Rehabilitation is a structured program that results in controlling the alcohol or drug use and in replacing alcohol or drug dependence with activities that are nonchemical in nature. Modalities may include methadone maintenance (for opiate dependents), therapeutic communities (residential), and long-term outpatient drug- or alcohol-free treatments.

Coding Therapies for Alcohol and Drug Dependence

The codes for therapies for alcohol and drug dependence are found in the Tabular List in volume 3 of ICD-9-CM.

Therapy for alcohol abuse and dependence is coded as follows:

94.61 **Alcohol rehabilitation**
94.62 **Alcohol detoxification**
94.63 **Alcohol rehabilitation and detoxification**

Therapy for drug abuse and dependence is coded as follows:

94.64 **Drug rehabilitation**
94.65 **Drug detoxification**
94.66 **Drug rehabilitation and detoxification**

Combined therapies for patients with both alcohol and drug dependence are coded as follows:

94.67 **Combined alcohol and drug rehabilitation**
94.68 **Combined alcohol and drug detoxification**
94.69 **Combined alcohol and drug rehabilitation and detoxification**

It may happen that a patient receives detoxification for either drug or alcohol dependence and rehabilitation for both alcohol and drug dependence. This would be coded as 94.62 for alcohol detoxification or 94.65 for drug detoxification, and 94.67 for combined alcohol and drug rehabilitation (*Coding Clinic*, 2nd Quarter 1991).

Review Exercise: Chapter 8

Assign ICD-9-CM codes to the following:

1. Drug withdrawal; diazepam dependence, continuous; patient underwent detox services

   292.0, 304.11, 94.65

2. Acute exacerbation of chronic undifferentiated schizophrenia

   (295.64)   295.94 ✓ .   chk.

3. Reactive depressive psychosis due to death of child

   298.0

4. Dissociative fugue

   300.13   '

5. Anxiety reaction manifested by fainting

   300.00   780.2

6. Alcoholic gastritis due to chronic alcoholism, episodic

   535.30   303.92

7. Disruptive behavior disorder

   312.9

8. Acute senile depression

   ✓296.20 (290.21)   ? chk

9. Hypochondriac with continuous laxative habit

   300.7 (305.91)

10. Psychogenic mucous colitis

    316, 564.9

11. Attention deficit disorder with hyperactivity (ADDH)

    314.01

12. Alcohol dependence syndrome in remission resulting in cirrhosis of liver   chk.

    571.2, 303.3

13. Cerebral arteriosclerotic vascular dementia   chk.

    290.40, 437.0

14. Bipolar II disease

    296.89

15. Acute reaction to stress secondary to death of spouse

    308.3

Chapter 9

Diseases of the Nervous System and Sense Organs

Chapter 6, Diseases of the Nervous System and Sense Organs (320–389)

Chapter 6, Diseases of the Nervous System and Sense Organs, in the Tabular List in volume 1 of ICD-9-CM classifies conditions affecting the brain and spinal cord, as well as the peripheral nervous system. In addition, it classifies a variety of eye and adnexal disorders, and diseases of the ear and mastoid process.

Chapter 6 is subdivided into the following categories and section titles:

Categories	Section Titles
320–326	Inflammatory Diseases of the Central Nervous System
330–337	Hereditary and Degenerative Diseases of the Central Nervous System
340–349	Other Disorders of the Central Nervous System
350–359	Disorders of the Peripheral Nervous System
360–379	Disorders of the Eye and Adnexa
380–389	Diseases of the Ear and Mastoid Process

Inflammatory Diseases of the Nervous System (320–326)

This subsection describes how to code for meningitis and the late effects of conditions within the description of inflammatory diseases of the nervous system.

Meningitis

Meningitis is the inflammation of the meninges, which cover the brain and the spinal cord. A variety of microorganisms or viruses can cause meningitis, which is classified in ICD-9-CM in chapter 6, Diseases of the Nervous System and Sense Organs, and chapter 1, Infectious and Parasitic Diseases. Because of this particular classification, the instructions provided in the Alphabetic Index to Diseases must be followed to ensure accurate code assignment.

> **Meningitis** . . . 322.9
>   abacterial NEC *(see also* Meningitis, aseptic) 047.9
>   actinomycotic 039.8 *[320.7]*
>   adenoviral 049.1
>   Aerobacter aerogenes 320.82
>   anaerobes (cocci) (gram-negative)
>   (gram-positive) (mixed) (NEC) 320.81
>   arbovirus NEC 066.9 *[321.2]*
>   specified type NEC 066.8 *[321.2]*

Note that in the preceding example two codes are required in some cases, and in other cases, one code is sufficient. However, accurate sequencing of the two codes is essential. The second code listed is in brackets and set in italic type, meaning that this code must always follow the code describing the underlying cause. (See the discussion on mandatory multiple coding in chapter 1 of this book.)

Category 326, Late Effects of Conditions

Category 326 is used to identify late effects of conditions classified in categories 320 through 325. The note under category 326 must be reviewed carefully because some codes in categories 320 through 325 are excluded. Instructions to "Use additional code to identify condition," such as hydrocephalus or paralysis, also must be reviewed.

> **EXAMPLE:** Residual hemiplegia due to late effect of encephalitis
>
> 342.90 Hemiplegia, unspecified, affecting unspecified side
>
> 326 Late effects of intracranial abscess or pyogenic infection

Organic Sleep Disorders (327)

Sleep medicine is a new and growing specialty within medicine. The American Academy of Sleep Medicine has published the *International Classification of Sleep Disorders,* which contains diagnostic, severity, and duration criteria to aid clinical diagnosis and treatment of sleep disorders. A new category 327, Organic sleep disorders, has been added to ICD-9-CM with fourth and fifth digit codes to classify various types of insomnia, hypersomnia, and sleep apnea. Several of the subclassification codes contain the direction "Code first underlying condition." Codes for unspecified forms of sleep disturbances (780.51–780.57) are included in chapter 16, Symptoms, Signs, and Ill-defined Conditions. Coders are likely to see additional modifications in ICD-9-CM for other sleep disorders in the future.

Other Disorders of the Nervous System (340–349)

The following subsections discuss the categories of other disorders of the nervous system, including paralytic conditions and epilepsy.

Categories 342–344, Paralytic Conditions

Categories 342–344 classify paralytic conditions such as hemiplegia, infantile cerebral palsy, and quadriplegia.

Category 342, Hemiplegia and Hemiparesis

The terms *hemiplegia* and *hemiparesis* both refer to the paralysis of one side of the body. Category 342 has fourth-digit subcategories that differentiate between flaccid and spastic hemiplegia. Flaccid refers to the loss of muscle tone in the paralyzed parts with the absence of tendon reflexes, while spastic refers to the spasticity of the paralyzed parts with increased tendon reflexes. The 342 codes often are assigned when the health record provides no further information, when the cause of the hemiplegia and hemiparesis is unknown, or as an additional code when the condition results from a specified cause.

A fifth-digit subclassification is included in category 342 to identify whether the dominant or nondominant side of the body is affected. This type of specificity may not be available in the health record; if not, assign the fifth digit 0.

Category 343, Infantile Cerebral Palsy

Infantile cerebral palsy is a nonprogressive, brain-damaging disturbance that originates during the prenatal and perinatal period. It is characterized by persistent, qualitative motor dysfunction, paralysis, and, in severe cases, mental retardation. Fourth-digit subcategories identify the different forms of infantile cerebral palsy.

Category 344, Other Paralytic Syndromes

Category 344 includes conditions such as quadriplegia, paraplegia, diplegia, and monoplegia. Also classified in this section are codes for cauda equina syndrome, with or without neurogenic bladder.

Category 345, Epilepsy

The term *epilepsy* denotes any disorder characterized by recurrent seizures. A seizure is a transient disturbance of cerebral function due to an abnormal paroxysmal neuronal discharge in the brain.

Physicians often document "recurrent seizure" or "seizure disorder" in a health record. These statements are not synonymous with epilepsy and do not warrant the assignment of code 345. In addition, the administration of certain anticonvulsive medication may or may not imply that a patient has epilepsy. Only when the documentation in the health record states "epilepsy" can code 345 be assigned.

ICD-9-CM identifies several types of epilepsy, including grand mal and petit mal status. Again, documentation in the health record provides direction as to what code to select. If the health record does not identify a particular form of epilepsy, assign code 345.9x, Epilepsy, unspecified.

Fifth digits are used with category 345 to identify the mention of intractable epilepsy as follows:

> **EXAMPLE:** The following fifth-digit subclassification is for use with categories 345.0, .1, .4–.9:
>
> **0** **without mention of intractable epilepsy**
> **1** **with intractable epilepsy**

A point to remember: The physician must state intractable epilepsy in the health record before the fifth digit 1 can be assigned. Never assume that the epilepsy is intractable based on generalities in the health record.

Category 357, Inflammatory and Toxic Neuropathy

Category 357 contains different forms of polyneuritis and polyneuropathy, some of which are the result of other diseases, such as diabetes, malignancy, and collagen vascular diseases.

Subcategories 357.1, 357.2, 357.3, and 357.4 include a direction to "code first underlying disease." Other forms of polyneuropathy included in this category can be coded as a first code or a single code, such as Guillain-Barré Syndrome or acute infective polyneuritis, 357.0.

Diabetic polyneuropathy or peripheral neuropathy is a serious and progressive complication of diabetes associated with significant morbidity, loss of quality of life, and increase in healthcare costs. Although there are different stages of diabetic peripheral neuropathy, a single code (357.2) is used to represent the entire spectrum. This italicized code contains a direction to "code first underlying disease (250.6)."

Critical Illness Neuropathy (357.82)

Critical illness neuropathy has two components: critical illness polyneuropathy (CIP) and critical illness myopathy (CIM). CIP is a major cause of prolonged morbidity associated with sepsis and multiple organ failure. The neuropathy produces severe weakness and causes difficulty in weaning from mechanical ventilation. CIM also causes difficulty in weaning from mechanical ventilation and prolonged recovery time after illness. CIM has also been described in patients receiving both neuromuscular blocking agents and corticosteroids in asthma and organ transplant patients. Two subclassification codes exist to describe these conditions: 357.82, Critical illness polyneuropathy, and 359.81, Critical illness myopathy.

Disorders of the Eye and Adnexa (360–379)

The "Disorders of the Eye and Adnexa" section in chapter 6 classifies conditions such as cataracts, retinal disorders, glaucoma, corneal ulcers, conjunctivitis, and disorders of the eyelids, orbits, and optic nerve.

Category 362, Other Retinal Disorders

Within category 362, various stages and severity of diabetic retinopathy are classified as 362.01–362.06. Diabetic retinopathy is a complication of diabetes that is caused by changes in the blood vessels of the eye. It is the leading cause of legal blindness among working-age Americans. Diabetic retinopathy in its earliest stages is called nonproliferative diabetic retinopathy (NPDR). As the disease advances, moderate or severe NPDR is diagnosed. The more advanced stage is known as proliferative diabetic retinopathy (PDR). In addition, a code exists for diabetic macular or retinal edema (362.06), which must be used with a code for diabetic retinopathy. Diabetic macular edema (DME) is swelling of the retina in diabetes mellitus due to leaking of fluid from the blood vessels within the macula. DME cannot occur in the absence of diabetic retinopathy. Subcategory 362.0, Diabetic retinopathy, is an italicized code that indicates the etiology, diabetes with ophthalmic complications (250.5x) must be listed first.

Category 365, Glaucoma

Glaucoma is a group of eye diseases characterized by an increase in intraocular pressure that causes pathological changes in the optic disk and typical visual field defects. Category 365 is subdivided to identify the various types of glaucoma. For example, patients developing glaucoma as a result of corticosteroid therapy are classified to subcategory 365.3. Glaucoma associated with a congenital anomaly, dystrophy, or systemic syndromes is classified to subcategory 365.4. The codes and code titles in subcategory 365.4 are set in italic type, with an instruction to first code the associated disease or disorder, such as neurofibromatosis, aniridia, Rieger's anomaly, and so forth. Subcategory 365.8 includes code 365.83, Aqueous misdirection, formerly known as malignant glaucoma. Aqueous misdirection usually requires surgical treatment. It is neither angle-closure or open-angle glaucoma. In this form of glaucoma, the aqueous flows into the vitreous instead of flowing into the anterior chamber. Finally, if documentation in the health record states glaucoma only, code 365.9, Unspecified glaucoma, should be assigned.

Category 366, Cataract

A cataract is the opacity of the crystalline lens of the eye, or its capsule, which results in a loss of vision. ICD-9-CM identifies many types of cataracts. However, the exclusion note under category 366 directs coders to codes 743.30 through 743.34 for congenital cataracts.

The first two subcategories of cataracts, 366.0 and 366.1, classify cataracts according to their onset in life. Subcategory 366.3 describes cataracts that are secondary to ocular disorders. Subcategory 366.4 describes cataracts associated with other disorders.

Codes 366.41 through 366.44 are set in italic type and, as such, are not used for primary coding. The underlying disease—such as calcinosis or craniofacial dysostosis—is coded first. If documentation in the health record states only cataract, assign code 366.9, Unspecified cataract.

Diseases of the Ear and Mastoid Process (380–389)

The "Diseases of the Ear and Mastoid Process" section in chapter 6 includes conditions such as otitis externa, otitis media, Meniere's disease, cholesteatoma, hearing loss, and tinnitus.

Otitis Externa

Otitis externa (external otitis, swimmer's ear) is an infection of the external auditory canal that may be classified as acute or chronic. Acute otitis externa is characterized by moderate to severe pain, fever, regional cellulitis, and partial hearing loss. Instead of pain, chronic otitis externa is characterized by pruritus, which leads to scaling and a thickening of the skin.

ICD-9-CM classifies otitis externa to subcategories 380.1, Infective otitis externa, and 380.2, Other otitis externa. When otitis externa is not further specified, the following codes may be reported: 380.10, Infective otitis externa, unspecified, and 380.23, Chronic otitis externa.

Otitis Media

Otitis media (OM) is an inflammation of the middle ear that may be further specified as suppurative or secretory, and acute or chronic. These variations and their symptoms follow:

- Acute suppurative OM is characterized by severe, deep, throbbing pain; sneezing and coughing; mild to high fever; hearing loss; dizziness; nausea; and vomiting.

- Acute secretory OM results in severe conductive hearing loss and, in some cases, a sensation of fullness in the ear with popping, crackling, or clicking sounds on swallowing or with jaw movement.

- Chronic OM has its origin in the childhood years but usually persists into adulthood. Cumulative effects of chronic OM include thickening and scarring of the tympanic membrane, decreased or absent tympanic mobility, cholesteatoma, and painless purulent discharge.

ICD-9-CM classifies OM to categories 381, Nonsuppurative otitis media and Eustachian tube disorders, and 382, Suppurative and unspecified otitis media. Both of these categories are subdivided to identify acute and chronic forms of OM and other specific types of OM. The following codes identify common forms of otitis media:

381.00 **Acute nonsuppurative otitis media, unspecified**
381.01 **Acute serous otitis media**
381.10 **Chronic serous otitis media**
381.3 **Chronic otitis media with effusion**
381.4 **Nonsuppurative otitis media**
382.00 **Acute suppurative otitis media**
382.3 **Chronic suppurative otitis media**
382.4 **Suppurative otitis media**
382.9 **Otitis media NOS**
      Acute otitis media NOS
      Chronic otitis media NOS

Review Exercise: Chapter 9

Assign ICD-9-CM codes to the following (no need to assign morphology codes):

1. Aerobacter aerogenes meningitis

          320.82

2. Intracranial abscess

          324.0

3. Fungal meningitis

          117.9, 321.1

4. Postviral encephalitis

          079.99, 323.6

5. Conjunctivochalasis; excision of redundant conjunctival tissue

          372.81, 10.31

6. Tay-Sachs disease with profound mental retardation

          330.1, 318.2

7. Partial retinal detachment with single retinal defect

          361.01

8. Congenital diplegic cerebral palsy

          343.0

9. Tic douloureux

          350.1

Review Exercise: Chapter 8 (Continued)

10. Infantile spastic quadriplegia

    343.2

11. Carpal tunnel syndrome with surgical release

    354.0 , 04.43

12. Tonic-clonic epilepsy

    345.10

13. Acute follicular conjunctivitis

    372.02

14. Communicating hydrocephalus; insertion of ventriculoperitoneal shunt

    331.3 , 02.34

15. Senile mature cataract; phacoemulsification and aspiration of cataract

    366.17 , 13.41

16. Chronic serous otitis media; bilateral myringotomy and placement of tubes

    381.10 , 20.01 (20.01 x2)

    Graded later

17. Cerebellar ataxia in alcoholism

    303.90 , 334.4

18. Classical migraine

    346.00

19. Cholesteatoma of middle ear with excision

    385.32 , 20.51

20. Type I diabetes mellitus with polyneuropathy

    250.61 , 357.2

Chapter 10

Diseases of the Circulatory System

Chapter 7, Diseases of the Circulatory System (390–459)

Chapter 7, Diseases of the Circulatory System, in the Tabular List in volume 1 of ICD-9-CM is subdivided into the following categories and section titles:

Categories	Section Titles
390–392	Acute Rheumatic Fever
393–398	Chronic Rheumatic Heart Disease
401–405	Hypertensive Disease
410–414	Ischemic Heart Disease
415–417	Diseases of Pulmonary Circulation
420–429	Other Forms of Heart Disease
430–438	Cerebrovascular Disease
440–448	Diseases of Arteries, Arterioles, and Capillaries
451–459	Diseases of Veins and Lymphatics, and Other Diseases of Circulatory System

Circulatory diagnoses are often difficult to code because a variety of nonspecific terminology is used to describe these conditions. All inclusion and exclusion notes within chapter 7 should be carefully reviewed prior to selecting a code.

In this chapter, the following conditions and procedures are highlighted: acute rheumatic fever and rheumatic heart disease, hypertension, myocardial infarction, angina, atherosclerosis, congestive heart failure, and cerebrovascular disease.

Acute Rheumatic Fever and Rheumatic Heart Disease

Acute and chronic diseases of rheumatic origin are classified in categories 390 through 398. This section also covers diseases of mitral and aortic valves, because when the ICD classification system was set up, clinicians believed that mitral stenosis was caused by rheumatic heart disease.

Categories 390–392, Acute Rheumatic Fever

Rheumatic fever occurs after a streptococcal sore throat (Group A streptococcus hemolyticus). The acute phase of the illness is marked by fever, malaise, sweating, palpitation, and polyarthritis, which varies from vague discomfort to severe pain felt chiefly in the large joints. Most patients have elevated titers of antistreptolysin antibodies and increased sedimentation rates.

The importance of rheumatic fever derives entirely from its capacity to cause severe heart damage. Salicylates markedly reduce fever, relieve joint pain, and may reduce joint swelling, if present. Because rheumatic fever often recurs, prophylaxis with penicillin is recommended and has markedly reduced the incidence of rheumatic heart disease in the general population.

Categories 393–398, Chronic Rheumatic Heart Disease

Rheumatic heart disease develops with an initial attack of rheumatic fever in about 30 percent of cases. The cardiac involvement may affect all three layers, causing pericarditis, scarring and weakening of the myocardium, and endocardial involvement of heart valves. The latter condition occurs in almost 66 percent of children who have had rheumatic fever and in about 20 percent of adults with rheumatic fever. A murmur heard over the heart is symptomatic of a valvular lesion. Rheumatic fever causes inflammation of the valves, thus damaging the valve cusps so that the opening may become permanently narrowed (stenosis). The mitral valve is involved in 75 percent to 80 percent of such cases; the aortic valve, in 30 percent; and the tricuspid and pulmonary valves, in less than 5 percent. In about 10 percent of patients, two of these valves are involved.

When stenosis affects the mitral valve, blood flow decreases from the left atrium into the left ventricle. As a result, blood is held back in the lungs, then in the right side of the heart, and, finally, in the veins of the body. Incompetence of a valve may also occur because the cusps will not retract. If the mitral valve cannot close, blood escapes back into the left atrium from the mitral valve. In the case of the aortic valve, blood escapes from the aorta into the left ventricle. In such cases, plastic and metal replacement valves that function as well as normal valves may be surgically inserted.

In coding diseases of the mitral valve and diseases affecting both the mitral and aortic valves, the Alphabetic Index to Diseases offers direction to codes from categories 393 through 398. Remember to always trust the Alphabetic Index to Diseases and assign the code it indicates.

Insufficiency, insufficient . . .
   mitral (valve) 424.0
      with
         aortic (valve) disease 396.3
            insufficiency, incompetence, or regurgitation 396.3
            stenosis or obstruction 396.2
         obstruction or stenosis 394.2
            with aortic valve disease 396.8
      congenital 746.6
      rheumatic 394.1
         with
            aortic (valve) disease 396.3
               insufficiency, incompetence, or regurgitation 396.3
               stenosis or obstruction 396.2
            obstruction or stenosis 394.2
               with aortic valve disease 396.8
      active or acute 391.1
         with chorea, rheumatic
           (Sydenham's) 392.0

The inclusion note under category 396 states that category 396 includes involvement of both mitral and aortic valves, whether specified as rheumatic or not.

Exercise 10.1

Assign ICD-9-CM codes to the following:

1. Congestive rheumatic heart failure

   398.91

2. Mitral valve stenosis with aortic valve insufficiency

   396.1

3. Chronic rheumatic endocarditis

   397.9

4. Mitral stenosis with regurgitation

   394.2

5. Acute rheumatic heart disease

   391.9

Hypertensive Disease

The Alphabetic Index to Diseases uses a table to display hypertensive diseases. This table provides a complete listing of all conditions due to, or associated with, hypertension. Part of the table for hypertensive diseases follows:

Hypertension	Index to Diseases		
	Malignant	Benign	Unspecified
Hypertension, hypertensive (arterial) (arteriolar) (crisis) (degeneration) (disease) (essential) (fluctuating) (idiopathic) (intermittent) (labile) (low renin) (orthostatic) (paroxysmal) (primary) (systemic) (uncontrolled) (vascular)...................................	401.0	401.1	401.9
with			
heart involvement (conditions classifiable to 429.0–429.3, 429.8, 429.9 due to hypertension) (*see also* Hypertension, heart)................	402.00	402.10	402.90
with kidney involvement—*see* Hypertension, cardiorenal			
renal involvement (*only* conditions classifiable to 585, 586, 587) (*excludes conditions classifiable to 584*) (*see also* Hypertension, kidney)...............	403.00	403.10	403.90
with heart involvement—*see* Hypertension, cardiorenal			
failure (and sclerosis) (*see also* Hypertension, kidney)..	403.01	403.11	403.91
sclerosis without failure (*see also* Hypertension, kidney).....................................	403.00	403.10	403.90
accelerated (*see also* Hypertension, by type, malignant)....	401.0	—	—
antepartum—*see* Hypertension, complicating pregnancy, childbirth, or the puerperium			
cardiorenal (disease)...............................	404.00	404.10	404.90
with			
heart failure (congestive)........................	404.01	404.11	404.91
and renal failure	404.03	404.13	404.93
renal failure.................................	404.02	404.12	404.92
and heart failure (congestive)	404.03	404.13	404.93

The first column in the table identifies the hypertensive condition, such as accelerated, antepartum, cardiovascular disease, cardiorenal, and cerebrovascular disease. The remaining three columns are titled "Malignant," "Benign," and "Unspecified," and they constitute the subcategories of hypertensive disease. The documentation in the patient's health record often will not specify a hypertensive condition as malignant or benign; therefore, the unspecified code to describe that hypertensive condition must be assigned.

Definition of Hypertension

A threshold of blood pressure that an individual could overshoot and then be considered hypertensive has not been defined. However, the standard commonly applied is that a sustained diastolic pressure above 90 mm Hg and a sustained systolic pressure above 140 mm Hg constitutes hypertension. The prevalence of hypertension increases with age. About 90 percent of hypertension is primary (essential hypertension), and its cause is unknown. The remaining 10 percent is secondary to renal disease. Both essential and secondary hypertension can be either benign or malignant. Complications of hypertension include left ventricular failure, arteriosclerotic heart disease, retinal hemorrhages, cerebrovascular insufficiency, and renal failure.

Benign Hypertension

In most cases, benign hypertension remains fairly stable over many years and is compatible with a long life. If untreated, however, it becomes an important risk factor in coronary heart disease and cerebrovascular disease. Benign hypertension is also asymptomatic until complications develop. Effective antihypertensive drug therapy is the treatment of choice.

Malignant Hypertension

Malignant hypertension is far less common, occurring in only about 5 percent of patients with elevated blood pressure. The malignant form is frequently of abrupt onset and runs a course measured in months. It often ends with renal failure or cerebral hemorrhage. Usually a person with malignant hypertension will complain of headaches and difficulties with vision. Blood pressures of 200/140 are common, and an abnormal protrusion of the optic nerve (papilledema) occurs with microscopic hemorrhages and exudates seen in the retina. The initial event appears to be some form of vascular damage to the kidneys. This may result from long-standing benign hypertension with damage of the arteriolar walls, or it may derive from arteritis of some form. The chances for long-term survival depend on early treatment before significant renal insufficiency has developed.

Hypertensive Heart Disease

Hypertensive heart disease refers to the secondary effects on the heart of prolonged sustained systemic hypertension. The heart has to work against greatly increased resistance in the form of high blood pressure. The primary effect is thickening of the left ventricle, finally resulting in heart failure. The symptoms are similar to those of heart failure from other causes. Many persons with controlled hypertension do not develop heart failure. However, when a patient has heart failure due to hypertension, an additional code is required to be used with category 402 codes to specify the type of heart failure that exists, such as 428.0, 428.20–428.23, 428.30–428.33, or 428.40–428.43, if known.

Official Coding Guidelines

The following guidelines are applicable in coding hypertensive diseases:

1. **Hypertension, essential or NOS:** Assign hypertension (arterial) (essential) (primary) (systemic) (NOS) to category 401, with the appropriate fourth digit to indicate malignant (.0), benign (.1), or unspecified (.9). Do not use either .0 (malignant) or .1 (benign) unless the documentation in the health record supports such a designation.

2. **Hypertension with heart disease:** Heart conditions (425.8, 429.0–429.3, 429.8, 429.9) are assigned to a code from category 402 when a causal relationship is stated

(due to hypertension) or implied (hypertensive). Use an additional code from category 428 to identify the type of heart failure in those patients with heart failure. More than one code from category 428 may be assigned if the patient has systolic or diastolic failure and congestive heart failure.

In ICD-9-CM, a stated causal relationship is usually documented using the term *due to* (for example, congestive heart failure *due to* hypertension). An implied causal relationship is documented using the term *hypertensive.* In ICD-9-CM, hypertensive is interpreted to mean "due to." Therefore, hypertensive cardiomegaly can also be described as cardiomegaly due to hypertension.

In category 402, Hypertensive heart disease, the fourth-digit subcategory describes whether the hypertensive condition is malignant, benign, or unspecified. The fifth-digit subclassification states the absence or presence of heart failure.

Certain heart conditions (425.8, 429.0–429.3, 429.8, 429.9) with hypertension, but without a stated causal relationship, are coded separately and sequenced according to the circumstances of the admission or encounter.

Although hypertension is frequently the cause of various forms of heart and vascular disease, ICD-9-CM does not presume a cause-and-effect relationship. The mention of "heart disease with hypertension only" should not be interpreted as a "due to" condition. Use of the terms *and* and *with* in the diagnostic statement does not imply cause and effect.

> **EXAMPLE:**   Cardiomegaly and hypertension
>
> 429.3   Cardiomegaly
> 401.9   Essential hypertension, unspecified

3. **Hypertensive kidney disease and chronic kidney disease:** Assign codes from category 403, Hypertensive kidney disease, when conditions classified to categories 585 through 587 are present. Unlike hypertension with heart disease, ICD-9-CM presumes a cause-and-effect relationship and classifies renal failure with hypertensive renal disease. As with hypertensive heart disease, the fourth-digit subcategory describes whether the hypertensive condition is malignant, benign, or unspecified. The fifth-digit subclassification identifies the presence or absence of chronic kidney disease. Under category 403 is the direction to "use additional code to identify the stage of chronic kidney disease (585.1–585.6), if known."

> **EXAMPLE:**   Hypertension and chronic kidney disease
>
> 403.91   Hypertensive renal disease, unspecified with chronic
>   kidney disease, stage 1 (585.1)

4. **Hypertensive heart and kidney disease:** Assign codes from category 404, Hypertensive heart and kidney disease, when both hypertensive kidney disease and hypertensive heart disease are stated in the diagnosis. Assume a causal relationship between the hypertension and the kidney disease, whether or not the condition is designated that way. Remember, the fourth-digit subcategory describes whether the hypertensive condition is malignant, benign, or unspecified. The fifth-digit subclassification identifies the presence, absence, or combination of heart failure and/or chronic kidney disease. An additional code from category 428 is required to identify the type of heart failure. More than one code from category 428 may be assigned if the patient has systolic or

diastolic failure and congestive heart failure. An additional code from 585.1–585.6 is required to identify the stage of chronic kidney disease.

> **EXAMPLE:** Hypertensive cardiomegaly and hypertensive kidney disease
>
> 404.92   Hypertensive heart and kidney disease, unspecified with chronic kidney disease, stage III (585.3)

In this example, the fifth digit 2 reflects the presence of chronic kidney disease alone. A second code indicates the form of chronic kidney disease.

5. **Hypertensive cerebrovascular disease:** Two codes are required to fully describe a hypertensive cerebrovascular condition. The first code assigned describes the cerebrovascular disease (430–438), followed by the appropriate code describing the hypertension (401–405).

> **EXAMPLE:** Cerebrovascular accident and benign hypertension
>
> 434.91   Acute, but ill-defined cerebrovascular disease
> 401.1   Benign essential hypertension

6. **Hypertensive retinopathy:** Two codes are required to identify the hypertensive retinopathy condition. First, assign code 362.11, Hypertensive retinopathy, followed by the appropriate code from categories 401 through 405 describing the hypertension (for example, 401.1, Benign essential hypertension).

7. **Hypertension, secondary:** When a physician documents that the hypertension is due to another disease (secondary hypertension), two codes are required to completely describe the condition. One code describes the underlying condition, and the other code is selected from category 405, Secondary hypertension. Sequencing of codes is determined by the reason for the admission or encounter.

Category 405 is subdivided at the fourth-digit level to describe whether the hypertensive condition is malignant, benign, or unspecified. The fifth-digit subclassification identifies the underlying condition of renovascular origin or of another origin.

Renovascular origin can include renal artery aneurysm, anomaly, embolism, fibromuscular hyperplasia, occlusion, stenosis, or thrombosis. Other types of diseases causing secondary hypertension can include a calculus of the ureter or kidney, a brain tumor, polycystic kidneys, or polycythemia.

> **EXAMPLE:** Hypertension due to a malignant neoplasm of the brain
>
> 191.9   Malignant neoplasm of brain, unspecified
> 405.99   Other unspecified secondary hypertension

8. **Hypertension, transient:** Assign code 796.2, Elevated blood pressure reading without diagnosis of hypertension, unless patient has an established diagnosis of hypertension. Assign code 642.3x for transient hypertension of pregnancy.

9. **Hypertension, controlled:** Assign the appropriate code from categories 401 through 405 to describe a diagnostic statement of controlled hypertension. This type of statement usually refers to an existing state of hypertension under control by therapy.

10. **Uncontrolled hypertension:** Uncontrolled hypertension may refer to untreated hypertension or to hypertension not responding to current therapeutic regimen. In either case, assign the appropriate code from categories 401 through 405 to designate the stage and type of hypertension, with the appropriate fourth and fifth digits.

11. **Elevated blood pressure:** For a statement of elevated blood pressure without further specificity, assign code 796.2, Elevated blood pressure reading without diagnosis of hypertension, rather than a code from category 401.

Exercise 10.2

Assign ICD-9-CM codes to the following:

1. Hypertensive cardiovascular disease, malignant

   402.00

2. Congestive heart failure; benign hypertension

   428.0, 401.1

3. Secondary benign hypertension; stenosis of renal artery

   440.1, 405.11

4. Malignant hypertensive nephropathy with chronic kidney disease, stage IV

   403.01, 585.4

5. Acute renal failure; essential hypertension

   584.9, 401.9

6. Congestive heart failure due to hypertensive heart disease

   402.91, 428.0

7. Hypertension with chronic kidney disease, stage I

   403.91 585.1

8. Hypertensive cardiorenal disease with congestive heart failure and chronic kidney disease, stage II

   404.93, 585.2 428.0

9. Hypertension due to Cushing's disease

   405.99, (255.0)

10. Congestive heart failure and chronic kidney disease due to accelerated hypertension with end-stage renal disease (ESRD)

    (404.03)404.3, 428.0, 585.6

Categories 410–414, Ischemic Heart Disease

Ischemic heart disease is synonymous with arteriosclerotic heart disease, coronary ischemia, and coronary artery disease. It is the generic name for three forms of heart disease: myocardial infarction, angina pectoris, and chronic ischemic heart disease. All three diseases result from an imbalance between the need of the myocardium for oxygen and the oxygen supply. Usually, the imbalance results from insufficient blood flow due to arteriosclerotic narrowing of the coronary arteries. These three forms of heart disease are discussed in this chapter.

At the beginning of the ischemic heart disease section, the inclusion note states that this section includes ischemic heart conditions with mention of hypertension. The statement "Use additional code to identify presence of hypertension" also appears at the beginning of this section as an instruction to assign an additional code to describe hypertension, if present.

Acute Myocardial Infarction

Acute myocardial infarction (AMI) usually occurs as a result of a sudden inadequacy of coronary flow. The first symptom of acute myocardial infarction is the development of deep substernal pain described as aching or pressure, often with radiation to the back or left arm. The patient is pale, diaphoretic (sweaty), and in severe pain. Peripheral or carotid cyanosis may be present, as well as arrhythmias. Treatment is designed to relieve the patient's distress, reduce cardiac work, and prevent and treat complications. Major complications include tachycardia, frequent ventricular premature beats, Mobitz II heart block, and ventricular fibrillation. Heart failure occurs in about two-thirds of hospitalized patients.

When the physician describes a condition as "aborted myocardial infarction," the code 411.1, Intermediate coronary syndrome, should be assigned. This condition usually means the patient did not have any myocardial damage and an acute myocardial infarction has not occurred.

Included under category 410, Acute myocardial infarction, is the terminology of "ST elevation (STEMI) and non-ST elevation (NSTEMI) myocardial infarction" that coders may see documented by physicians in the records of patients with acute myocardial infarction. Other terminology used by physicians for cardiac emergencies is "acute coronary syndrome," which ranges from STEMI to NSTEMI to unstable angina. A thorough review of the documentation in the record is required to clarify which condition is present prior to coding.

Diagnostic Tools

The diagnosis of acute myocardial infarction (AMI) depends on the patient's clinical history, the physical examination, interpretation of electrocardiogram (EKG), chest radiograph, and measurement of serum levels of cardiac enzymes, such as troponins or CK-MB.

Diagnostic uncertainty frequently arises because of various factors. Many patients with AMI have atypical symptoms. Other people with typical physical symptoms do not have AMI. Electrocardiograms may also be nondiagnostic. Laboratory tests known as biochemical or serum markers of cardiac injury are commonly relied upon to diagnose or exclude an acute myocardial infarction.

Creatine kinase and lactate dehydrogenase have been the "gold standard" for the diagnosis of AMI for many years. However, single values of these tests have limited sensitivity and specificity. Newer serum markers in use today are Troponin T and I, myoglobin, and the MB isoenzyme of creatine kinase. These new markers are now being used instead of, or along with, the standard markers.

The various proteins are released from myocardial cells after an infarct or ischemia has occurred and can be detected in the serum within hours. Recent research has found that an elevation in cardiac Troponin T (cTnT) has excellent sensitivity for diagnosing acute myocardial infarction (Rice and MacDonald 1999; Johnson et al. 1999).

Electrocardiograms (EKGs) also prove useful in diagnosing myocardial infarctions. The initial EKG may be diagnostic in acute transmural myocardial infarction, but serial EKGs may be necessary to confirm the diagnosis for other myocardial infarction sites.

Fourth-Digit Subcategories and Fifth-Digit Subclassifications

ICD-9-CM classifies myocardial infarction to category 410, with the following fourth-digit subcategories describing the specific site involved:

410.0   **Of anterolateral wall**
        ST elevation myocardial infarction of anterolateral wall
410.1   **Of other anterior wall**
        ST elevation myocardial infarction of other anterior wall
410.2   **Of inferolateral wall**
        ST elevation myocardial infarction of inferolateral wall
410.3   **Of inferoposterior wall**
        ST elevation myocardial infarction of inferoposterior wall
410.4   **Of other inferior wall**
        ST elevation myocardial infarction of other inferior wall
410.5   **Of other lateral wall**
        ST elevation myocardial infarction of other lateral wall
410.6   **True posterior wall infarction**
        ST elevation of true posterior wall myocardial infarction
410.7   **Subendocardial infarction**
        Non-ST elevation myocardial infarction
410.8   **Of other specified sites**
        ST elevation myocardial infarction of other specified sites
410.9   **Unspecified site**
        Myocardial infarction NOS

Effective October 1, 1989, revisions to ICD-9-CM added the following fifth-digit subclassifications to category 410, Acute myocardial infarction, to indicate the episode of care:

---

0   **episode of care unspecified**
Use fifth digit 0 when the source document does not contain sufficient information for the assignment of fifth digit 1 or 2.

1   **initial episode of care**
Use fifth digit 1 to designate the first episode of care (regardless of facility site) for a newly diagnosed myocardial infarction. The fifth digit 1 is assigned regardless of the number of times a patient may be transferred during the initial episode of care.

2   **subsequent episode of care**
Use fifth digit 2 to designate episode of care following the initial episode when the patient is admitted for further observation, evaluation, or treatment for a myocardial infarction that has received initial treatment but is still less than 8 weeks old.

EXAMPLE: A male patient was admitted to Hospital A with the diagnosis of acute anterolateral wall myocardial infarction. The patient was transferred to Hospital B four days later. The patient was discharged from Hospital B after undergoing cardiac catheterization.

Principal diagnosis code for Hospital A: 410.01
Principal diagnosis code for Hospital B: 410.01

EXAMPLE: A female patient was admitted to University Hospital for aorto-coronary bypass six weeks after experiencing a myocardial infarction that was treated at a community hospital.

MI diagnosis code for University Hospital: 410.92

EXAMPLE: An 80-year-old female was admitted to the skilled nursing facility after a total hip replacement to treat a fractured hip. Seven weeks ago, the patient was treated for an acute inferolateral wall myocardial infarction.

MI diagnosis code for the skilled nursing facility: 410.22

EXAMPLE: A 65-year-old man was admitted to Community Medical Center and treated for an anterior wall myocardial infarction. Subsequent coronary angiography demonstrated four-vessel coronary artery disease. The patient was discharged home to contemplate future coronary artery bypass surgery. Four weeks later, the patient was readmitted to Community Medical Center for the coronary artery bypass surgery.

MI diagnosis for first hospital stay: 410.11
MI diagnosis for second hospital stay: 410.12

Old Myocardial Infarction

Code 412, Old myocardial infarction, is assigned when the diagnostic statement mentions the presence of a healed MI presenting no symptoms during the current episode of care.

Angina

There are two types of angina: unstable angina and angina pectoris.

Category 411.1, Unstable Angina

Unstable angina, also known as crescendo and preinfarction angina, is defined as the development of prolonged episodes of anginal discomfort, usually occurring at rest and requiring hospitalization to rule out a myocardial infarction.

ICD-9-CM classifies unstable angina under code 411.1, Intermediate coronary syndrome, which includes the types of angina just discussed, as well as impending or aborted myocardial infarction. Code 411.1 is assigned when a patient is admitted to the hospital and treated for unstable angina without documentation of infarction, occlusion, or thrombosis.

Category 413, Angina Pectoris

Angina pectoris refers to chest pain due to ischemia (loss of blood supply to a part) of the heart. The blood flow, with its supply of oxygen, is reduced because of atherosclerosis (hardening of arteries). Immediate causes of angina pectoris are exertion, stress, cold weather, or digestion of a large meal. The discomfort of angina is highly variable. Pain is most commonly felt beneath the sternum, and a vague or a sharp pain sometimes radiates down the left arm. Blood pressure and heart rate are increased during an attack; however, angina lasts only a few minutes and is relieved by rest and/or sublingual nitroglycerin. Angina pectoris is a warning of more severe heart disease, such as myocardial infarction or congestive heart failure.

ICD-9-CM classifies angina pectoris to category 413. The fourth-digit subcategories identify specific types of angina pectoris, such as angina decubitus and Prinzmetal angina.

Sequencing of Angina and Coronary Disease

Keep in mind the definition of principal diagnosis: "the condition established after study to be chiefly responsible for occasioning the admission of the patient to the hospital for care." This definition must be used when a patient suffers from angina.

EXAMPLE: A patient was admitted with angina. Diagnostic cardiac catheterizations determined that the angina was due to coronary atherosclerosis of the native vessels. The patient was discharged on antianginal medications.

The coronary atherosclerosis, 414.01, is listed as the principal diagnosis. Angina, 413.9 is listed as an additional diagnosis.

EXAMPLE: A patient was admitted with symptomatic angina that evolved into an acute myocardial infarction.

The acute myocardial infarction is sequenced as the principal diagnosis, 410.91, and no additional code is assigned for angina as it is an inherent part of the condition.

EXAMPLE: A patient with unstable angina was admitted to the hospital for left heart cardiac catheterization. He was found to have significant four-vessel coronary atherosclerosis. He had four-native-vessel coronary artery bypass surgery performed during the same admission.

The principal diagnosis is the coronary atherosclerosis, 414.01. The diagnosis of unstable angina, 411.1, may be listed as an additional diagnosis.

EXAMPLE: A patient who experienced an acute myocardial infarction five weeks ago was admitted with unstable angina. The angina was treated and no further infarction occurred.

The principal diagnosis is the unstable angina, 411.1. An additional diagnosis of the acute myocardial infarction, subsequent episode of care, 410.92, is also used.

Further examples of coding and sequencing of angina and coronary heart disease can be found in *Coding Clinic* 1993, 10:5, 17–24.

Category 414, Chronic Ischemic Heart Disease

ICD-9-CM classifies chronic ischemic heart disease to category 414. Chronic ischemic heart disease (arteriosclerotic heart disease) refers to those cases where ischemia has induced general myocardial atrophy and scattered areas of interstitial scarring. Scarring from past myocardial infarctions may also be present. Generally, chronic ischemic heart disease results from slow, progressive narrowing of the coronary arteries. This course, however, may be altered by episodes of sudden severe coronary insufficiency. The patient with chronic ischemic heart disease may develop angina or an acute myocardial infarction.

Atherosclerosis

Atherosclerosis is the formation of lesions on the inside of arterial walls from the accumulation of fat cells and platelets. The gradual enlargement of the lesion eventually weakens the arterial wall and narrows the lumen, or channel of the blood vessel, decreasing the volume of blood flow. The large arteries—the aorta and its main branches—are primarily affected, but smaller arteries such as the coronary and cerebral arteries can also be affected. In such a case, the patient experiences chest pain, shortness of breath, and sweating. Blood pressure is high; pulse is rapid and weak. An x-ray reveals cardiomegaly and narrowing, or occlusion, of the affected vessel wall. Blood tests may show hypercholesterolemia.

Atherosclerosis is the major cause of ischemia of the heart, brain, and extremities. Its complications include stroke, congestive heart failure, angina pectoris, myocardial infarction, and kidney failure. Treatment is directed toward the specific manifestation.

Subcategories of 414, Other Forms of Chronic Ischemic Heart Disease

ICD-9-CM classifies chronic ischemic heart disease to category 414, Other forms of chronic ischemic heart disease. The fourth-digit subcategories describe specific types of ischemic heart diseases, such as coronary atherosclerosis (414.0) and aneurysm of the heart (414.1).

Subcategory code 414.0 is further expanded to fifth-digit subclassifications to identify whether the atherosclerosis is present in a native artery, in a bypass graft, or in a coronary artery of a transplanted heart. These fifth-digit codes are vessel specific and should be assigned when the physician's documentation states that atherosclerosis has been found in that specific vessel. A fifth-digit code should not be assigned based solely on the fact that a patient has atherosclerosis and a history of bypass surgery. An explanation of these fifth-digit codes follows:

1. Code 414.00 is assigned when there is no information in the health record as to whether the disease is present in a native vessel or a graft.

2. Code 414.01 is assigned to show coronary artery disease in a native coronary artery. This code is used when a patient has coronary artery disease and no history of coronary artery bypass (CABG) surgery. This code may be used if a patient, who in the past had a percutaneous transluminal coronary angioplasty (PTCA), has vessels that have reoccluded as demonstrated by a recent cardiac catheterization.

3. Code 414.02 is assigned to show coronary artery disease in an autologous vein bypass graft. Vein bypass grafts have been the most commonly performed coronary bypass grafts in the past. Patients who had a CABG procedure several years ago probably had saphenous veins used for graft material. Often these patients are readmitted for a "redo" CABG procedure.

4. Code 414.03 is assigned to show coronary artery disease in a nonautologous biological bypass graft.

5. Code 414.04 is assigned if the physician documents the diagnosis of coronary atherosclerosis in an internal mammary artery used for a bypass graft.

6. Code 414.05 is assigned if the physician documents the diagnosis of coronary atherosclerosis in a bypass graft and the patient has a history of CABG surgery. This code is used when there is no further documentation of the type of bypass graft used.

7. Code 414.06 is assigned when atherosclerosis develops in the native coronary artery of a transplanted heart. It is presumed that the development of atherosclerosis is a natural process and not a complication of the transplant.

8. Code 414.07 is assigned when coronary atherosclerosis is present in the artery or vein bypass graft(s) of the transplanted heart.

Subcategory code 414.1 was recently revised to differentiate between aneurysms and dissections of the heart. Code 414.12 is included for dissection of the coronary artery. An arterial dissection is characterized by blood coursing within the layers of the arterial wall and is not an aneurysm. The term *dissecting aneurysm* has been removed from code 441.0, Dissection of aorta. Arterial dissections are a common complication of interventional radiology procedures.

Although the aorta is the most common site for dissections, they can occur in other arteries in the body. A new subcategory, 443.2, Other arterial dissection, was added with fifth-digit sub-classifications to describe dissections of the carotid, iliac, renal, vertebral, and other arteries.

Subcategory code 414.8, Other specified forms of chronic ischemic heart disease, includes an important note:

414.8   Other specified forms of chronic ischemic heart disease

Chronic coronary insufficiency
Ischemia, myocardial (chronic)
Any condition classifiable to 410 specified as chronic, or
    presenting with symptoms after 8 weeks from date of infarction

Excludes: coronary insufficiency (acute) (411.89)

The preceding note advises that code 414.8 should be assigned if a diagnosis states chronic myocardial infarction with symptoms presenting eight weeks after the date of the infarction.

Exercise 10.3

Assign ICD-9-CM codes to the following:

1. Acute myocardial infarction of inferolateral wall, initial episode of care
   _____410.21_____

2. Arteriosclerotic heart disease (native coronary artery) with angina pectoris
   _____414.01, 413.9_____

3. Old myocardial infarction
   _____412_____

4. Coronary arteriosclerosis involving an autologous vein bypass graft
   _____414.02_____

5. Preinfarction syndrome
   _____411.1_____

Category 428, Heart Failure

Heart failure is the heart's inability to contract with enough force to properly pump blood. This may be caused by coronary artery disease (usually in a patient with a previous myocardial infarction), cardiomyopathy, hypertension, or heart valve disease. Sometimes the exact cause of heart failure is not found. Heart failure may develop gradually or occur acutely.

Heart failure has the following three effects:

- **Pressure in the lungs is increased.** Fluid collects in the lung tissue, inhibiting O_2 and CO_2 exchange.

- **Kidney function is hampered.** Blood does not filter well, and body sodium and water retention increase, resulting in edema.

- **Blood is not properly circulated throughout the body.** Fluid collects in tissues, resulting in edema of the feet and legs.

Symptoms of heart failure include:

- Difficulty breathing, especially with exertion or when lying flat in bed

- Waking up breathless at night

- Frequent dry, hacking cough, especially when lying down

- Fatigue and weakness

- Dizziness or fainting

- Swollen feet, ankles, and legs

- Nausea with abdominal swelling, pain and tenderness

The symptoms are caused by the inability of the heart to pump with adequate strength. When the heart cannot pump enough blood to organs and muscles, the body becomes fatigued. Blood and fluids may collect in the lungs and this causes breathing problems. Fluid also collects in other parts of the body including the feet, ankles, legs, and abdomen.

The term *heart failure* is not synonymous with *congestive heart failure.* Many patients with heart failure do not manifest pulmonary or systemic congestion. Guidelines from the Agency for Healthcare Research and Quality define systolic and diastolic dysfunction with heart failure. Recently, ICD-9-CM category 428 was expanded to distinguish between congestive heart failure (428.0), systolic heart failure (428.2), diastolic heart failure (428.3), and combined systolic and diastolic heart failure (428.4.) With the exception of 428.0, the subcategories require a fifth digit to describe the acute, chronic, acute on chronic, and unspecified forms of heart failure that can exist.

Diagnostic Tests

Several diagnostic tests are important in diagnosing congestive heart failure in a patient. Typical remarks on a chest x-ray indicating heart failure include hilar congestion, "butterfly" or "batwing" appearance of vascular markings, bronchial edema, Kerley B lines signifying chronic elevation of left atrial pressure, and heart enlargement. An echocardiograph measures the amount of blood pumped from the heart with each beat. This measurement is known as the ejection fraction. A normal heart pumps one-half (50 percent) or more of the blood in the left ventricle with each heartbeat. With heart failure, the weakened heart may pump 40 percent or less, and less blood is pumped with less force to all parts of the body.

Vital capacity (amount of air that can be expelled from the lungs) is reduced. Oxygen content of blood is reduced, and circulation time is longer (normal circulation time from arm to lung is 4 to 8 seconds).

Urinalysis results show slight albuminuria, increased concentration with specific gravity of 1.020, and urine sodium decreased. Laboratory findings may include BUN 60 mg/100 ml; acidosis -pH 7.35 due to increased CO_2 in blood from pulmonary insufficiency; blood volume increased with decrease in chloride, albumin, and total protein.

For most patients, heart failure is a chronic condition, which means it can be treated and managed, but not cured. Usually the patient's management plan consists of medications, such as ACE inhibitors, diuretics and digitalis, low sodium diet, possibly some modifications in daily activities, regular exercise such as walking and swimming, and other changes in lifestyle and health habits such as reducing alcohol consumption and quitting smoking.

Cardiac Arrhythmias and Conduction Disorders

Cardiac arrhythmias identify disturbances or impairments of the normal electrical activity of heart muscle excitation. ICD-9-CM classifies cardiac arrhythmias to several categories depending on the specific type. Without further specification as to the type of cardiac arrhythmia, code 427.9 may be reported. A discussion of common arrhythmias follows:

Atrial fibrillation (427.31) is commonly associated with organic heart diseases, such as coronary artery disease, hypertension and rheumatic mitral valve disease, thyrotoxicosis, pericarditis, and pulmonary embolism. Treatment includes pharmacologic therapy (verapamil, digoxin, or propranolol) and cardioversion.

Atrial flutter (427.32) is associated with organic heart diseases, such as coronary artery disease, hypertension, and rheumatic mitral valve disease. Treatment is similar to that for atrial fibrillation.

Ventricular fibrillation (427.41) involves no cardiac output and is associated with cardiac arrest. Treatment is consistent with that for cardiac arrest.

Paroxysmal supraventricular tachycardia (427.0) is associated with congenital accessory atrial conduction pathway, physical or psychological stress, hypoxia, hypokalemia, caffeine and marijuana use, stimulants, and digitalis toxicity. Treatment includes pharmacologic therapy (quinidine, propranolol, or verapamil) and cardioversion.

Sick sinus syndrome (SSS) (427.81) is an imprecise diagnosis with various characteristics. SSS may be diagnosed when a patient presents with sinus arrest, sinoatrial exit block, or persistent sinus bradycardia. This syndrome is often the result of drug therapy, such as digitalis, calcium channel blockers, beta-blockers, sympatholytic agents, or antiarrhythmics. Another presentation includes recurrent supraventricular tachycardias associated with bradyarrhythmias. Prolonged ambulatory monitoring may be indicated to establish a diagnosis of sick sinus syndrome. Treatment includes insertion of a permanent cardiac pacemaker.

Various forms of conduction disorders may be classified in ICD-9-CM. Conduction disorders are disruptions or disturbances in the electrical impulses that regulate the heartbeats.

Wolff-Parkinson-White (WPW) syndrome (426.7) is caused by conduction from the sinoatrial node to the ventricle through an accessory pathway that bypasses the atrioventricular node. Patients with WPW syndrome present with tachyarrhythmias, including supraventricular tachycardia, atrial fibrillation, or atrial flutter. Treatment includes catheter ablation following electrophysiologic evaluation.

Atrioventricular (AV) heart blocks are classified as first, second, or third degree.

- **First-degree AV block** is associated with atrial septal defects or valvular disease. ICD-9-CM classifies first-degree AV block to code 426.11.

- **Second-degree AV block** is further classified as follows:

  —**Mobitz type I (Wenckebach)** is associated with acute inferior wall myocardial infarction or with digitalis toxicity. Treatment includes discontinuation of digitalis and administration of atropine. ICD-9-CM classifies Mobitz type I AV block to code 426.13.

  —**Mobitz type II** is associated with anterior wall or anteroseptal myocardial infarction and digitalis toxicity. Treatment includes temporary pacing and, in some cases, permanent pacemaker insertion, as well as discontinuation of digitalis and administration of atropine. ICD-9-CM classifies Mobitz type II AV block to code 426.12.

- **Third-degree heart block,** also referred to as complete heart block, is associated with ischemic heart disease or infarction, postsurgical complication of mitral valve replacement, digitalis toxicity, and Stokes-Adams syndrome. Treatment includes permanent cardiac pacemaker insertion. ICD-9-CM classifies third-degree heart block to code 426.0. When this type of heart block is congenital in nature, code 746.86 is reported rather than 426.0.

Without further specification, atrioventricular block is reported with code 426.10.

Long Q-T syndrome is suspected in patients with a prolonged Q-T interval on an electrocardiogram. It is associated with recurrent syncope and sudden death. Various forms of the syndrome exist. A number of specified genetic defects have been identified as causes, such as genes for ion channels that control repolarization of the heart. This condition is usually diagnosed in childhood and is more commonly found in Asians but may be present in people of any genetic background. Treatment may include an implantable cardioverter-defibrillator. The syndrome is reported with code 426.82.

Sinus tachycardia is associated with normal physiologic response to fever, exercise, anxiety, pain, and dehydration. It may also accompany shock, left ventricular failure, cardiac tamponade, anemia, hyperthyroidism, hypovolemia, pulmonary embolism, and anterior myocardial infarction. Treatment is geared toward correcting the underlying cause. ICD-9-CM classifies sinus tachycardia, as well as supraventricular tachycardia, to code 427.89.

Cardiac Arrest

Cardiac arrest, code 427.5 (excluding cardiac arrest that occurs with pregnancy, anesthesia overdose or wrong substance given, and postoperative complications), may be assigned as a principal diagnosis under the following circumstance:

- The patient arrives in the hospital in a state of cardiac arrest and cannot be resuscitated or is only briefly resuscitated, and is pronounced dead with the underlying cause of the cardiac arrest not established or unknown. This applies whether the patient is only seen in the emergency department or is admitted to the hospital and the underlying cause is not determined prior to death.

Cardiac arrest may be used as a secondary diagnosis in the following situations:

- The patient arrives at the hospital's emergency department in a state of cardiac arrest and is resuscitated and admitted with the condition prompting the cardiac arrest known, such as trauma or ventricular tachycardia. The condition causing the cardiac arrest is sequenced first with the cardiac arrest code listed as a secondary code.

- When cardiac arrest occurs during the course of the hospital stay and the patient is resuscitated, code 427.5 may be used as a secondary code except as outlined in the exclusion note under category 427.

When the physician documents cardiac arrest to describe an inpatient death, code 427.5 should not be assigned when the underlying cause or contributing cause of death is known. The patient's discharge disposition as expired will be collected as a data element required under the Uniform Hospital Discharge Data Set (UHDDS.)

Exercise 10.4

Assign ICD-9-CM codes to the following:

1. Atrial fibrillation

   427.31

2. Pulmonary hypertension

   416.8

3. Alcoholic cardiomyopathy

   425.5

4. Chronic cor pulmonale

   416.9

5. Acute endocarditis due to streptococcus infection

   (421.0) 421.9   041.00

6. Atrioventricular block, Mobitz type II

   426.12

7. Cardiac arrest, etiology unknown

   427.5

8. Sick sinus syndrome

   427.81

9. Acute pulmonary edema with left ventricular failure

   428.1

10. Benign hypertensive cardiomegaly

    402.90 (402.10)

Cerebrovascular Disease (430–438)

Cerebrovascular disease is an insufficient blood supply to a part of the brain and is usually secondary to atherosclerotic disease, hypertension, or a combination of both.

At the beginning of the "Cerebrovascular Disease" section, the inclusion note states that this section includes cerebrovascular diseases with mention of hypertension. The statement "Use additional code to identify presence of hypertension" also appears at the beginning of this section as an instruction to assign an additional code to describe hypertension, if present.

ICD-9-CM classifies cerebrovascular disease according to the following types of conditions:

430 **Subarachnoid hemorrhage**
431 **Intracerebral hemorrhage**
432 **Other and unspecified intracranial hemorrhage**
433 **Occlusion and stenosis of precerebral arteries**

434 Occlusion of cerebral arteries
435 Transient cerebral ischemia
436 Acute, but ill-defined cerebrovascular disease
437 Other and ill-defined cerebrovascular disease
438 Late effects of cerebrovascular disease

Categories 433 and 434 provide a fifth-digit subclassification that identifies the presence or absence of cerebral infarction.

This chapter highlights cerebrovascular diseases in categories 434 and 438.

Code 434.91, Default Code for Acute Cerebrovascular Accident

Code 434.91, Cerebral artery occlusion, unspecified, with cerebral infarction, is assigned when the diagnosis states stroke, cerebrovascular or cerebral vascular accident (CVA) without further specification. The health record should be reviewed to make sure nothing more specific is available.

Conditions resulting from an acute cerebrovascular disease, such as aphasia or hemiplegia, should be coded only if stated to be residual or present at the time of discharge. Do not code if these conditions are transient and resolved by the time of discharge.

> **EXAMPLE:** Patient was admitted with aphasia and hemiplegia due to an acute CVA. On discharge, the aphasia had cleared; however, the hemiplegia is still present and will require outpatient physical therapy. Codes include 434.91, default code for acute cerebrovascular accident (CVA); 342.90, Hemiplegia and hemiparesis, unspecified.

The aphasia is not coded because it cleared during admission.

Category 438, Late Effects of Cerebrovascular Disease

Category 438 codes identify late effects of cerebrovascular disease. Category 438 is used to indicate conditions classifiable to categories 430 through 437 as the causes of late effects (neurologic deficits), themselves classified elsewhere. These late effects include neurologic deficits that persist after initial onset of conditions classifiable to 430 through 437. The neurologic deficits caused by cerebrovascular disease may be present from the onset or may arise at any time after the onset of the condition classifiable to 430 through 437.

> **EXAMPLE:** Patient was admitted for physical therapy for monoplegia of the leg affecting the nondominant side due to an old CVA. Codes include V57.1, Other physical therapy; 438.42, Late effect of cerebrovascular disease, monoplegia of lower limb affecting nondominant side.

The documentation in the health record may state the late effect in any of the following ways:

- 438.11, Aphasia, late effect of a CVA

- 438.21, Hemiplegia of the dominant side following a CVA one year ago

- 438.82, Dysphagia, sequelae of old CVA

When the health record documentation indicates an old cerebrovascular accident with no neurologic deficits, assign code V12.59, Personal history of other diseases of circulatory system. In this circumstance, it is incorrect to assign a code from category 438.

The code V12.59 is located in the Alphabetic Index under "History (personal), disease (of) circulatory system, V12.50." When referencing the Tabular List, the coder will note V12.50 is for unspecified circulatory disease. Because the diagnosis is specifically old cerebrovascular accident with no neurologic deficits, code V12.59, Personal history of other diseases of circulatory system, other, would be more appropriate to use.

Codes from category 438 may be assigned on a healthcare record with codes from 430 through 437, if the patient has a current CVA and deficits from an old CVA.

> **EXAMPLE:** Patient was admitted with occlusion of cerebral arteries resulting in infarction. Patient has a history of old CVA one year ago with residual hemiplegia affecting the dominant side. Codes include 434.91, Cerebral artery occlusion, unspecified, with cerebral infarction; 438.21, Late effect of cerebrovascular disease, hemiplegia affecting dominant side.

Deep Vein Thrombosis of Lower Extremity

The term *deep vein thrombosis* (DVT) is commonly documented in health records. Until recently, a unique code for DVT did not exist in ICD-9-CM, although interest in tracking patients with this condition has greatly increased over the past several years. Venous thromboembolism (VTE) refers to the occlusion within the venous system. It includes DVT, typically of the lower extremities, and embolism to the pulmonary vascular system. A new subcategory, 453.4, Venous embolism and thrombosis of deep vessels of lower extremity, was created to capture the DVT information. Recently, codes 453.40–453.41 and 453.42 were added to describe DVT, not otherwise specified, as well as DVT when it occurs in the deep vessels of the proximal lower extremity (femoral, iliac, popliteal, upper leg, and thigh) and in the distal lower extremity (calf, lower leg, peroneal, and tibial vessels).

Exercise 10.5

Assign ICD-9-CM codes to the following:

1. Bilateral thrombosis of carotid artery; bilateral endarterectomy

   433.10   38.12(x2)

2. Generalized cerebral ischemia

   437.1

3. Insufficiency of precerebral arteries

   435.9

4. Deep vein thrombosis of the iliac vein

   453.40   (453.41)

5. Atherosclerosis of lower extremity with intermittent claudication and gangrene; right femoropopliteal artery bypass graft

   440.24, 440.30   (39.29)

Exercise 10.5 (Continued)

6. Thrombotic infarction of brain; no residuals

   434.01

7. Nontraumatic subdural hematoma

   432.1

8. Ruptured berry aneurysm

   430

9. Varicose veins of lower extremities with stasis dermatitis

   454.1

10. Bleeding esophageal varices in patient with portal hypertension

    572.3, 456.20

11. Mitral valve insufficiency, nonrheumatic

    424.0

12. Acute nontransmural myocardial infarction, initial episode; ventricular fibrillation

    (410.71) 410.91   427.41

13. Congestive heart failure with severe pleural effusion; diabetes mellitus, type I; thoracentesis

    428.1 (511.9) 250.1   34.91

14. Congestive heart failure; malignant hypertension

    428.0   401.0

15. Internal hemorrhoids with bleeding and prolapse; hemorrhoidectomy by ligation

    455.2   49.45

16. Chronic kidney disease, stage II with benign hypertension

    585.2   401.1   (403.11, 585.2)

17. Endocarditis in patient due to disseminated lupus erythematosus

    424.91   710.0   (710.0, 424.91)

18. Thrombophlebitis of deep femoral vein

    453.41   (451.11)

19. Hypertension due to kidney stone; percutaneous kidney stone removal

    (592.0) 405.99, 55.03

20. Wolff-Parkinson-White syndrome

    426.7

Cardiovascular Procedures

This section highlights several cardiovascular procedures.

Cardiac Catheterization (37.21–37.23)

Cardiac catheterization is a common diagnostic test used to identify, measure, and verify almost every type of intracardiac condition. The technique includes the passage of a flexible catheter through the arteries or veins into the heart chambers and vessels. Cardiac catheterizations can determine the size and location of a coronary lesion, evaluate left and right ventricular function, and measure heart pressures. Cardiac catheterization is often performed prior to coronary artery bypass graft (CABG) surgery to determine the patient's left ventricular function.

In addition to serving as a diagnostic tool, cardiac catheterizations may be therapeutic in nature. For example, both percutaneous transluminal coronary angioplasties (PTCAs) and intracoronary streptokinase injections can be performed via cardiac catheterization.

Cardiac catheterization can be performed on the left or right side of the heart, using the antecubital and femoral vessels. In a right heart catheterization, a catheter is inserted through the femoral or antecubital vein, advanced first into the superior or inferior vena cava, then into the right atrium, the right ventricle, and, finally, into the pulmonary artery.

In a left heart catheterization, a catheter enters the body through either the brachial artery or the femoral artery. The catheter is advanced into the aorta, through the aortic valve, and then into the left ventricle.

ICD-9-CM provides the following codes to describe cardiac catheterizations:

37.21   Right heart catheterization
37.22   Left heart catheterization
37.23   Combined right and left heart catheterization

Cardiac Angiography

Cardiac angiography can be performed on the right or left side of the heart, or in a combined process including both the right and left sides of the heart. Right-side cardiac angiography is useful in detecting pericarditis and congenital lesions, such as Ebstein's malformation of the tricuspid valve. Left-side cardiac angiography reveals congenital and acquired lesions affecting the mitral valve, including mitral stenosis and mitral regurgitation.

In ICD-9-CM, cardiac or coronary angiograms are assigned to the following codes:

88.52   Angiocardiography of right heart structures
88.53   Angiocardiography of left heart structures
88.54   Combined right and left heart angiocardiography

Percutaneous Transluminal Coronary Angioplasty

Percutaneous transluminal coronary angioplasty (PTCA) is used to relieve obstruction of coronary arteries. PTCA is performed to widen a narrowed area of a coronary artery by employing a balloon-tipped catheter. The catheter is passed to the obstructed area, and the balloon is inflated one or more times to exert pressure on the narrowed area. A thrombolytic agent may be infused into the heart.

Recent revisions have been made to the coding of PTCA and coronary stent insertions. At one time, angioplasty and stents were focused on treating single, short coronary obstructions. More extensive lesions were treated with coronary artery bypass grafts. Now, with advances in the devices used, it is possible to insert stents in several different vessels during the same operative episode. It is also possible to insert multiple adjoining or overlapping stents.

Under the category heading, 36, Operations on vessels of heart, three "code also" notes are included:

- Code also any injection or infusion of platelet inhibitor (99.20)

- Code also any injection or infusion of thrombolytic agent (99.10)

- Code also cardiopulmonary bypass, if performed [extracorporeal circulation] [heart-lung machine] (39.61)

The percutaneous transluminal coronary angioplasty (PTCA) or coronary atherectomy is identified with procedure code 36.01. It may also be referred to as a balloon angioplasty of a coronary artery. Beneath code 36.01 are directional notes to "code also":

- Insertion of drug-eluting coronary artery stent(s) 36.07

- Insertion of non-drug-eluting coronary artery stent(s) 36.06

- Number of vascular stents inserted (00.45–00.48

- Number of vessels treated (00.40–00.43)

Note: PTCA with atherectomy involving different coronary arteries should be coded individually on the basis of the procedure performed.

> **EXAMPLE:** PTCA of left anterior descending artery with insertion of single drug-eluting stent: 36.01, 36.07, 00.40, 00.45
>
> **EXAMPLE:** PTCA of left anterior descending artery and circumflex vessels with insertion of three non-drug-eluting stents: 36.01, 36.06, 00.41, 00.47

A point to remember: Percutaneous transluminal angioplasty may also be performed on other arteries, such as renal, femoral, femoropopliteal, and vertebral. Code 39.50, Angioplasty or atherectomy of noncoronary vessel, is available for classifying angioplasty of these vessels. Insertion of stents into noncoronary vessels is reported with code 39.90, Insertion of noncoronary artery stent or stents. You also code the number of vascular stents inserted (00.45–00.48) and the number of vessels treated (00.40–00.43).

Code 36.06 is used for the insertion of a non-drug-eluting coronary artery stent(s), while 36.07 is used for the insertion of a drug-eluting coronary artery stent(s).

Coronary Artery Bypass Graft

Category 36.1, Bypass anastomosis for heart revascularization, includes codes for the CABG procedure.

The coronary circulation consists of two main arteries, the right and the left, that are further subdivided into several branches:

Right coronary artery
    Right marginal
    Right posterior descending
Left main coronary artery
    Left anterior descending branch
        Diagonal
        Septal
    Left circumflex
        Obtuse marginal
        Posterior descending
        Posterolateral

The following three surgical approaches are used in CABG procedures:

1. Aortocoronary bypass uses the aorta to bypass the occluded coronary artery.

2. Internal mammary-coronary artery bypass uses the internal mammary artery to bypass the occluded coronary artery.

3. Abdominal-coronary artery bypass uses an abdominal artery.

Aortocoronary Bypass or Coronary Artery Bypass Graft (CABG)

Aortocoronary bypass brings blood from the aorta into the obstructed coronary artery using a segment of the saphenous vein or a segment of the internal mammary artery for the graft. The procedure is commonly referred to as coronary artery bypass graft(s) or by the abbreviation CABG, pronounced "cabbage." ICD-9-CM provides the following codes to classify aorto-coronary bypass, depending on the number of coronary arteries involved:

36.10   **Aortocoronary bypass for heart revascularization, not otherwise specified**
36.11   **Aortocoronary bypass of one coronary artery**
36.12   **Aortocoronary bypass of two coronary arteries**
36.13   **Aortocoronary bypass of three coronary arteries**
36.14   **Aortocoronary bypass of four or more coronary arteries**

Internal Mammary-Coronary Artery Bypass

Internal mammary-coronary artery bypass is accomplished by loosening the internal mammary artery from its normal position and using the internal mammary artery to bring blood from the subclavian artery to the occluded coronary artery. Codes are selected based on whether one or both internal mammary arteries are used, regardless of the number of coronary arteries involved. ICD-9-CM provides the following two codes to classify internal mammary-coronary artery bypass:

36.15   **Single internal mammary-coronary artery bypass**
36.16   **Double internal mammary-coronary artery bypass**

Abdominal-Coronary Artery Bypass

A new code was added in 1996 to describe abdominal-coronary artery bypass. This type of procedure involves creating an anastomosis between an abdominal artery, commonly the gastroepiploic, and a coronary artery beyond the occluded portion, for example, 36.17, Abdominal-coronary artery bypass (*Coding Clinic* 1991, 1996).

Cardiac Pacemakers

A cardiac pacemaker has the following three basic components:

- The pulse generator is the pacing system that contains the pacemaker battery (power source) and the electronic circuitry.

- The pacing lead carries the stimulating electricity from the pulse generator to the stimulating electrode.

- The electrode is the metal portion of the lead that comes in contact with the heart.

There are different types of pacemakers:

- Single-chamber pacemakers use a single lead that is placed in the right atrium or the right ventricle.

- Dual-chamber pacemakers use leads that are inserted into both the atrium and the ventricle.

- Rate-responsive pacemakers have a pacing rate modality that is determined by physiological variables other than the atrial rate.

- Cardiac resynchronization pacemaker without a defibrillator (CRT-P), also known as biventricular pacing without internal cardiac defibrillator.

ICD-9-CM Coding Format for Pacemakers

ICD-9-CM classifies cardiac pacemakers to code 37.8, Insertion, replacement, removal, and revision of pacemaker device. The note at the beginning of this subcategory states: Code also any lead insertion, lead replacement, lead removal, and/or lead revision (37.70–37.77). Therefore, a second code must be assigned to describe the insertion, replacement, removal, or revision of a lead by using codes 37.70 through 37.77. For example:

- In coding initial insertion of a permanent cardiac pacemaker, two codes are required: one for the pacemaker (37.80–37.83) and one for the lead (37.70–37.74).

- When a pacemaker is replaced with another pacemaker, only the replaced pacemaker is coded (37.85–37.87). Removal of the old pacemaker is not coded.

- Removal of a pacemaker is assigned code 37.89, Revision or removal of pacemaker device.

Also note the exclusion note in subcategory 37.8, which states that these codes exclude implantation of cardiac resynchronization pacemaker (00.50) and implantation or replacement of cardiac resynchronization pacemaker pulse generator only (00.53). Replacement of cardiac resynchronization devices or the component parts are classified with codes 00.52, 00.53, or 00.54.

Reprogramming of Cardiac Pacemakers

Patients admitted for reprogramming of a cardiac pacemaker are assigned diagnostic code V53.31, Fitting and adjustment of cardiac pacemaker. No procedure code in ICD-9-CM exists to describe reprogramming.

Automatic Implantable Cardioverter-Defibrillators

The automatic implantable cardioverter-defibrillator (AICD) is a special type of pacemaker that proves effective for patients with recurring, life-threatening dysrhythmias, such as ventricular tachycardia or fibrillation.

The AICD is an electronic device consisting of a pulse generator and three leads. The pulse generator is implanted into the abdomen of the patient. The first lead senses heart rate at the right ventricle; the second lead, sensing morphology and rhythm, defibrillates at the right atrium; the third lead defibrillates at the apical pericardium. The AICD can be programmed to suit each patient's needs, and it uses far less energy than an external defibrillator.

ICD-9-CM classifies the AICD to code 37.9, Other operations on heart and pericardium, and to 00.5, Other cardiovascular procedures, with the following codes available:

37.94 **Implantation or replacement of automatic cardioverter/defibrillator, total system (AICD)**—Assign this code when a total system AICD is inserted. Total system refers to the implantation of the defibrillator with leads, formation of pocket, and any transvenous lead.

37.95 **Implantation of automatic cardioverter/defibrillator lead(s) only**

37.96 **Implantation of automatic cardioverter/defibrillator pulse generator only**

37.97 **Replacement of automatic cardioverter/defibrillator lead(s) only**

37.98 **Replacement of automatic cardioverter/defibrillator pulse generator only**

37.99 **Operations on heart and pericardium**—Assign this code when only the lead(s) or only the pulse generator requires revision or repositioning.

86.09 **Other incision of skin and subcutaneous tissue**—Assign this code when the pacemaker pocket requires revision or repositioning.

00.51 Implantation of cardiac resynchronization defibrillator, total system (CRT-D)

00.54 Implantation or replacement of cardiac resynchronization defibrillator, pulse generator device only (CRT-D)

Diagnostic Procedures

The following procedures are often performed during a cardiac catheterization:

- Cardiac angiography
- Coronary arteriography
- Ventriculography

Cardiac Angiography

Cardiac angiography can be performed on the right or left side of the heart, or in a combined process including both the right and left sides of the heart. Right-side cardiac angiography is useful in detecting pericarditis and congenital lesions, such as Ebstein's malformation of the tricuspid valve. Left-side cardiac angiography reveals congenital and acquired lesions affecting the mitral valve, including mitral stenosis and mitral regurgitation.

In ICD-9-CM, cardiac or coronary angiograms are assigned to the following codes:

88.52   **Angiocardiography of right heart structures**
88.53   **Angiocardiography of left heart structures**
88.54   **Combined right and left heart angiocardiography**

Coronary Arteriography

Coronary arteriography serves as a diagnostic tool in detecting obstruction within the coronary arteries. The following two techniques are used in performing a coronary arteriography:

- Sones technique uses a single catheter inserted via a brachial arteriotomy.

- Judkins technique uses two catheters inserted percutaneously through the femoral artery.

ICD-9-CM provides the following codes to describe coronary arteriograms:

88.55   **Coronary arteriography using a single catheter (Sones technique)**
88.56   **Coronary arteriography using two catheters (Judkins technique)**
88.57   **Other and unspecified coronary arteriography**

Ventriculography

Ventriculograms measure stroke volume and ejection fraction. The ejection fraction is the amount of blood ejected from the left ventricle per beat; it is presented as a percentage of the total ventricular volume. The fraction is usually about 65 percent, plus or minus 8 percent. A fraction below 50 percent is usually a sign of severe ventricular dysfunction; a fraction below 35 percent signals profound dysfunction.

The Alphabetic Index in volume 3 of ICD-9-CM offers directions for coding ventriculograms. Use codes 88.52 through 88.54 for cardiac angiograms.

Exercise 10.6

Assign ICD-9-CM procedure codes to the following:

1. Insertion of dual-chamber cardiac pacemaker and atrial and ventricular leads

   _00.50_   _(37.83, 37.72)_

2. Coronary artery bypass graft of four vessels with cardiopulmonary bypass

   _36.14   39.61_

3. Insertion of total system automatic implantable cardioverter-defibrillator

   _37.94_

4. Right and left cardiac catheterization with Judkins coronary arteriogram and right and left ventriculogram

   _37.23   88.56   88.54_

5. Percutaneous transluminal angioplasty of single coronary artery with thrombolytic agent

   _00.66   00.40 99.10   (00.66, 99.10, 00.40)_

Review Exercise: Chapter 10

Assign the appropriate ICD-9-CM codes to the following diagnoses and procedures:

1. Right bundle branch block

2. Acute pericardial effusion; pericardiocentesis

3. Atrial fibrillation; insertion of single-chamber, rate-responsive cardiac pacemaker with ventricular lead

4. Arteriosclerotic heart disease of autologous vein bypass graft; left cardiac catheterization, left ventriculogram, Sones arteriogram

5. Endocardial fibroelastosis

6. Thoracic aortic aneurysm; aneurysmectomy with graft replacement

7. Mitral valve insufficiency with prosthetic mitral valve replacement; cardiopulmonary bypass

8. Acute myocardial infarction of the posterolateral wall, initial episode; triple coronary artery bypass using saphenous vein graft to diagonal branch and circumflex, and left internal mammary artery to left anterior descending; cardiopulmonary bypass

9. Subacute bacterial endocarditis secondary to staphylococcal aureus; ventricular tachycardia

10. Acute myocardial infarction, anterior wall (initial episode); percutaneous transluminal coronary angioplasty (PTCA) of two vessels with infusion of thrombolytic agent

11. Arteriosclerosis of the right lower extremity (native arteries) with rest pain, right popliteal-tibial bypass

12. End-stage renal disease (ESRD) with hypertension; venous catheterization for dialysis; renal dialysis

13. Infected varicose veins of the lower extremity with development of ulcer

14. Occlusive disease of iliac artery; percutaneous angioplasty of iliac artery with drug-eluting stent insertion

15. Raynaud's disease with gangrene

Chapter 11

Diseases of the Respiratory System

Chapter 8, Diseases of the Respiratory System (460–519)

Chapter 8, Diseases of the Respiratory System, of the Tabular List in volume 1 of ICD-9-CM is subdivided into the following categories and section titles:

Categories	Section Titles
460–466	Acute Respiratory Infections
470–478	Other Diseases of the Upper Respiratory Tract
480–487	Pneumonia and Influenza
490–496	Chronic Obstructive Pulmonary Disease and Allied Conditions
500–508	Pneumoconioses and Other Lung Diseases Due to External Agents
510–519	Other Diseases of the Respiratory System

This chapter highlights coding instructions for specific respiratory conditions.

Bronchitis

Bronchitis is an inflammation of the bronchi and can be acute or chronic in nature. Acute bronchitis is an inflammation of the tracheobronchial tree with a short and more or less severe course. It is often due to exposure to cold, inhalation of irritant substances, or acute infections. Chronic bronchitis is a condition associated with prolonged exposure to nonspecific bronchial irritants and is accompanied by mucus hypersecretion and certain structural changes in the bronchi. Usually associated with cigarette smoking, one form of bronchitis is characterized clinically by a chronic productive cough.

ICD-9-CM provides separate codes to describe acute and chronic bronchitis. The following acute conditions of bronchitis are classified to code 466.0:

> **466.0 Acute bronchitis**
> Bronchitis, acute or subacute:
> fibrinous
> membranous
> pneumococcal
> purulent
> septic
> viral
> with tracheitis
> Croupous bronchitis
> Tracheobronchitis, acute

Code 490, Bronchitis, not specified as acute or chronic, is assigned when the specific type of bronchitis is not documented in the health record. Chronic bronchitis is included in the section titled "Chronic Obstructive Pulmonary Disease and Allied Conditions." Category 491, Chronic bronchitis, is subdivided to describe the types of chronic bronchitis, such as simple, mucopurulent, and obstructive.

A point to remember: When chronic bronchitis is described as obstructive or is associated with chronic obstructive pulmonary disease (COPD), codes 491.20 through 491.21 should be reported.

Pneumonia

The third and fifth sections of chapter 8 include codes for pneumonias, with the following separate categories identifying the underlying organism or site:

480	**Viral pneumonia**
481	**Pneumococcal pneumonia [Streptococcus pneumoniae pneumonia]**
482	**Other bacterial pneumonia**
483	**Pneumonia due to other specified organism**
484	**Pneumonia in infectious diseases classified elsewhere**
485	**Bronchopneumonia, organism unspecified**
486	**Pneumonia, organism unspecified**
487.0	**Influenza with pneumonia**
507	**Pneumonitis due to solids and liquids**

Category 480, Viral Pneumonia

Category 480, Viral pneumonia, is subdivided to fourth-digit subcategories that identify the specific virus. Viral pneumonia is a highly contagious disease affecting both the trachea and the bronchi of the lungs. Inflammation destroys the action of the cilia and causes hemorrhage. Isolation of the virus is difficult, and x-rays do not reveal any pulmonary changes.

Category 481, Pneumococcal Pneumonia

Category 481, Pneumococcal pneumonia [Streptococcus pneumoniae pneumonia], describes pneumonia caused by the pneumococcal bacteria. The bacteria lodge in the alveoli and cause an inflammation. If the pleura are involved, the irritated surfaces rub together and cause painful breathing. On examination, pleural friction can be heard. A chest x-ray demonstrates a consolidation of the lungs that results from pus forming in the alveoli and replacing the air. Approximately 90 percent of lobar pneumonia is due to pneumococcal bacteria.

Category 482, Other Bacterial Pneumonia

Category 482, Other bacterial pneumonia, is subdivided to fourth-digit subcategories that identify specific bacteria, such as Klebsiella pneumoniae (482.0), Pseudomonas (482.1), Hemophilus influenzae (482.2), Streptococcus (482.3x), and Staphylococcus (482.4x). Bacteria are the most common cause of pneumonia in adults. Gram staining is a rapid and cost-effective method for diagnosing bacterial pneumonia, if a good sputum sample is available.

Category 483, Pneumonia Due to Other Specified Organism

Category 483 includes codes for pneumonia due to other specified organisms, including Mycoplasma pneumoniae (483.0). The fourth digit identifies the specific organism.

Category 484, Pneumonia in Infectious Diseases Classified Elsewhere

Category 484, Pneumonia in infectious diseases classified elsewhere, is subdivided to fourth-digit subcategories that identify the specific infectious disease. These codes are set in italic type and thus are not meant for primary tabulation. In addition, instructional notations in this category direct coders to assign an additional code to describe the underlying disease.

Category 485, Bronchopneumonia, Organism Unspecified

Category 485, Bronchopneumonia, organism unspecified, is a three-digit code that describes the site of the pneumonia. Bronchopneumonia usually begins in the terminal bronchioles of the lung and causes the air space to become filled with exudates.

Category 486, Pneumonia, Organism Unspecified

Category 486, Pneumonia, organism unspecified, is a three-digit code that should be assigned only when the health record does not identify the causative organism.

Category 487, Influenza

Influenza with respiratory manifestations is classified to 487.0–487.8. A "use additional code" note is included under code 487.0, Influenza with pneumonia, to identify the type of pneumonia (480.0–480.9, 482.0–482.9, 483.0–483.8, 485). Code 486, Pneumonia, organism unspecified, would be inappropriate to use with code 487.0 because the connection has been made between the influenza and the resulting pneumonia. An excludes note appears under code 487.8, Influenza with other manifestations. Intestinal flu [viral gastroenteritis] would not be coded here, but instead to code 008.8. Influenzal conditions classified to category 487 are respiratory conditions.

Category 507, Pneumonitis Due to Solids and Liquids

Category 507, Pneumonitis due to solids and liquids, is subdivided to fourth-digit subcategories that describe the causative agent. This category also is referred to as aspiration pneumonia. If the causative agent is unspecified, the Alphabetic Index to Diseases offers direction to code 507.0.

A point to remember: In cases where the patient develops both aspiration pneumonia and bacterial pneumonia, codes for both types of pneumonia should be assigned.

> **EXAMPLE:** Patient was admitted with aspiration pneumonia, as well as Klebsiella pneumonia: 507.0, Pneumonitis due to inhalation of food or vomitus; 482.0, Pneumonia due to Klebsiella pneumoniae

Exercise 11.1

Assign ICD-9-CM codes to the following:

1. Aspiration pneumonia due to regurgitated food

   507.0

2. Streptococcal group B pneumonia

   482.32

3. Staphylococcal bronchopneumonia

   ~~485~~ 482.40

4. Allergic pneumonitis

   495.9

5. Pneumonia in cytomegalic inclusion disease

   078.5, 484.1

Category 493, Asthma

Asthma is a condition marked by recurrent attacks of paroxysmal dyspnea, with wheezing due to spasmodic contraction of the bronchi. In some cases, it is an allergic manifestation in sensitized persons. The term *reactive airway disease* is considered synonymous with asthma.

Fourth-Digit Subcategories

ICD-9-CM classifies asthma to category 493, with the following subcategories that describe the specific types of asthma:

493.0   **Extrinsic asthma** (an asthmatic condition caused by environmental allergen factors)
493.1   **Intrinsic asthma** (a form of asthma caused by the body's own immunological response)
493.2   **Chronic obstructive asthma** (a chronic form of asthma coexisting with chronic obstructive pulmonary disease [COPD] that includes chronic asthmatic bronchitis)
493.81 **Exercise induced bronchospasm**
493.82 **Cough variant asthma**
493.9   **Asthma, unspecified** (the subcategory used when the documentation does not specify one of the types listed above)

Fifth-Digit Subclassification

The fifth-digit subclassifications of category 493 apply to subcategory codes 493.0, 493.1, 493.2, and 493.9 only. The fifth-digit subclassifications describe whether the patient was in status asthmaticus or suffered what may be described as an exacerbation or acute exacerbation of the asthma. Status asthmaticus (fifth digit 1) is an acute asthmatic attack in which the degree of bronchial obstruction is not relieved by usual treatments such as epinephrine or aminophylline. A patient in status asthmaticus fails to respond to therapy administered during an asthmatic attack. This is a life-threatening complication that requires emergency care and, most likely, inpatient hospitalization. If status asthmaticus is documented as occurring in a patient with any type of COPD or with acute bronchitis, the status asthmaticus is sequenced first. It supersedes any type of COPD. An acute exacerbation or with exacerbation (fifth digit 2) is an increase in the severity of the disease or any of its signs or symptoms, such as wheezing or shortness of breath. Chronic obstructive asthma is another form of the disease. A physician may document that the patient has COPD and asthma. Following the Alphabetic Index entries, these two conditions combine into one code, 493.2, Chronic obstructive asthma, which requires a fifth digit. An acute exacerbation of this type of asthma is a worsening or a decompensation of a chronic condition.

A fifth digit of 0, 1, or 2 must be added as applicable to subcategories 493.0, 493.1, 493.2, and 493.9 only. Fifth digit 0, unspecified, indicates that there is no mention of status asthmaticus. Fifth digit 1 indicates that status asthmaticus is mentioned. Fifth digit 2 describes the asthma as having an acute exacerbation or with exacerbation (the term *acute* does not need to be stated).

0   unspecified
1   with status asthmaticus
2   with (acute) exacerbation

Keep in mind that documentation in the health record must support the use of the fifth digits 1 and 2. In a patient where the physician describes the condition as both acute exacerbation and status asthmaticus, only the fifth digit 1, with status asthmaticus, should be assigned.

Bronchiectasis

Bronchiectasis is a chronic, congenital, or acquired disease characterized by irreversible dilation of the bronchi with secondary infection. The incidence of bronchiectasis has decreased with the widespread use of antibiotics and immunizations in pediatrics. In adults, the condition may develop following a necrotizing pneumonia or lung abscess. Recently, category 494 was expanded to describe bronchiectasis without acute exacerbation (494.0) and bronchiectasis with acute exacerbation or acute bronchitis with bronchiectasis (494.1).

Chronic Obstructive Pulmonary Disease

Chronic obstructive pulmonary disease (COPD) is a diffuse obstruction of the smaller bronchi and bronchioles that results in coughing, wheezing, shortness of breath, and disturbances of gas exchange. Exacerbations of COPD, such as episodes of increased shortness of breath and cough, often are treated on an outpatient basis. More severe exacerbations, such as pneumonia, bronchitis, or other infections, usually result in admission to the hospital. When acute bronchitis is documented with COPD, code 491.22, Obstructive chronic bronchitis with acute bronchitis, should be assigned. It is not necessary to assign code 466.0 with 491.22. Code 491.22 supersedes code 491.21, Chronic obstructive bronchitis with (acute) exacerbation. Code 491.21 is used when the medical record includes documentation of COPD with acute exacerbation, without mention of acute bronchitis.

Code 496, Chronic airway obstruction, not elsewhere classified, should not be used with any code from categories 491 through 493 because these codes all are specific forms of COPD, such as bronchitis, emphysema, and asthma. Code 496 is an unspecified form of COPD.

ICD-9-CM classifies COPD to the following codes:

496	**COPD without further specification**
491.2x	**COPD with chronic bronchitis**
491.20	**Obstructive chronic bronchitis without exacerbation**
	Emphysema with chronic bronchitis
491.21	**Chronic obstructive bronchitis with (acute) exacerbation**
491.22	**Obstructive chronic bronchitis with acute bronchitis**
492.8	**COPD with emphysema**
493.2x	**COPD with asthma**

Respiratory Failure

Respiratory failure is the inability of the respiratory system to supply adequate oxygen to maintain proper metabolism and/or to eliminate carbon dioxide (CO_2). ICD-9-CM classifies different forms of respiratory failure to the following codes in category 518, Other diseases of lung:

518.81	**Acute respiratory failure**
	Respiratory failure, not otherwise specified
518.83	**Chronic respiratory failure**
518.84	**Acute and chronic respiratory failure**

Respiratory failure is assigned when documentation in the health record supports its use. It may be due to, or associated with, other respiratory conditions such as pneumonia, chronic bronchitis, or COPD. Respiratory failure also may be due to, or associated with, nonrespiratory conditions such as myasthenia gravis, congestive heart failure, myocardial infarction, or cerebrovascular accident.

Arterial blood gases may be useful in diagnosing respiratory failure; however, normal values may vary from person to person depending on individual health status. Coders should not assume the condition of respiratory failure exists based solely on laboratory and radiology test findings.

Coding and Sequencing of Acute Respiratory Failure

The coding and sequencing of acute respiratory failure presents many challenges to both the new and the experienced clinical coder. Various coding rules and guidelines must be considered.

Acute respiratory failure, code 518.81, may be assigned as a principal or secondary diagnosis depending on the circumstances of the inpatient admission. It may be the principal diagnosis when it is the condition established after study to be chiefly responsible for occasioning the admission of the patient to the hospital for care. This selection would have to be supported by the Alphabetic Index and the Tabular List as well. However, chapter-specific coding guidelines (obstetrics, poisoning, HIV, newborn) that provide specific sequencing direction take precedence. In those cases, respiratory failure may be listed as a secondary diagnosis. In addition, if respiratory failure occurs after admission, it may be listed as a secondary diagnosis.

When a patient is admitted in respiratory failure with another acute condition, the principal diagnosis will not be the same in every situation. There is not one respiratory failure coding rule. Selection of the principal diagnosis will depend on the circumstances of the admission. If both the respiratory failure and the other acute condition are responsible for the patient's admission, the guidelines regarding two or more diagnoses that equally meet the definition for principal diagnosis (Section II, C) may be applied.

Respiratory failure never exists as a single condition. It is a life-threatening condition that is always caused by an underlying condition. It is usually the terminal phase of a disease or a combination of diseases. It may be caused by diseases of the circulatory system, respiratory system, central nervous system, peripheral nervous system, respiratory muscles, and chest wall muscles. The primary goal of the treatment of acute respiratory failure is to assess the severity of underlying disease and to correct the inadequate oxygen delivery and tissue hypoxia.

The following are examples of the appropriate coding and sequencing of acute respiratory failure in association with the underlying disease.

EXAMPLE 1: A patient with chronic myasthenia gravis suffers an acute exacerbation and develops acute respiratory failure. The patient is admitted to the hospital to treat the respiratory failure.

Principal diagnosis: 518.81, Acute respiratory failure
Secondary diagnosis: 358.01, Myasthenia gravis with (acute) exacerbation

EXAMPLE 2: A patient with emphysema develops acute respiratory failure. The patient is admitted to the hospital for treatment of the respiratory failure.

Principal diagnosis: 518.81, Acute respiratory failure
Secondary diagnosis: 492.8, Emphysema

EXAMPLE 3: A patient with congestive heart failure is brought to the emergency department in acute respiratory failure. The patient is intubated and admitted to the hospital. The physician documents that acute respiratory failure is the reason for the admission.

Principal diagnosis: 518.81, Acute respiratory failure
Secondary diagnosis: 428.0, Congestive heart failure

In the above example, the physician has stated that the reason for the admission is to treat the respiratory failure. If the documentation is not clear regarding whether the congestive heart failure or the acute respiratory failure was the reason for admission, the coder should ask the physician for clarification.

EXAMPLE 4: A patient with asthma in status asthmaticus develops acute respiratory failure and is admitted to the hospital for treatment of the acute respiratory failure.

Principal diagnosis: 518.81, Acute respiratory failure
Secondary diagnosis: 493.91, Asthma, unspecified, with status asthmaticus

EXAMPLE 5: A patient is admitted to the hospital during the postpartum period as a result of developing pulmonary embolism leading to respiratory failure.

Principal diagnosis: 673.24, Obstetrical blood-clot embolism, postpartum condition or complication
Secondary diagnosis: 518.81, Acute respiratory failure

The above example is one of a chapter-specific guideline. The obstetric code is sequenced first because chapter 11 (obstetric) codes have sequencing priority over codes from other ICD-9-CM chapters (Guideline Section I. C. 11. a. 1).

EXAMPLE 6: A patient who is diagnosed as having overdosed on crack cocaine is admitted to the hospital with respiratory failure.

Principal diagnosis: 970.8, Poisoning by other specified central nervous system stimulant

Secondary diagnosis: 518.81, Acute respiratory failure

This is another example of a chapter-specific guideline. The poisoning code is sequenced first because a chapter-specific guideline (Section I. C. 17. e. 2. d) provides sequencing directions specifying that the poisoning code is listed first, followed by a code for the manifestation of the poisoning. In example 6, the respiratory failure is a manifestation of the poisoning or overdose.

EXAMPLE 7: A patient is admitted with respiratory failure due to Pneumocystis carinii pneumonia, which is associated with AIDS.

Principal diagnosis: 042, Human immunodeficiency virus (HIV) disease

Secondary diagnosis: 518.81, Acute respiratory failure; 136.3, Pneumocystosis

In example 7, the AIDS code (042) is listed as the principal diagnosis with the respiratory failure and pneumonia listed as secondary diagnoses according to the chapter-specific guidelines regarding HIV-related conditions. In this case, the pneumocystosis is the HIV-related condition that caused the respiratory failure. The guidelines in Section I. C. 1. a. 2. a. state that if a patient is admitted for an HIV-related condition, the principal diagnosis should be 042, AIDS, followed by additional diagnosis codes for all reported HIV-related conditions.

EXAMPLE 8: A patient is admitted to the hospital with severe staphylococcal aureus sepsis and acute respiratory failure.

Principal diagnosis: 038.11, Staphylococcus aureus septicemia

Secondary diagnosis: 995.92, Systemic inflammatory response syndrome due to infectious process with organ dysfunction; 518.81, Acute respiratory failure

In this example, the severe sepsis is sequenced first because there is an instructional note under subcategory 995.92 indicating to "code first" the underlying systemic infection. In addition, code 995.92 has a "use additional code" note to specify organ dysfunction and lists acute respiratory failure (518.81.) This instruction would indicate that the respiratory failure would be a secondary diagnosis. This is an example of code selection based on the Alphabetic Index and Tabular List directions.

Exercise 11.2

Assign ICD-9-CM codes to the following:

1. Respiratory failure due to myasthenia gravis with exacerbation (patient admitted to the hospital to treat the respiratory failure)

   _518.81, 358.01_

2. Intrinsic asthma in status asthmaticus

   _493.11_

3. COPD with emphysema   *Chk*

   _496, 492.8_

4. Obstructive chronic bronchitis

   _491.20_

5. Acute respiratory failure due to emphysema (patient admitted to the hospital to treat the respiratory failure)   (518.84)   *Chk,*

   _518.81, 492.8_

6. Pneumococcal pneumonia due to HIV infection/AIDS   *CK*

   _042 V08 481_

7. Acute bronchiolitis due to respiratory syncytial virus   (466.1)   *Chk*

   _466.19 079.6_

8. Pansinusitis with hypertrophy of nasal turbinates

   _473.8 478.0_

9. Pneumonia with whooping cough   *Chk*

   _486, 033.9 (484.3)_

10. Emphysema with acute exacerbation of obstructive bronchitis

    _491.21_

Respiratory Procedures

This section describes the coding of two respiratory procedures: closed endoscopic biopsy and endoscopic excision of lesions.

Closed Endoscopic Biopsy

When coding closed endoscopic biopsies, take special note of the existence of combination codes that describe both the endoscopy and the biopsy. For example:

31.43   Closed [endoscopic] biopsy of larynx
31.44   Closed [endoscopic] biopsy of trachea
33.24   Closed [endoscopic] biopsy of bronchus
33.27   Closed [endoscopic] biopsy of lung

Endoscopic Excision of Lesions

Because many lesions in the respiratory tract can be removed by endoscopic means that do not require opening the chest, ICD-9-CM provides codes for this type of procedure. For example:

32.01   **Endoscopic excision or destruction of lesion or tissue of bronchus**
32.28   **Endoscopic excision or destruction of lesion or tissue of lung**

In both of the above cases, it would be inaccurate to assign two separate codes to identify the endoscopy and the excision because one code describes both procedures.

Mechanical Ventilation

Mechanical ventilation is clinically indicated for patients with apnea, acute respiratory failure, and impending acute respiratory failure. Subcategory 96.7 is used to classify other continuous mechanical ventilation. Code 96.7 is subdivided to classify the number of hours a patient is on continuous mechanical ventilation. A note at the beginning of this subcategory describes how to calculate the number of hours a patient was on continuous mechanical ventilation. Coders should review this note. Additional codes should be assigned, when applicable, to describe endotracheal tube insertion (96.04) and tracheostomy (31.1–31.29).

Review Exercise: Chapter 11

Assign ICD-9-CM diagnosis and procedure codes to the following:

1. Respiratory failure following surgery

    518.81   518.5 ?

2. Hypertrophy of tonsils and adenoids; tonsillectomy and adenoidectomy

    474.10 , 28.3

3. Hay fever due to pollen

    477.0

4. Vocal cord paralysis, complete; diagnostic laryngoscopy

    (478.34) 478.32   31.42

5. Acute respiratory failure; COPD; continuous mechanical ventilation for 20 hours; endotracheal intubation (patient admitted to the hospital to treat the acute respiratory failure)

    518.81 , 496 , 96.71 , (96.04)

6. Chronic simple bronchitis; closed biopsy of the bronchus

    491.0 , 33.24

7. Tension pneumothorax with thoracentesis

    512.0   34.91

8. Carcinoma of left upper lobe of the lung with endoscopic excision of lesion in left upper lobe

    162.3   32.28

9. Frontal sinus polyp with excision of polyp

    471.8 , 21.31 (22.42)

10. Chronic laryngotracheitis; endoscopic biopsy of larynx

    (476.1) 464.20 , 31.43

11. Gram-negative bacterial pneumonia

    482.83

12. Pneumonia due to influenza

    487.0

13. Viral pneumonia due to SARS-associated coronavirus

    480.3

14. Black lung disease

    500

15. Postoperative pneumothorax

    512.1

chk
chk   Graded Later
chk

Chapter 12

Diseases of the Digestive System

Chapter 9, Diseases of the Digestive System (520–579)

Chapter 9, Diseases of the Digestive System, in the Tabular List in volume 1 of ICD-9-CM contains the following categories and section titles:

Categories	Section Titles
520–529	Diseases of Oral Cavity, Salivary Glands, and Jaws
530–537	Diseases of Esophagus, Stomach, and Duodenum
540–543	Appendicitis
550–553	Hernia of Abdominal Cavity
555–558	Noninfectious Enteritis and Colitis
560–569	Other Diseases of Intestine and Peritoneum
570–579	Other Diseases of Digestive System

Diseases of Oral Cavity, Salivary Glands, and Jaws

Until recently, there were no comprehensive ICD-9-CM codes to describe oral health concerns. The codes that were created with ICD-9-CM in the late 1970s had not been updated to meet the existing standards of care in dentistry today. As a result, diagnostic coding has not been widely used in dentistry. However, the need for dental codes has become urgent with the advent of electronic health records and the desire of dentists to track patient conditions with their outcomes. Updated codes would also support educational and research needs of dentistry. Expanded codes more accurately describe types of dental caries, abrasions and erosions, gingival and periodontal disease, dentofacial anomalies, diseases of supporting structures, and diseases of oral soft tissues.

Gastrointestinal Ulcers

Ulcers of the gastrointestinal tract can be found in the following categories:

531 Gastric ulcer
532 Duodenal ulcer
533 Peptic ulcer, site unspecified
534 Gastrojejunal ulcer

The preceding categories are subdivided to fourth-digit subcategories that describe acute and chronic conditions and the presence of hemorrhage or perforation. The bleeding ulcer or hemorrhage does not have to be actively bleeding at the time of the examination procedure, such as an endoscopy, to use the code for ulcer with hemorrhage. A statement by the physician that bleeding has occurred and it is attributed to the ulcer is sufficient. The fifth-digit subclassification identifies the presence or absence of obstructions.

Category 535, Gastritis and Duodenitis

ICD-9-CM classifies gastritis and duodenitis to category 535, which is subdivided to fourth-digit subcategories that describe types of gastritis and duodenitis. The fifth-digit subclassification identifies the presence or absence of hemorrhage. Active bleeding during the current examination or procedure does not have to be present to use the fifth digit to describe the hemorrhage. It may be diagnosed clinically by the physician based on the patient's history and/or physical examination.

Categories 550–553, Hernias

Hernias of the abdominal cavity are classified to categories 550 through 553. A fifth digit is used to describe whether the hernia is unilateral, bilateral, or unspecified as to one- or two-sided and whether it is recurrent.

A hernia is the protrusion of a loop or knuckle of an organ or tissue through an abdominal opening. Many different types of hernias exist, including the following:

- An inguinal hernia is a hernia of an intestinal loop into the inguinal canal. An inguinal hernia may also be referred to as "direct" or "indirect," which describes the anatomical location more precisely but cannot be coded as specifically in ICD-9-CM.

- A femoral hernia is a hernia of a loop of intestine into the femoral canal.

- A hiatal hernia is usually the herniation of the stomach through the esophageal hiatus of the diaphragm.

- A ventral hernia, or abdominal hernia, is a herniation of the intestine or some other internal body structure through the abdominal wall.

- An incisional hernia is an abdominal hernia at the site of a previously made incision.

- An umbilical hernia is a type of abdominal hernia in which part of the intestine protrudes at the umbilicus and is covered by skin and subcutaneous tissue. This type may also be described as an omphalocele.

- A hernia may be described as "reducible." This means the physician can manipulate the displaced structure(s) back into position.

- An "irreducible" hernia is also known as an "incarcerated" hernia. An incarcerated hernia is a hernia of intestine that cannot be returned or reduced by manipulation; it may or may not be strangulated.

- A strangulated hernia is an incarcerated hernia that is so tightly constricted as to restrict the blood supply to the contents of the hernial sac and possibly cause gangrene of the contents, such as the intestine. This represents a medical emergency requiring surgical correction.

- ICD-9-CM uses the term *obstruction* to indicate that incarceration, irreducibility, or strangulation is present with the hernia.

550   **Inguinal hernia**
551   **Other hernia of abdominal cavity, with gangrene**
552   **Other hernia of abdominal cavity, with obstruction, but without mention of gangrene**
553   **Other hernia of abdominal cavity without mention of obstruction or gangrene**

Categories 555–558, Noninfectious Enteritis and Colitis

ICD-9-CM classifies noninfectious enteritis and colitis to categories 555 through 558 in chapter 9. Infectious enteritis and colitis are classified in chapter 1, Infectious and Parasitic Diseases.

Regional Enteritis (555)

Regional enteritis, also known as Crohn's disease and granulomatous enteritis, is defined as a chronic inflammatory disease commonly affecting the distal ileum and colon. Regional enteritis is characterized by chronic diarrhea, abdominal pain, fever, anorexia, weight loss, right lower quadrant mass or fullness, and lymphadenitis of the mesenteric nodes.

ICD-9-CM classifies regional enteritis to category 555, with the fourth digit identifying the specific site affected, such as the large intestine. Without further specification as to site, assign code 555.9.

Gastroenteritis

Gastroenteritis is characterized by diarrhea, nausea and vomiting, and abdominal cramps. It can be caused by bacteria, amoebae, parasites, viruses, ingestion of toxins, reaction to drugs, or enzyme deficiencies. Food allergy, hypersensitivity or sensitivity to a food, can be described as an abnormal immunologic reaction in which the body's immune system overacts to harmless things. Irritating, uncomfortable symptoms may result after eating a food or food additive. Allergic reactions as a response to food allergens may manifest as gastrointestinal reactions, the most common of which are nausea, vomiting, diarrhea, and abdominal cramping. Recently, a new code was added to describe allergic and dietetic gastroenteritis and colitis.

Gastroenteritis is classified by cause in chapters 1 and 9 in the Tabular List in volume 1 of ICD-9-CM.

003.0   **Salmonella gastroenteritis**
005.9   **Gastroenteritis due to food poisoning**
008.8   **Viral gastroenteritis, NEC**
009.0   **Infectious gastroenteritis**
556.9   **Ulcerative gastroenteritis**
558.3   **Allergic gastroenteritis and colitis**
558.9   **Other and unspecified noninfectious gastroenteritis and colitis**
       Colitis, enteritis, gastroenteritis, ileitis, jejunitis, and sigmoiditis, NOS, dietetic or noninfectious

Categories 567 and 568, Peritonitis and Retroperitoneal Infections and Other Disorders of Peritoneum

Peritonitis is inflammation of the peritoneum, usually accompanied by abdominal pain and tenderness, constipation, vomiting, and moderate fever. It may be caused by a bacteria, such as staphylococcus, pseudomonas, or mycobacterium; it may be fungal, most commonly Candida peritonitis, or caused by other factors, such as trauma or childbirth.

ICD-9-CM codes distinguish between generalized (acute) peritonitis, code 567.21, and peritoneal abscess of a specific location, such as mesenteric or subphrenic, code 567.22. Similarly, a retroperitoneal abscess (567.31) is coded differently than other forms of retroperitoneal infections (567.39.) Unique codes exist for spontaneous bacterial peritonitis as well as other acute bacterial forms of the disease. Choleperitonitis, code 567.81, occurs as the result of bile in the peritoneal cavity. Sclerosing mesenteritis, code 567.82, refers to a number of inflammatory processes involving the mesenteric fat, including fat necrosis and fibrosis. Each condition requires specific treatment.

Cholecystitis and Cholelithiasis

Two categories are available to classify cholecystitis and cholelithiasis:

574   **Cholelithiasis**
575   **Other disorders of gallbladder**

Category 574 is divided into the following four-digit subcategories to describe the existence of calculus or stones with acute or chronic cholecystitis:

574.0   **Calculus of gallbladder with acute cholecystitis**
574.1   **Calculus of gallbladder with other cholecystitis**
574.2   **Calculus of gallbladder without mention of cholecystitis**
574.3   **Calculus of bile duct with acute cholecystitis**
574.4   **Calculus of bile duct with other cholecystitis**
574.5   **Calculus of bile duct without mention of cholecystitis**
574.6   **Calculus of gallbladder and bile duct with acute cholecystitis**
574.7   **Calculus of gallbladder and bile duct with other cholecystitis**
574.8   **Calculus of gallbladder and bile duct with acute and chronic cholecystitis**
574.9   **Calculus of gallbladder and bile duct without cholecystitis**

In category 574, the fifth-digit subclassification describes the presence or absence of obstructions.

Category 575 contains the following two codes relating to cholecystitis:

575.0   **Acute cholecystitis**
575.1   **Other cholecystitis**

In subcategory 575.1, the fifth-digit subclassification indicates severity.

575.10   **Cholecystitis, unspecified**
575.11   **Chronic cholecystitis**
575.12   **Acute and chronic cholecystitis**

Category 578, Gastrointestinal Hemorrhage

Category 578 includes subcategories for hematemesis (578.0), blood in stool or melena (578.1), and unspecified gastrointestinal hemorrhage (578.9).

The use of category 578 is limited to cases where a GI bleed is documented, but no bleeding site or cause is identified. A hemorrhage in the GI tract may produce either dark black, tarry, clotted stools (also referred to as melena) or bright red blood in the stool or vomitus. This is not the same as "occult blood," which is invisible and only detected by microscopic exam or by a guaiac test. Occult blood is a small amount of blood coming from the GI tract. Occult blood or guaiac-positive stool is reported with ICD-9-CM diagnosis code 792.1, Nonspecific abnormal findings in other body substances, stool contents.

Note the lengthy excludes note under the category 578. This note identifies a number of gastrointestinal conditions that can be coded with the presence of hemorrhage or bleeding. The use of the 578 category code is not appropriate when one of the conditions listed under the excludes note is present. ICD-9-CM assumes that the GI bleeding results from the GI lesion identified (angiodysplasia, diverticulitis, diverticulosis, gastritis and duodenitis, and ulcer) and the combination code should usually be applied. Active bleeding does not have to be occurring at the time of the examination or procedure, but it does have to be identified in the patient's history. Two codes should be assigned when—and only when—the physician explicitly states that the GI hemorrhage is unrelated to a coexisting GI condition: one for the GI hemorrhage and one for the GI condition without hemorrhage.

Exercise 12.1

Assign ICD-9-CM diagnosis and procedure codes to the following:

1. Mesio-occlusion dentofacial anomaly

   524.23   ~~524.89~~

2. Unilateral femoral hernia with gangrene; repair of hernia with graft

   551.00   ~~53.69~~ (53.21

3. Cholesterolosis of gallbladder

   575.6

4. Regional enteritis of large intestine

   555.1

5. Allergic diarrhea

   558.3

6. Melena; esophagogastroduodenoscopy with biopsy

   578.1   45.16

7. Acute perforated peptic ulcer

   533.10

8. Acute hemorrhagic gastritis with acute blood loss anemia

   535.01 , 285.1

9. Acute appendicitis with perforation and peritoneal abscess; open appendectomy

   540.1   ~~47.9~~ (47.09

10. Acute cholecystitis with cholelithiasis; laparoscopic cholecystectomy

    574.00 , 51.23

11. Temporomandibular joint disorder with clicking sounds when moving the jaw

    524.64

12. Diverticulosis and diverticulitis of colon; flexible fiber-optic colonoscopy

    562.11   45.23

13. Esophageal reflux with esophagitis

    530.11

14. Infection of colostomy

    569.61

15. Small bowel obstruction with peritoneal adhesions; lysis peritoneal adhesions

    560.81 ,(54.59)

Gastrointestinal Procedures

This section highlights coding for gastrointestinal procedures such as:

- Closed endoscopic biopsies
- Endoscopic excisions of lesions
- Gastrointestinal ostomies

Closed Endoscopic Biopsies

In coding closed endoscopic biopsies, note the following combination codes that describe both the endoscopy and the biopsy:

42.24	Closed [endoscopic] biopsy of esophagus
44.14	Closed [endoscopic] biopsy of stomach
45.14	Closed [endoscopic] biopsy of small intestine
45.16	Esophagogastroduodenoscopy [EGD] with closed biopsy
45.25	Closed [endoscopic] biopsy of large intestine
48.24	Closed [endoscopic] biopsy of rectum
51.14	Other closed [endoscopic] biopsy of biliary duct or sphincter of Oddi
52.14	Closed [endoscopic] biopsy of pancreatic duct

Endoscopic Excision of Lesions

Many lesions in the digestive tract can be removed using endoscopic methods so that opening the abdomen is not required. ICD-9-CM provides the following codes for this type of procedure:

42.33	Endoscopic excision or destruction of lesion or tissue of esophagus
43.41	Endoscopic excision or destruction of lesion or tissue of stomach
45.30	Endoscopic excision or destruction of lesion of duodenum
45.42	Endoscopic polypectomy of large intestine
45.43	Endoscopic destruction of other lesion or tissue of large intestine
49.31	Endoscopic excision or destruction of lesion or tissue of anus
51.64	Endoscopic excision or destruction of lesion of biliary ducts or sphincter of Oddi
52.21	Endoscopic excision or destruction of lesion or tissue of pancreatic duct

Gastrointestinal Ostomies

Notations must be reviewed carefully when coding gastrointestinal ostomies because additional codes are required to describe the performance of any synchronous resection.

Gastrostomy

A gastrostomy involves making an incision into the stomach to permit insertion of a synthetic feeding tube. This surgery is performed on patients who are unable to ingest food normally because of stricture or lesion of the esophagus. ICD-9-CM classifies gastrostomy to code 43.19, Other gastrostomy. Code 43.11 describes percutaneous [endoscopic] gastrostomy [PEG].

Colostomy

A colostomy is the creation of an artificial opening of the colon through the abdominal wall. ICD-9-CM classifies all types of colostomies to subcategory 46.1. However, loop colostomy is assigned to code 46.03, and a colostomy performed with synchronous anterior rectal resection is assigned to code 48.62.

Code 46.03, Exteriorization of large intestine (a loop colostomy), involves bringing a loop of the large intestine out through a small abdominal incision, suturing it to the skin, and opening it. This resulting colostomy provides a temporary channel for the emptying of feces. This procedure is performed to give the bowel a rest following a colon resection. When the bowel is able to return to normal functioning, the loop colostomy is closed.

Ileostomy

An ileostomy is the creation of an opening of the ileum through the abdominal wall. ICD-9-CM classifies ileostomy to subcategory 46.2; however, loop ileostomy is assigned to code 46.01, Exteriorization of small intestine. A loop ileostomy involves transposing a segment of the small intestine to the exterior of the body.

Other Enterostomies

Other enterostomies are classified to subcategory 46.3. This subcategory includes percutaneous (endoscopic) jejunostomy, duodenostomy, and feeding enterostomy.

Revision and Closure of Intestinal Stoma

Subcategory 46.4, Revision of intestinal stoma, includes codes for the revision of both the small and large intestinal stoma. Subcategory 46.5, Closure of intestinal stoma, includes codes for the closure of both the small and large intestinal stoma.

Intestinal Resection and Anastomosis

When coding partial excision of the small and large intestine, note the following instructions:

> **45.5 Isolation of intestinal segment**
> Code also any synchronous:
> anastomosis other than end-to-end (45.90–45.94)
> enterostomy (46.10–46.39)
>
> **45.6 Other excision of small intestine**
> Code also any synchronous:
> anastomosis other than end-to-end (45.90–45.93, 45.95)
> colostomy (46.10–46.13)
> enterostomy (46.10–46.39)
>
> **45.7 Partial excision of large intestine**
> Code also any synchronous:
> anastomosis other than end-to-end (45.90–45.94)
> enterostomy (46.10–46.39)

The codes for anastomosis other than end-to-end or colostomy are appropriate to code when the procedures were performed in addition to the bowel resection.

Laparotomy

Laparotomy is an incision into the abdominal wall. ICD-9-CM classifies laparotomy to subcategory 54.1, which is further subdivided to describe exploratory laparotomy, reopening of a recent laparotomy, and drainage of intraperitoneal abscess or hematoma.

A point to remember: Take special note of the exclusion note in code 54.11, Exploratory laparotomy: "exploration incidental to intra-abdominal surgery—omit code." In such a case, the laparotomy is the surgical approach and, as such, should not be coded.

Application of Adhesion Barrier

In many categories of codes in this section, a note instructs that an additional code is to be assigned for any application or administration of an adhesion barrier substance (99.77).

The adhesion barrier is a temporary bioresorbable membrane used during the primary surgical procedure to assist in the prevention of postoperative adhesions following abdomino-pelvic procedures.

To place the adhesion barrier, a significant change in operative technique is required. The product is customized to fit the desired application site, and once prepared, the abdominal wall and organs are retracted. The product is placed at the site of trauma, and an average procedure requires the preparation and placement of multiple adhesion barriers.

Review Exercise: Chapter 12

Assign ICD-9-CM diagnosis and procedure codes to the following:

1. Chronic gastric ulcer with proximal gastrectomy

   531.70   43.5

2. Chronic ulcerative enterocolitis; colonoscopy with biopsy

   (556.0 556.9   45.25

3. Right inguinal hernia, recurrent; repair of direct inguinal hernia

   550.91   53.01

4. Hepatitis due to infectious mononucleosis

   075, 573.2   (573.1)

5. Chronic duodenal ulcer with hemorrhage; esophagogastroduodenoscopy

   532.40   45.13

6. Acute cholecystitis with choledocholithiasis; percutaneous removal of common bile duct calculi

   574.30   , 51.98   (51.96)

7. Adenocarcinoma of the sigmoid colon; resection of the sigmoid colon with end-to-end anastomosis

   (153.3) 239.0   45.76

8. Rectal ulcer; colonoscopy with biopsy of the rectum

   569.41   45.25   (48.24)

9. Irritable bowel syndrome (IBS)

   564.1

10. Polyp of the distal colon; endoscopic polypectomy

    211.3   42.33   (45.42)

11. Severe dysphagia secondary to old cerebrovascular accident; percutaneous endoscopic gastrostomy (PEG)

    438.82   43.11

12. Incarcerated incisional hernia; repair of hernia

    553.21,   53.9 (53.51)

13. Acute and chronic pancreatitis with atrophic gastritis

    577.0 577.1   535.10

14. Postsurgical malabsorption syndrome

    579.3

15. Chronic active hepatitis

    571.49

Chapter 13

Diseases of the Genitourinary System

Chapter 10, Diseases of the Genitourinary System (580–629)

Chapter 10, Diseases of the Genitourinary System, in the Tabular List in volume 1 of ICD-9-CM contains the following categories and section titles:

Categories	Section Titles
580–589	Nephritis, Nephrotic Syndrome, and Nephrosis
590–599	Other Diseases of Urinary System
600–608	Diseases of Male Genital Organs
610–611	Disorders of Breast
614–616	Inflammatory Disease of Female Pelvic Organs
617–629	Other Disorders of Female Genital Tract

Nephritis, Nephrotic Syndrome, and Nephrosis (580–589)

The exclusion note at the beginning of the section "Nephritis, Nephrotic Syndrome, and Nephrosis" states "hypertensive kidney disease" (403.00–403.91). As discussed in chapter 10, Diseases of the Circulatory System, when hypertension and chronic kidney disease exist in a patient, a causal relationship is presumed unless documentation in the health record states that the hypertension is secondary.

Renal failure and renal insufficiency represent a range of disease processes that occur when the kidneys have problems eliminating metabolic products from the blood. These problems can by caused by various underlying conditions such as hypertension and diabetes, or they may affect patients with a single kidney or those with a family history of kidney disease. There are both acute and chronic renal failure and acute and chronic renal insufficiency, which are identified as separate conditions with different codes in ICD-9-CM.

Proper terminology, as used in ICD-9-CM, is chronic kidney disease (CKD), rather than the vague terms of chronic renal failure and chronic renal insufficiency. CKD has five stages based on the glomerular filtration rate (GFR.) Care of patients with stage IV and V is intensive and complicated. For any patient, the goal is to slow the progression of CKD or better prepare the patient for renal replacement therapy. The determination of GFR is based on a well-established formula. Only patients on dialysis or receiving kidney transplants may be considered as having end-stage renal disease (ESRD.) Actually, ESRD terminology is mandated by Congress for insurance benefits. It is a federal government term that indicates chronic treatment by dialysis or transplantation.

Chronic renal insufficiency is a form of CKD classified with code 585.9, Chronic kidney disease, unspecified. Also included in this unspecified code are the vague diagnoses of chronic kidney disease and chronic renal failure. A specific form of CKD and chronic renal insufficiency should not be coded in the same record. Acute renal insufficiency, a vague but different condition from CKD, is classified to code 593.9, Unspecified disorder of kidney and ureter, with other vague descriptions such as acute renal disease or renal disease unspecified.

Acute renal failure (ARF) is assigned to category 584, with the fourth-digit subcategories identifying the location of the lesion. ARF occurs suddenly, usually as the result of physical trauma, infection, inflammation, or toxicity. Symptoms include oliguria or anuria with hyperkalemia and pulmonary edema. Physicians may identify ARF with more specificity by referring to it as prerenal, intrarenal, or postrenal, which more specifically identifies underlying causes such as congestive heart failure (prerenal), acute nephritis or nephrotoxicity (intrarenal), or obstruction of urine flow out of the kidneys (postrenal). ARF is treated differently from chronic kidney disease and is classified to category 584, Acute renal failure.

Other Diseases of Urinary System (590–599)

The section "Other Diseases of Urinary System" classifies many genitourinary infections, such as pyelonephritis, urinary tract infection, and cystitis, as well as other disorders of the bladder, ureter, and urethra. It is important to read all the notes at the beginning of the categories and subcategories in chapter 10 because many conditions in this chapter require assignment of an additional code to identify the organism involved.

EXAMPLE: Chronic pyelitis due to E. coli: 590.00, Chronic pyelonephritis without lesion of renal medullary necrosis; 041.4, Escherichia [E. coli] infection in conditions classified elsewhere and of unspecified site

Cystitis

Cystitis is a bacterial infection of the urinary bladder. Most common in women, this condition is often recurrent. Most cases are due to a vaginal infection that extends through the urethra to the bladder. Cystitis in men is due to urethral or prostatic infections or catheterizations. Symptoms include burning or painful urination, urinary urgency and frequency, nocturia, suprapubic pain, and lower back pain.

A diagnosis of cystitis is made by obtaining a urine specimen from the bladder by either catheterization or a clean-catch midstream sample. A bacterial colony count of >1,000 colonies/ml in a catheterized specimen indicates cystitis, as does a bacterial count of >100,000/ml in a midstream sample. Urine also may be positive for pyuria and hematuria. Therapy with antibiotics is prescribed for uncomplicated infections.

Note: The coder should not arbitrarily record an additional diagnosis on the basis of an abnormal lab finding alone. The physician should always be queried if the specific diagnosis is not clearly stated in the health record (Coding Clinic 1993).

ICD-9-CM classifies cystitis to category 595, with the fourth-digit subcategories describing type, severity, and location. An instruction at the beginning of this category advises that an additional code from chapter 1, Infectious and Parasitic Diseases, should be assigned to identify the organism involved.

595.0	**Acute cystitis**
595.1	**Chronic interstitial cystitis**
595.2	**Other chronic cystitis**
595.3	**Trigonitis**
595.4	**Cystitis in diseases classified elsewhere**
595.8x	**Other specified types of cystitis**
595.9	**Cystitis, unspecified**

Diseases of Male Genital Organs (600–608)

The section "Diseases of Male Genital Organs" also has notes requiring the use of an additional code to identify the organism involved.

> **EXAMPLE:** Infected hydrocele; organism involved—staphylococcus:
> 603.1, Infected hydrocele; 041.10, Unspecified staphylococcus infection in conditions classified elsewhere and of unspecified site

Benign Prostatic Hypertrophy

Benign prostatic hypertrophy (BPH) is a condition commonly occurring in men over sixty years old. The prostate gland, which encircles the urethra at the base of the bladder, becomes enlarged and presses on the urethra, obstructing the flow of urine from the bladder. Symptoms of BPH include urinary frequency, urgency, nocturia, incontinence, and hesitancy; decreased size and force of stream; and/or complete urinary retention. Straining to void may rupture veins of the prostate, causing hematuria.

A diagnosis of BPH is made by a rectal examination that finds the prostate enlarged and with a rubbery texture. Urinalysis shows WBC, RBC, albumin, bacteria, and blood. Cystoscopy reveals the extent of enlargement. A postvoiding cystogram shows the amount of residual urine in the bladder.

ICD-9-CM classifies many forms of hyperplasia of the prostate to category 600. Some forms of hyperplasia may be indicative of the need for further testing due to the increased risk for prostatic cancer. Hyperplasia of the prostate often produces the symptom of urinary obstruction or the inability to urinate. The urinary obstruction is the problem that typically brings the patient to the physician or to the hospital emergency department. Admission to the hospital is usually to relieve the obstruction. Coding of hyperplasia of the prostate has been a problem due to the fact that the urinary obstruction is a routine symptom of the condition. The debate in the past has been whether to code the urinary obstruction or the underlying cause of hyperplasia as the first-listed code. Recently, new combination codes have been created to resolve the debate.

Category 600 is expanded to the fifth-digit subclassification level to describe the type of hyperplasia of prostate and whether or not urinary obstruction is present. For example:

600.00 Hypertrophy (benign) of prostate without urinary obstruction

The category has been further expanded to the fifth-digit level to show the presence of urinary retention. These combination codes will solve sequencing problems.

Disorders of Breast (610–611)

Disorders such as gynecomastia, fibroadenosis, inflammatory disease, and solitary cyst of the breast are included in this section. Fibrocystic disease of the breast is classified to code 610.1, Diffuse cystic mastopathy.

Certain signs and symptoms of breast disease, such as mastodynia, breast lump, and nipple discharge, are included in category 611, rather than in chapter 16, with other symptoms, signs, and ill-defined conditions. Neoplasms of the breast are classified in chapter 2, Neoplasms, in ICD-9-CM.

Inflammatory Disease of Female Pelvic Organs (614–616)

This section includes infections of the female pelvic organs. The note at the beginning of the section indicates to "Use additional code to identify organism, such as staphylococcus or streptococcus."

EXAMPLE: Acute salpingitis; organism involved—streptococcus: 614.0, Acute salpingitis and oophoritis; 041.00, Unspecified streptococcus infection in conditions classified elsewhere and of unspecified site

Disorders of Female Genital Tract (617–629)

The "Disorders of Female Genital Tract" section includes conditions such as the following:

- Endometriosis, which occurs when endometrial glands or stroma are present outside the uterine cavity; for example, in the ovaries, uterine ligaments, rectovaginal septum, and pelvic peritoneum. Many women in the United States suffer from endometriosis, and it is one of the most common causes of infertility in women.

- Genital prolapse, or prolapse of the vaginal walls with and without uterine prolapse, can be described with recently revised ICD-9-CM codes to identify precise forms of these conditions.

- Ovarian cysts of a variety of types are the most common pelvic masses diagnosed in women.

Other gynecological conditions described in this chapter of ICD-9-CM include:

- Noninflammatory disorders of the female genital organs, including dysplasia of the cervix and vulva

- Disorders of menstruation

- Menopausal and postmenopausal disorders

- Infertility

Abnormal Pap Smear Findings

The classifying of abnormal cervical Papanicolaou (Pap) smears has become more sophisticated over time. Over 90 percent of the laboratories in the United States use the Bethesda system for reporting the results of Pap smears. This system was first published in 1989, and it was revised in 1991 and 2001. The ICD-9-CM classification system has been updated to be consistent with the Bethesda terminology. The descriptive diagnoses included in the Bethesda system include benign cellular changes, reactive cellular changes, and epithelial cell abnormalities. These abnormalities include:

- Nonneoplastic findings such as reactive cellular changes

- Epithelial cell abnormalities such as: atypical squamous cells, low-grade and high-grade squamous intraepithelial lesions including mild to severe cervical dysplasia, and squamous cell carcinoma

- Glandular cell abnormalities that include endocervical adenocarcinoma in situ and other adenocarcinomas

ICD-9-CM codes 622.10–622.12 describe mild dysplasia of the cervix or cervical intraepithelial neoplasia I (CIN I), moderate dysplasia of cervix (CIN II), and unspecified dysplasia of cervix. However, if the condition is described as carcinoma in situ of the cervix, or CIN III, it is classified in subcategory 233.1.

Codes under subcategory 795.0 are used to describe the results of other abnormal Pap smears of the cervix. The following codes describe various ways to explain why results were not available and why a Pap smear must be repeated:

- Abnormal glandular Pap smear of cervix (795.00)

- Squamous cell abnormalities (705.01–795.04)

- Cervical high-risk human papillomavirus (HPV) DNA test positive (795.05)

- Unsatisfactory smear or inadequate sample (795.08)

ICD-9-CM codes 622.11 and 622.12 describe mild dyplasia of the cervix (CIN I) and moderate dysplasia of cervix (CIN II). CIN III and carcinoma in situ of the cervix are classified in subcategory 233.1. Subcategory 795.0 is used to describe nonspecific abnormal Pap smear of the cervix. Diagnoses such as atypical squamous cells of undetermined significance, as well as low-grade squamous intraepithelial lesion (LGSIL) or high-grade squamous intraepithelial lesion (HGSIL), are included here. Terminology that is out of date today but may be seen in older health records is "ASCUS favor benign" (for atypical squamous cells of undetermined significance, once coded to 795.01) and ASCUS favor dysplasia (for atypical squamous cells, high grade, once coded to 795.02). These same conditions today are described as ASC-US and ASC-H. Also within this subcategory, codes exist to describe a Pap smear of cervix with high-risk human papilloma virus (HPV) DNA test positive (795.95) and Pap smear of cervix with low-risk HPV DNA test positive.

Finally, a code exists to describe an unsatisfactory smear or inadequate sample (795.08) to explain why results were not available and why a Pap smear must be repeated.

Menopause

The diagnosis of menopause or menopausal syndrome often needs to be more specific. ICD-9-CM includes several options for coding. Codes exist for both symptomatic menopausal syndrome and asymptomatic menopausal status. A crucial factor is whether the menopause is the result of the natural aging process or whether surgical intervention or other treatment such as radiation has created artificially induced menopause. The patient who has a menopausal disorder or symptom associated with artificial or postsurgical menopause may be coded with:

256.2   **Postablative ovarian failure**
627.4   **Symptomatic states associated with artificial menopause**

The patient who is menopausal as a result of having her ovaries removed surgically but is asymptomatic may be coded with:

256.2   **Postablative ovarian failure**
V45.77   **Acquired absence of genital organ (ovary)**

The patient who has a menopausal disorder or symptoms associated with age-related or naturally occurring menopause may be coded with:

256.39   **Other ovarian failure**
627.2   **Symptomatic menopausal or female climacteric states**

Other codes in the 627 category may also be used to describe menopausal-related disorders such as bleeding, atrophic vaginitis, and so forth. Other symptoms may be classified with codes from other chapters.

The patient who is postmenopausal as a result of the natural or age-related process and is asymptomatic is coded with:

V49.81   **Postmenopausal status (age-related) (natural)**

Review Exercise: Chapter 13

Assign ICD-9-CM diagnosis and procedure codes to the following:

1. Vesicoureteral reflux with bilateral reflux nephropathy

   ~~593.73~~ (593.72)

2. Acute glomerulonephritis with necrotizing glomerulitis

   580.4

3. Actinomycotic cystitis

   039.8   595.4

4. Subserosal uterine leiomyoma, cervical polyp, and endometriosis of uterus; total abdominal hysterectomy with bilateral salpingo-oophorectomy

   218.2   622.7   617.0   68.4   65.61

5. Moderate dysplasia of the cervix (CIN II); biopsy of cervix

   622.12   67.12

Review Exercise: Chapter 13 (Continued)

6. Absence of menstruation

   626.0

7. Symptomatic menopausal symptoms associated with ovarian failure as the result of age-related menopause

   627.2   256.39

8. Fibrocystic disease of the breast; needle biopsy of the breast

   610.1   85.11

9. Benign prostatic hypertrophy with urinary obstruction; transurethral resection of prostate

   600.01   60.29

10. Unilateral gynecomastia in male patient with reduction mammoplasty

    611.1   85.31

11. Wilms' tumor; right radical nephrectomy

    189.0   55.51

12. Left ureteral stone; ureteral stent insertion

    (592.1)594.2   59.8

13. Infected hydrocele with hydrocelectomy (spermatic cord)

    (603.1) +603.01   63.1

14. Diabetic nephrotic syndrome, type I

    250.41   581.81

15. Benign hyperplasia of prostate with urinary obstruction; transurethral microwave thermo-therapy (TUMT) of prostate

    (600.01+600.21   60.96

16. Midline cystocele, rectocele with pelvic muscle wasting; repair of cystocele and rectocele

    618.01 (618.04)618.83   70.50

17. Female infertility secondary to Stein-Leventhal syndrome

    +628.9   256.4 (628.0)

18. Acute abscess of breast with incision and drainage of abscess

    611.0   85.0

19. Acquired multiple cysts of the kidney

    753.19 (593.2)

20. Acute pyelonephritis due to Pseudomonas

    590.10 (041.7)

Chapter 14

Complications of Pregnancy, Childbirth, and the Puerperium

Chapter 11, Complications of Pregnancy, Childbirth, and the Puerperium (630–677)

Chapter 11, Complications of Pregnancy, Childbirth, and the Puerperium, in the Tabular List in volume 1 of ICD-9-CM includes the following categories and section titles:

Categories	Section Titles
630–633	Ectopic and Molar Pregnancy
634–639	Other Pregnancy with Abortive Outcome
640–648	Complications Mainly Related to Pregnancy
650–659	Normal Delivery, and Other Indications for Care in Pregnancy, Labor, and Delivery
660–669	Complications Occurring Mainly in the Course of Labor and Delivery
670–677	Complications of the Puerperium

Abortion

Abortion is the expulsion or extraction from the uterus of all or part of the products of conception: an embryo or a nonviable fetus weighing less than 500 gm. When a fetus's weight cannot be determined, an estimated gestation of less than twenty-two completed weeks is considered an abortion.

Abortions, as well as complications following abortion and ectopic and molar pregnancies, are classified to categories 634 through 639 in ICD-9-CM.

634   **Spontaneous abortion**
635   **Legally induced abortion**
636   **Illegally induced abortion**
637   **Unspecified abortion**
638   **Failed attempted abortion**
639   **Complications following abortion and ectopic and molar pregnancies**

Fourth-Digit Subcategories

The fourth digits used with categories 634 through 638 indicate the presence or absence of a complication arising during an admission or an encounter for an abortion. The following list of fourth-digit subcategories is at the beginning of the section "Other Pregnancy with Abortive Outcome" (634–639):

.0 Complicated by genital tract and pelvic infection
Endometritis
Salpingo-oophoritis
Sepsis NOS
Septicemia NOS
Any condition classifiable to 639.0, with condition classifiable to 634–638

| *Excludes:* | urinary tract infection (634–638 with .7) |

.1 Complicated by delayed or excessive hemorrhage
Afibrinogenemia
Defibrination syndrome
Intravascular hemolysis
Any condition classifiable to 639.1, with condition classifiable to 634–638

.2 Complicated by damage to pelvic organs and tissues
Laceration, perforation, or tear of:
    bladder
    uterus
Any condition classifiable to 639.2, with condition classifiable to 634–638

.3 Complicated by renal failure
Oliguria
Uremia
Any condition classifiable to 639.3, with condition classifiable to 634–638

.4 Complicated by metabolic disorder
Electrolyte imbalance with conditions classifiable to 634–638

.5 Complicated by shock
Circulatory collapse
Shock (postoperative) (septic)
Any condition classifiable to 639.5, with condition classifiable to 634–638

.6 Complicated by embolism
Embolism:
    NOS
    Amniotic fluid
    Pulmonary
Any condition classifiable to 639.6, with condition classifiable to 634–638

.7 With other specified complications
Cardiac arrest or failure
Urinary tract infection
Any condition classifiable to 639.8, with condition classifiable to 634–638

.8 With unspecified complication

.9 Without mention of complication

Fifth-Digit Subclassification

Abortion

The following three fifth digits are available for use with categories 634 through 637:

0   **unspecified**
1   **incomplete**
2   **complete**

ICD-9-CM uses the following definitions for complete and incomplete abortions:

- A complete abortion is the expulsion of all of the products of conception from the uterus prior to the episode of care.

- An incomplete abortion is the expulsion of some, but not all, of the products of conception from the uterus. If placenta or secundines remain, the abortion is considered incomplete. A subsequent admission for retained products of conception following a spontaneous or legally induced abortion is assigned the appropriate code from category 634, Spontaneous abortion, or 635, Legally induced abortion, with a fifth digit of 1 for incomplete. This advice is appropriate even when the patient was discharged previously with a discharge diagnosis of complete abortion.

A review of the pathology report will confirm a complete or an incomplete abortion.

Category 638 does not require the use of a fifth digit because the code describes a failed attempted abortion and, as such, the abortion did not occur.

Complications

Complications are classified according to the body system involved, such as "complicated by genital tract and pelvic infection" or by the specific type, such as "complicated by shock."

The fourth digit 7 is assigned when a specific complication is stated in the health record but cannot be classified to the previous six subcategories. In these cases, the abortion code is listed first, followed by a code specifying the complication.

The fourth digit 8 is assigned when the documentation indicates the presence of a complication of an abortion without further specification as to type of complication. Avoid assigning the fourth digit 8. The physician should be queried in these situations. The fourth digit 9 is assigned when a complication is not mentioned.

As shown in the preceding examples, codes from categories 640 through 648 and 651 through 657 may be used as additional codes with an abortion code to indicate the complication that resulted in the abortion. When a complication of pregnancy is the known cause of the abortion, the fifth digit 3, antepartum condition or complication, should be assigned with the pregnancy code. This advice differs from the instruction given in past years to use the fifth digit 0 for pregnancy codes used with an abortion code.

A point to remember: Codes from the 660 through 669 series must not be used for complications of abortion. Other codes in the pregnancy chapter may be used and reported with the fifth digit 3, antepartum condition or complication.

Category 639

Category 639, Complications following abortion and ectopic and molar pregnancies, is used when a complication occurs after the abortion itself was completed during a previous admission. The category is provided for use when it is required to classify separately the complications classifiable to the fourth-digit level in categories 634 through 638. For example, category 639 is used when (1) the complication itself was responsible for an episode of medical care (the abortion or ectopic or molar pregnancy itself having been dealt with at a previous episode) and (2) there are immediate complications of ectopic or molar pregnancies classifiable to 630 through 633 that cannot be identified at the fourth-digit level. Note that the fourth-digit subcategories in category 639 parallel those in categories 634 through 638.

A point to remember: A code from categories 634 through 638 cannot be assigned with a code from category 639.

Early Onset of Delivery (644.21) Resulting in Live Fetus

The National Center for Health Statistics (NCHS), in consultation with the American College of Obstetricians and Gynecologists (ACOG), has confirmed that code 644.21, Early onset of delivery, should be assigned for the delivery of a liveborn infant weighing less than 500 grams or having completed less than an estimated twenty-two weeks of gestation. If the infant was not liveborn, the situation would be diagnosed as an abortion because of the infant's weight and the term of pregnancy. By definition, an abortion (fetus weighing less than 500 grams or gestation less than 22 completed weeks) cannot result in a liveborn infant. Therefore, this guideline was introduced in 1991 (*Coding Clinic* 1991). In addition to code 644.21, a code to describe the outcome of delivery (V27) must be assigned. If the delivery was induced, a code for the procedure performed for the termination of pregnancy also should be assigned.

> **EXAMPLE:** Spontaneous abortion resulting in liveborn fetus: 644.21, Early onset of delivery; V27.0, Outcome of delivery, single liveborn

> **EXAMPLE:** Induced abortion resulting in liveborn fetus; aspiration and curettage: 644.21, Early onset of delivery; V27.0, Outcome of delivery, single liveborn; 69.51, Aspiration curettage of uterus for termination of pregnancy

Missed Abortion (632)

A missed abortion occurs when the fetus has died before completion of twenty-two weeks' gestation, with retention in the uterus. ACOG defines a missed abortion as an empty gestational sac, blighted ovum, or a fetus or fetal pole without a heartbeat prior to completion of 20 weeks 0 days of gestation. ACOG acknowledges the ICD-9-CM definition of missed abortion as any fetal death prior to completion of twenty-two weeks. The assignment of the ICD-9-CM code follows the coding definition.

After six weeks in the uterus, dead fetus syndrome (641.3x) may develop, with disseminated intravascular coagulation (DIC) and progressive hypofibrinogenemia. Massive bleeding may occur when delivery is finally completed. During this time, symptoms of pregnancy disappear. A brownish vaginal discharge may occur, but no bleeding.

Missed abortions should be completed by physician intervention as soon as a diagnosis with Doppler ultrasound or other methods is certain. A common method of terminating the pregnancy involves the insertion of laminaria stents to dilate the cervix (69.93), followed by aspiration.

Coders frequently confuse the clinical condition of missed abortion with a different clinical state: spontaneous abortion. A missed abortion is the retention in the uterus of a fetus that has died. The death is indicated by cessation of growth, hardening of the uterus, loss of size of the uterus, and absence of fetal heart tones after they have been heard on previous examinations. In contrast to a spontaneous abortion, no products of conception, fetal parts, or tissue is expelled from the uterus when the patient has a missed abortion. All of the uterine contents remain in the uterus. When a spontaneous abortion occurs, the woman experiences one or more of the classic symptoms, such as uterine contractions, uterine hemorrhage, dilation of the cervix, and presentation or expulsion of all or part of the products of conception.

Threatened Abortion (640.0)

A threatened abortion is characterized by bleeding of intrauterine origin occurring before the twenty-second completed week of gestation, with or without uterine colic, without expulsion of the products of conception, and without dilatation of the cervix. Generally, the pregnancy continues.

Habitual or Recurrent Abortion (646.3 and 629.9)

A habitual or recurrent abortion is the spontaneous expulsion of a dead or nonviable fetus in three or more consecutive pregnancies at about the same period of development. Coding guidelines for this condition include:

- If the recurrent abortion is current, that is, the patient's admission or encounter is for an abortion, ICD-9-CM offers direction to the abortion codes (634–638).

- If the current hospital admission or encounter involves a pregnancy, assign code 646.3x, Habitual aborter.

- If the current hospital admission or encounter does not involve a pregnancy, assign code 629.9, Unspecified disorder of female genital organ.

Exercise 14.1

Assign ICD-9-CM diagnosis and procedure codes to the following:

1. Defibrination syndrome following induced abortion two weeks ago

    _____

2. Missed abortion, 19 weeks' gestation

    _____ 632 _____

3. Complete legal abortion performed by dilation and curettage (D&C), complicated by excessive hemorrhage

    _____

4. Incompetent cervix resulting in incomplete spontaneous abortion; D&C performed to remove products of conception

    _____

5. Spontaneous abortion, complete, during the 22nd week of pregnancy, with liveborn infant

    _____

Pregnancy

Pregnancy is the state of a female after conception until the birth (delivery) of the child. Normal pregnancies are intrauterine and the duration of pregnancy from conception to delivery is about 266 days. The following guidelines may be used in determining preterm, term, and post-term pregnancies:

- Preterm: Delivery before thirty-seven completed weeks of gestation (Patient is in her 37th or earlier week of pregnancy.)

- Term: Delivery between thirty-eight and forty completed weeks of gestation (Patient is in her 38th, 39th, or 40th week of pregnancy.)

- Postterm: Delivery between forty-one and forty-two completed weeks of gestation (Patient is in her 41st or 42nd week of pregnancy.)

- Prolonged: Delivery for a pregnancy that has advanced beyond forty-two completed weeks of gestation (Patient is in her 43rd or later week of pregnancy.)

The postpartum period, or puerperium, begins immediately after delivery and continues for six weeks. In the Alphabetic Index to Diseases, long listings of conditions appear under the following main terms:

Pregnancy
Labor
Delivery
Puerperium/Puerperal/Postpartum

Indentations are often used in the Alphabetic Index under these main terms, so extreme care should be taken in locating and selecting the appropriate code.

Exercise 14.2

Using *only* the Alphabetic Index (volume 2), assign diagnostic codes to the following (*excluding* fifth digits and outcome of delivery):

1. Postpartum varicose veins of legs

   _____

2. Spontaneous breech delivery

   _____

3. Twenty-four-week gestation with bleeding

   _____

4. Spontaneous abortion followed by a D&C

   _____

5. Triplet pregnancy, delivered spontaneously

   _____

Classification of Pregnancy

Pregnancies are classified to the following categories and sections:

633	Ectopic Pregnancy
640–648	Complications Mainly Related to Pregnancy
650–659	Normal Delivery, and Other Indications for Care in Pregnancy, Labor, and Delivery
660–669	Complications Occurring Mainly in the Course of Labor and Delivery
670–677	Complications of the Puerperium

Typically, obstetrical cases require assigning codes 630 through 677 from chapter 11, which describe complications of pregnancy, childbirth, and the puerperium. However, if the condition being treated is not affecting the pregnancy, assign code V22.2, Incidental pregnancy, rather than a code from chapter 11. Coders should note that the physician is responsible for indicating that a condition is not affecting the pregnancy.

Guidelines for Sequencing Codes Related to Pregnancy

In sequencing codes for conditions related to pregnancy, list codes from chapter 11 first, followed by other codes that further specify the condition or disease.

The following guidelines should be reviewed when selecting the principal diagnosis:

- The circumstances of the encounter or admission should determine the principal diagnosis.

- When an admission does not involve a delivery, the principal diagnosis should identify the principal complication that necessitated the admission. When more than one complication exists that equally meets the definition for principal diagnosis, any one of the complications may be sequenced first.

- When an admission involves delivery, the principal diagnosis should identify the main circumstance or complication of the delivery. In cases where a cesarean delivery was performed, the principal diagnosis should reflect the reason for it.

- In encounters for routine prenatal visits without the presence of any complication, the following codes are appropriate: V22.0, Supervision of normal first pregnancy, and V22.1, Supervision of other normal pregnancy. These codes are not to be assigned with codes from chapter 11.

- In encounters for prenatal visits in high-risk pregnancies, a code from category V23, Supervision of high-risk pregnancy, should be sequenced first. Additional codes from chapter 11 should be assigned to describe specific complications.

Ectopic Pregnancy (633)

An ectopic pregnancy is a pregnancy arising from implantation of the ovum outside the uterine cavity. About 98 percent of ectopic pregnancies are tubal (occurring in the fallopian tube). Other sites include the peritoneum or abdominal viscera, ovary, or cervix. ICD-9-CM classifies ectopic pregnancy to category 633, with fourth digits identifying the site of the ectopic pregnancy. The fifth digit of zero (0) or one (1) indicates whether or not an intrauterine pregnancy is present with the ectopic pregnancy. With the use of reproductive technology there appears to have been an increase in multiple gestation pregnancies with ectopic pregnancies coexisting with intrauterine pregnancies.

Fifth-Digit Subclassification

Assignment of the fifth digit centers on the episode of care. An episode of care is an encounter in which a patient receives care. Generally, an inpatient episode of care extends from the time of admission until the time of discharge. An outpatient episode of care involves a visit to a clinic or physician's office, or a home healthcare visit.

The following fifth-digit subclassification is required for use in categories 640–648, 651–659, 660–669, and 670–676:

---

0   **unspecified as to episode of care or not applicable**

1   **delivered, with or without mention of antepartum condition**

     Antepartum condition with delivery
     Delivery NOS   ⎫   (with mention of
     Intrapartum   ⎬   antepartum complication
       obstetric condition   ⎬   during current
     Pregnancy, delivered   ⎭   episode of care)

2   **delivered, with mention of postpartum complication**
     Delivery with mention of puerperal complication
       during current episode of care

3   **antepartum condition or complication**
     Antepartum obstetric condition, not delivered
       during the current episode of care

4   **postpartum condition or complication**
     Postpartum or puerperal obstetric condition or complication
       following delivery that occurred:
     during previous episode of care
     outside hospital, with subsequent admission for observation or care

---

The fifth digit 0 is for the rare occurrence in which the episode of care is unspecified and/or not applicable. Note that the fifth digit 0 is applicable with all the categories (excluding those so stated).

Fifth digits 1 and 2 indicate that the delivery occurred during the same admission. Fifth digit 1 is assigned whenever an antepartum complication is present; fifth digit 2 is assigned when a postpartum complication exists. Because these digits indicate that delivery occurred during the current episode of care, they may be used together on the same record if both an antepartum and a postpartum condition are present.

Fifth digits 3 and 4 both indicate that the delivery did not occur during the current episode of care. Fifth digit 3 is assigned when an antepartum condition is present; fifth digit 4 is assigned when a postpartum condition exists. Because these digits indicate that delivery did not occur during the current admission, they can never be combined with fifth digits 1 and 2. Moreover, they cannot be assigned together because the patient cannot be in both the antepartum state and the postpartum state during the same episode of care.

A point to remember: More than one fifth digit can occur in the same patient's health record, but only in the following combinations:

     1 only, or with 2, but *never* with 0, 3, or 4
     2 only, or with 1, but *never* with 0, 3, or 4
     3 only, *never* with 0, 1, 2, or 4
     4 only, *never* with 0, 1, 2, or 3

Note: All categories requiring the use of the fifth-digit subclassification have a section marker appearing directly before the category.

Exercise 14.3

Determine the appropriate fifth digit for the following:

1. Retained placenta without hemorrhage, delivery this admission   _____

2. Pyrexia of unknown origin during the puerperium (postpartum), delivery during previous admission   _____

3. Late vomiting of pregnancy, undelivered   _____

4. Prolonged first-stage labor, delivery this admission   _____

5. Shock during labor and delivery   _____

Normal Delivery (650)

Category 650, Normal delivery, is assigned when all the following criteria are met:

- Delivery of a full-term, single, healthy liveborn infant

- Delivery without prenatal or postpartum complications classifiable to categories 630 through 676 (This includes ante- and postpartum conditions such as multiple gestation and breast abscess. Code 650 may be used if the patient had a complication at some point during her pregnancy, but at the time of the admission for the delivery, the complication had been resolved.)

- Cephalic or occipital presentation with spontaneous, vaginal delivery requiring minimal or no assistance, with or without episiotomy, without fetal manipulation (for example, rotation, version) or instrumentation (forceps)

A point to remember: Because of these specific criteria, many deliveries cannot be assigned to category 650. No fourth or fifth digits apply to code 650. Code 650 is always a principal diagnosis code. It is not to be used if any other code from chapter 11 is needed to describe a current complication of the antenatal, delivery, or perinatal period. Additional codes from other chapters may be used with code 650 if they are not related to or are not in any way complicating the pregnancy.

The following procedure codes may be reported with code 650:

73.09   **Artificial rupture of membranes**
73.59   **Other manually assisted delivery**
73.6   **Episiotomy with repair**
75.34   **Other fetal monitoring**
03.91   **Injection into spinal canal, anesthetic agent for anesthesia**

Various procedure codes for sterilization, such as 66.21 through 66.29 or 66.31 through 66.39, can also be used with code 650.

Exercise 14.4

Which of the following obstetrical cases qualify for a code 650 assignment? Delivery of:

1. Liveborn infant, 35 weeks' gestation _____

2. Liveborn infant, full-term, with cephalic presentation _____

3. Liveborn infant, full-term, transverse presentation switched to cephalic by physician before delivery _____

4. Liveborn infant, full-term, cephalic presentation with fetal monitoring and epidural block _____

5. Liveborn infant, twin, with breaking of the water bag to facilitate delivery _____

6. Premature liveborn infant, delivered by low transverse cesarean delivery _____

7. Liveborn infant with artificial rupture of the membranes at 44 weeks' gestation _____

8. Vaginal birth after cesarean, normal liveborn infant _____

9. Normal full-term liveborn infant, cephalic presentation with midline episiotomy with repair _____

10. Stillborn infant, cephalic presentation, unassisted delivery _____

Outcome of Delivery (V Codes)

The outcome of delivery, as indicated by a code from category V27, should be included on all maternal delivery records (*Coding Clinic* 1996). This is always an additional, not a principal, diagnosis code used to reflect the number and status of babies delivered. Many hospitals rely on these codes to provide more information on obstetrical outcomes. Code V27 is referenced in the Alphabetic Index to Diseases under the main term "Outcome of delivery."

> **EXAMPLE:** Normal delivery and pregnancy, single liveborn: 650, Normal delivery; V27.0, Outcome of delivery, single liveborn

Obstetrical and Nonobstetrical Complications

Many preexisting conditions, including diabetes, hypertension, and anemia, may affect or complicate the pregnancy or its management. In addition, the pregnancy may aggravate the preexisting condition.

For this reason, if the pregnancy aggravates the preexisting or nonobstetrical condition or vice versa, the condition is reclassified to chapter 11 of ICD-9-CM. The categories representing such conditions are 642–643, 645, 646–648, 671, and 673–676. In some cases, the code in the obstetrical chapter is all that is required to completely describe the condition. In other situations, a secondary code is needed to specify the condition further.

Category 642

Category 642, Hypertension complicating pregnancy, childbirth, and the puerperium, provides specific subcategories for the type of hypertension; therefore, a secondary code from category 401, Essential hypertension, is not required.

> **EXAMPLE:** Term pregnancy complicated by benign essential hypertension, delivered: 642.01, Benign essential hypertension complicating pregnancy, childbirth, and the puerperium

Category 643

Category 643, Excessive vomiting in pregnancy, also provides specific subcategories; therefore, additional codes are not required unless ICD-9-CM notations instruct otherwise. For example, code 643.8 has the note to "Use additional code to specify the cause."

Category 645

The American College of Obstetricians and Gynecologists (ACOG) recently requested a code for women who are between 40 and 42 weeks' gestation. A pregnancy is not considered post-dates until after 42 completed weeks. Women in this group are considered potentially high risk for pregnancy complications.

In the past, category 645, Prolonged pregnancy, did not have fourth digits but, rather, required the use of the common fifth digits of the obstetrical codes.

The title of category 645 was changed from prolonged pregnancy to late pregnancy. Subcategory 645.1 was added to describe postterm pregnancy or pregnancy over 40 completed weeks to 42 completed weeks of gestation. Subcategory 645.2 was added to describe prolonged pregnancy or pregnancy that has advanced beyond 42 completed weeks of gestation.

Categories 646–648

For the most part, codes in categories 646 through 648 require the assignment of an additional code to further specify the condition. For example:

- Subcategory 646.2, Unspecified renal disease in pregnancy, without mention of hypertension, requires assignment of an additional code to specify the type of renal disease.

  > **EXAMPLE:** Term pregnancy with chronic nephropathy, delivered: 646.21, Unspecified renal disease in pregnancy, without mention of hypertension; 582.9, Chronic glomerulonephritis with unspecified pathological lesion in kidney

- Subcategory 646.6, Infections of genitourinary tract in pregnancy, requires assignment of an additional code to specify the infection.

- Subcategory 646.8, Other specified complications of pregnancy, is used when the complication is not classified elsewhere in chapter 11.

- Category 647, Infectious and parasitic conditions in the mother classifiable elsewhere, but complicating pregnancy, childbirth, or the puerperium, is further subdivided to identify the type of infectious or parasitic condition. A second code may be assigned to describe the infectious or parasitic condition.

EXAMPLE: Intrauterine pregnancy, 18 weeks with chronic gonorrhea: 647.13, Gonorrhea in the mother classifiable elsewhere, but complicating pregnancy, childbirth, or the puerperium; 098.2, Chronic gonococcal infection of lower genitourinary tract

- Category 648, Other current conditions in the mother classifiable elsewhere, but complicating pregnancy, childbirth, or the puerperium, is further subdivided to include a variety of conditions. This category is quite broad and requires assignment of an additional code to further specify the condition.

  EXAMPLE: Intrauterine pregnancy, 20 weeks, active cocaine abuse: 648.43, Mental disorders in the mother complicating pregnancy, childbirth, or the puerperium; 305.60, Nondependent cocaine abuse

  EXAMPLE: Intrauterine pregnancy, 20 weeks, dependence on cocaine: 648.33, Drug dependence in the mother complicating pregnancy, childbirth, or the puerperium; 304.20, Cocaine dependence

Note that ICD-9-CM reclassifies abuse of a drug to mental disorders and dependence on a drug to drug dependence in chapter 11. This is another example of why the health record must be reviewed carefully to ensure accurate code assignments.

Other conditions included in category 648 are diabetes mellitus in pregnancy and gestational diabetes. Pregnant women who are diabetic should be assigned code 648.0x with an additional code from category 250, Diabetes mellitus, to identify the type of diabetes present. Another code, V58.67, Long-term (current) use of insulin, should also be assigned if the type II diabetes is being treated with insulin. Gestational diabetes can occur during the second and third trimester of pregnancy in women who were not diabetic prior to pregnancy. Gestational diabetes can cause complications in pregnancy similar to those of preexisting diabetes mellitus. It also puts the woman at greater risk of developing diabetes mellitus after the pregnancy. Gestational diabetes is coded to 648.8x, Abnormal glucose tolerance. Codes 648.0x and 648.8x are never used on the same patient's record. In addition, code V58.67, Long-term (current) use of insulin, should also be assigned if the gestational diabetes is being treated with insulin.

Category 671

Category 671, Venous complications in pregnancy and the puerperium, is subdivided to identify the types of venous conditions/complications; therefore, no additional code assignment is required.

EXAMPLE: 26-week intrauterine pregnancy, varicose veins of legs: 671.03, Varicose veins of legs complicating pregnancy and the puerperium

Categories 673–676

For the most part, categories 673–676 also represent conditions or complications that are specific; therefore, no additional codes are required to further specify the conditions. However, subcategory 674.0, Cerebrovascular disorders in the puerperium, requires an additional code to describe the specific cerebrovascular disorder.

Exercise 14.5

Assign ICD-9-CM codes to the following:

1. Hyperemesis gravidarum with dehydration, 12 weeks' gestation

2. Uterine pregnancy, undelivered, with thyrotoxic crisis due to toxic diffuse goiter

3. Uterine pregnancy, delivered this admission, with postpartum superficial thrombophlebitis; single full-term liveborn male infant

4. Failure of lactation, delivered 1 week ago (patient discharged from hospital 5 days ago)

5. Mild preeclampsia complicating pregnancy, delivered this admission; single full-term liveborn female infant

Labor and Delivery

Labor and delivery refers to the way the female organism functions to expel the product of conception from the uterus through the vagina to the outside world. Labor is divided into four stages:

1. The first stage (stage of dilation) begins with the onset of regular uterine contractions and ends when the os is completely dilated and flush with the vagina, thus completing the birth canal.

2. The second stage (stage of expulsion) extends from the end of the first stage until the expulsion (delivery) of the infant is completed.

3. The third stage (placental stage) extends from the expulsion of the child until the placenta and membranes are expelled.

4. The fourth stage denotes the hour or two after delivery when uterine tone is reestablished.

Classification of Obstetrical Procedures

Obstetrical procedures are classified in chapter 13 of the Tabular List in volume 3 of ICD-9-CM. The codes for obstetrical procedures are listed under "Delivery" in the Alphabetic Index to Procedures. A partial listing appears in the following example:

Delivery (with)
    assisted spontaneous 73.59
    breech extraction (assisted) 72.52
        partial 72.52
            with forceps to aftercoming head 72.51
        total 72.54
            with forceps to aftercoming head 72.53
        unassisted (spontaneous delivery)
            —*omit code*
    cesarean section—*see* cesarean section
    Credé maneuver 73.59
    De Lee maneuver 72.4

ICD-9-CM classifies delivery procedures to the following categories:

72   **Forceps, vacuum, and breech delivery**
73   **Other procedures inducing or assisting delivery**
74   **Cesarean section and removal of fetus**
75   **Other obstetric operations**

Category 72, Forceps, Vacuum, and Breech Delivery

Category 72 is subdivided to describe the use of high, mid, or low forceps, the type of breech delivery, and vacuum extraction.

        EXAMPLE: Delivery with low forceps with episiotomy: 72.1, Low forceps operation with episiotomy

        EXAMPLE: Partial breech delivery: 72.52, Other partial breech extraction

Category 73, Other Procedures

Category 73 is subdivided to describe procedures that induce or assist the delivery process. The subdivisions include:

- Code 73.0, Artificial rupture of membranes, is further subdivided to describe induction or augmentation of labor.

- Code 73.1, Other surgical induction of labor, is assigned to indicate all other methods used to surgically induce labor, excluding artificial rupture of membranes.

- Code 73.2, Internal and combined version and extraction, is assigned when the physician externally and internally manipulates the fetus.

- Code 73.3, Failed forceps, is assigned when the physician uses forceps to assist in the delivery of the fetus, but delivery does not result.

- Code 73.4, Medical induction of labor, is assigned when a chemical substance (such as Pitocin) is introduced into the mother's body to stimulate labor. An exclusion note under this code states "medication to augment labor—omit code." In other words, if a chemical substance is administered to augment or "move along" the labor, the code is to be omitted.

- Code 73.5, Manually assisted delivery, is assigned when the hands of the physician or practitioner assist the head of the fetus through the birth canal. This code is further subdivided to specify codes for manual rotation of the fetal head (73.51) and other manually assisted delivery (73.59).

- Code 73.6, Episiotomy, is assigned when the vulvar orifice is incised to facilitate the birthing process. The exclusion note in this code indicates that episiotomies performed with vacuum extraction or forceps are assigned to codes in category 72.

- Code 73.8, Operations on fetus to facilitate delivery, is used to indicate when such procedures are necessary.

- Code 73.9, Other operations assisting delivery, includes external version, replacement of prolapsed umbilical cord, incision of cervix, and pubiotomy.

Category 74, Cesarean Section

Cesarean section (C-section) is the extraction of the fetus, placenta, and membranes through an incision in the abdominal and uterine walls. ICD-9-CM classifies C-sections to category 74, which is subdivided to describe two types of C-sections: classical and low cervical. In addition, code 74.3, Removal of extratubal ectopic pregnancy, is assigned for removal of an ectopic pregnancy.

Category 75, Other Obstetric Operations

The most commonly used procedure codes within this category are for diagnostic amniocentesis (75.1), other fetal monitoring (75.34), and repair of current obstetric lacerations (75.50–75.69) other than repair of routine episiotomy.

Exercise 14.6

Assign procedure codes to the following:

1. Low cervical cesarean delivery

   _____

2. Low forceps delivery with episiotomy

   _____

3. Total breech delivery

   _____

4. Manually assisted delivery

   _____

5. Medical induction of labor

   _____

Normal Delivery, and Other Indications for Care in Pregnancy, Labor, and Delivery (650–659)

Assignment of the codes in this category is as follows:

- Category 650, Normal delivery, is assigned for deliveries requiring minimal or no assistance.

- Category 651, Multiple gestation, is subdivided to fourth-digit subcategories that identify the number of fetuses.

- Category 652, Malposition and malpresentation of fetus, is subdivided to fourth-digit subcategories that identify the types of malposition and malpresentation.

- Category 653, Disproportion, addresses the difference in size between the fetal head and the pelvis. The fourth-digit subcategories identify the type of disproportion and the site.

- Category 654, Abnormality of organs and soft tissues of pelvis, classifies any abnormalities, congenital or acquired, affecting the delivery process.

- Category 655, Known or suspected fetal abnormality affecting management of mother, is subdivided to fourth-digit subcategories that describe the type of abnormality.

  EXAMPLE: Patient admitted at 38 weeks' gestation for a scheduled cesarean delivery (classical) for known fetal hydrocephalus confirmed on ultrasound: 655.01, Central nervous system malformation in fetus; 74.0, Classical cesarean section

- Category 656, Other fetal and placental problems affecting management of mother, is subdivided to fourth-digit subcategories that describe the specific problem.

  EXAMPLE: Patient admitted at 38 weeks' gestation in fetal distress; emergency cesarean delivery performed: 656.31, Fetal distress affecting management of mother; 74.99, Other cesarean section of unspecified type

A point to remember: Codes from categories 655 and 656 are assigned only when the fetal condition is actually responsible for modifying the management of the mother, that is, by requiring diagnostic studies, additional observation, special care, or termination of the pregnancy. The fact that a fetal condition exists does not justify assigning a code from this series to the mother's health record.

- Category 658, Other problems associated with amniotic cavity and membranes, is subdivided to fourth-digit subcategories that identify the types of conditions, such as polyhydramnios and infection of the amniotic cavity.

- Category 659, Other indications for care or intervention related to labor and delivery, not elsewhere classified, includes several conditions, including:

    —Subcategory 659.0, Failed mechanical induction, is the failure of induction by surgical or other instrumental methods, such as forceps.

    —Subcategory 659.1, Failed medical or unspecified induction, is the failure of the medical induction to stimulate the labor process.

Complications Occurring Mainly in the Course of Labor and Delivery

Complications that can occur in the course of labor and delivery include obstructed labor and trauma to the perineum and vulva, among others.

Obstructed Labor (660)

Category 660, Obstructed labor, is subdivided to describe the following types of obstructed labor:

- Subcategory 660.0, Obstruction caused by malposition of fetus at onset of labor, includes a note to assign an additional code from 652.0 through 652.9 to describe the malposition.

- Subcategory 660.1, Obstruction by bony pelvis, includes a note to assign an additional code from 653.0 through 653.9 to describe the disproportion.

- Subcategory 660.2, Obstruction by abnormal pelvic soft tissues, includes a note to assign an additional code from 654.0 through 654.9 to describe the abnormality.

Trauma to Perineum and Vulva during Delivery (664)

Category 664, Trauma to perineum and vulva during delivery, includes perineal lacerations. This category is subdivided into eight fourth-digit subcategories. The following five subcategories identify laceration degrees:

- Subcategory 664.0, First-degree perineal laceration, includes lacerations, ruptures, or tears involving the fourchette, hymen, labia, skin, vagina, and/or vulva.

- Subcategory 664.1, Second-degree perineal laceration, includes lacerations, ruptures, or tears (following episiotomy) that involve the pelvic floor, perineal muscles, and/or vaginal muscles.

- Subcategory 664.2, Third-degree perineal laceration, includes lacerations, ruptures, or tears (following episiotomy) that involve the anal sphincter, rectovaginal septum, and/or sphincter, not otherwise specified.

- Subcategory 664.3, Fourth-degree perineal laceration, includes lacerations, ruptures, or tears of sites classifiable to subcategory 664.2 and also involving the anal mucosa and/or the rectal mucosa.

- Subcategory 664.4, Unspecified perineal laceration, is available for use when the extent of the laceration is not specified in the health record.

Other Complications of Labor and Delivery (669)

Category 669, Other complications of labor and delivery, not elsewhere classified, includes the following three fourth-digit subcategories:

- Subcategory 669.5, Forceps or vacuum extractor delivery without mention of indication, is assigned when the reason for the forceps or vacuum extraction is not indicated.

- Subcategory 669.6, Breech extraction without mention of indication, is assigned when the reason for the breech extraction is not indicated.

- Subcategory 669.7, Cesarean delivery without mention of indication, is assigned when the reason for the cesarean delivery is not indicated.

A point to remember: If the specific reason is documented for the breech extraction or cesarean, forceps, or vacuum extractor delivery, that code is assigned rather than the preceding nonspecific codes.

A point to remember: Inexperienced coders often confuse conditions that affect the health of the mother with the conditions that affect the health of the newborn infant. Chapter 11 codes 630–677 are used to describe maternal conditions and are reported only on the mother's record.

Codes from chapter 15, Certain Conditions Originating in the Perinatal Period (760–779), are used to describe the fetus, newborn, or infant's conditions. The perinatal period is generally accepted as the first 28 days of life. Codes 760–763, Maternal causes of perinatal morbidity and mortality, are reported on the infant's record only when a maternal condition affects the infant's health and treatment. Codes 764–779 reflect other conditions that originate in the infant's perinatal period. These describe conditions that the infant may acquire before birth, at birth, or within the 28 days after birth.

Review Exercise: Chapter 14

Assign ICD-9-CM diagnosis, V, and procedure codes (if applicable) to the following:

1. Intrauterine death at 21 weeks' gestation, undelivered

    632

2. Spontaneous vaginal cephalic delivery of full-term live infant twins

    651.01   V27.2

3. Obstructed labor due to a large baby, single liveborn male; classic cesarean delivery

    660.81   653.51   V27.0   74.0

4. Normal pregnancy with spontaneous delivery; first-degree perineal laceration with repair; single liveborn

    650, 664.01   71.71   V27.0

5. Pregnancy, 26 weeks' gestation, with known Down's syndrome of the fetus; patient admitted for further management and evaluation, undelivered

    655.13, 758.0

6. 25-week pregnancy with urinary tract infection secondary to E. coli; patient went home undelivered

    041.4   646.63

7. Blighted ovum

    631

8. Tubal pregnancy (with no mention of concurrent intrauterine pregnancy); unilateral salpingectomy with removal of tubal pregnancy

    633.10, 66.62, 65.31, 65.39

9. Term pregnancy with placenta previa and hemorrhage; single liveborn male; repeat low cervical cesarean section

    641.11, V27.0, 74.1

10. Threatened abortion with hemorrhage at 15 weeks; home undelivered

    640.03

11. Term pregnancy with failure of cervical dilation; lower uterine segment cesarean delivery with single liveborn female

    661.11   V27.0, 74.1

12. 25-week pregnancy with internal hemorrhoids; home undelivered

    648.91   455.0   V22.0

13. Term pregnancy with cephalic presentation and normal spontaneous vaginal delivery of single liveborn

    650   V27.0

(Continued on next page)

Review Exercise: Chapter 14 (Continued)

14. 30-week pregnancy with uncontrolled type I diabetes mellitus; home undelivered

    648.03

15. Postpartum deep thrombophlebitis, developing three weeks following delivery

    671.44, 677

16. Admission for sterilization with multiparity; tubal ligation with Falope ring

    V25.2   66.39

17. Term pregnancy with postpartum pyrexia; single liveborn male; normal spontaneous vaginal delivery with low midline episiotomy with repair

    672.04, V27.0, 73.6

18. Low forceps delivery with episiotomy of term pregnancy; single liveborn female

    650   72.1, V27.0

19. Elective abortion (complete) complicated by excessive hemorrhage with acute blood loss anemia; elective abortion via dilation and curettage

    635.12   285.1   69.01

20. 35-week pregnancy with fetal distress; classical cesarean section with delivery of single stillborn

    656.81   74.0   V27.1

Chapter 15

Diseases of the Skin and Subcutaneous Tissue

Chapter 12, Diseases of the Skin and Subcutaneous Tissue (680–709)

Chapter 12, Diseases of the Skin and Subcutaneous Tissue, in the Tabular List in volume 1 of ICD-9-CM includes conditions such as dermatitis, cellulitis, ulcers of the skin and subcutaneous tissue, urticaria, and diseases of the nail and hair. Chapter 12 of ICD-9-CM contains the following categories and section titles:

Categories	Section Titles
680–686	Infections of Skin and Subcutaneous Tissue
690–698	Other Inflammatory Conditions of Skin and Subcutaneous Tissue
700–709	Other Diseases of Skin and Subcutaneous Tissue

Cellulitis and Abscess (681 and 682)

Cellulitis is an acute inflammation of a localized area of superficial tissue. Predisposing conditions are open wounds, ulcerations, tinea pedis, and dermatitis, but these conditions need not be present for cellulitis to occur. Physical findings of cellulitis reveal red, hot skin with edema at the site of the infection. The area is tender, and the skin surface has a *peau d'orange* (skin of an orange) appearance with ill-defined borders. Nearby lymph nodes often become inflamed.

A cutaneous or subcutaneous abscess is a localized collection of pus causing fluctuant soft-tissue swelling surrounded by erythema. These abscesses usually follow minor skin trauma, and the organisms isolated are typically bacteria infection indigenous to the skin of the involved area. Abscesses may occur internally in tissues, organs, and confined spaces. An abscess begins as cellulitis.

Cellulitis will clear within a few days with antibiotic treatment. Although drainage of abscesses may occur spontaneously, some abscesses may require incision and drainage, and possibly antibiotic therapy.

ICD-9-CM classifies cellulitis to categories 681 and 682. Category 681, Cellulitis and abscess of finger and toe, is subdivided to fourth-digit subcategories that identify the site. Category 682, Other cellulitis and abscess, also is subdivided to identify the site. An additional code should be assigned to identify the organism involved.

EXAMPLE: Cellulitis of the upper arm due to streptococcus: 682.3, Other cellulitis and abscess of upper arm and forearm; 041.00, Streptococcus infection in conditions classified elsewhere and of unspecified site

Dermatitis (690–694)

Dermatitis is an inflammation of the skin. ICD-9-CM classifies contact dermatitis, which is caused by a reaction to substances, to category 692. Fourth-digit subcategories include specific substances such as detergents, solvents, oils and greases, drugs and medicines in contact with the skin, other chemical products, foods, and plants.

EXAMPLE: Contact dermatitis due to detergents: 692.0, Contact dermatitis and other eczema due to detergents

Sunburn and other ultraviolet burns in ICD-9-CM are included in a dermatitis category. Sunburn and tanning bed burns can be equal in severity to second- and third-degree burns. In keeping with the intent of the ICD to separate sunburn from other burns, fifth-digit codes were added in 2001 to subcategory 692.7, Contact dermatitis and other eczema, due to solar radiation. The codes are 692.71, which includes sunburn, first-degree sunburn, and sunburn NOS; 692.76, Sunburn of second degree; and 692.77, Sunburn of third degree.

Another code, 692.82, was revised to describe dermatitis due to other (ultraviolet) radiation, such as from a tanning bed.

ICD-9-CM classifies dermatitis due to substances taken internally to category 693.

Decubitus Ulcer (707.00–707.09)

Decubitus ulcers are caused by tissue hypoxia secondary to pressure-induced vascular insufficiency, and they may become secondarily infected with components of the skin and gastrointestinal flora. The ulceration of tissue usually is at the location of a bony prominence that has been subjected to prolonged pressure against an external object, such as a bed, wheelchair, cast, or splint. Tissues over the elbows, sacrum, ischia, greater trochanters of the hip, external malleoli of the ankle, and heels are most susceptible. Other sites may be involved depending on the patient's positions. Patients may have more than one decubitus, located at different sites on the body. Decubitus ulcers may extend into deeper tissue including muscle and bone. The ulcers may also be referred to as pressure ulcers, pressure sores, or bedsores. Clinically, decubitus ulcers may be graded as to the severity of the condition and referred to by *stage* (1 through 4), but ICD-9-CM does not allow for separate classification of the ulcer by the different stages. ICD-9-CM contains codes at the fifth-digit level for the more common body sites where decubitus ulcers may occur.

Chronic Ulcer of Skin, Lower Limbs (707.1)

A patient may have a chronic ulcer of the skin of the lower limbs as a sole problem or the ulcer may be the result of another condition. Codes 707.10 through 707.19 may be used alone when there is no known underlying condition or cause. However, when the causal condition is known, that condition should be coded first with an additional code from the 707.1 subcategory. Common underlying causes may be diabetes, atherosclerosis, chronic venous hypertension, and postphlebetic syndrome.

Exercise 15.1

Assign ICD-9-CM codes to the following:

1. Diaper rash

   691.0

2. Acne vulgaris

   706.1

3. Postinfectional skin cicatrix

   709.2

4. Cellulitis of the foot; cellulitis due to streptococcus infection

   682.7   041.00

5. Infected ingrowing nail

   703.0

6. Pilonidal cyst with abscess; incision and drainage

   685.0   86.03

7. Allergic urticaria

   708.0

8. Circumscribed scleroderma

9. Erythema multiforme

10. Acute lymphadenitis due to staphylococcal infection

11. Dermatitis due to animal dander

12. Dermatitis attributed to eating strawberries

Operations on the Integumentary System (Breast, Skin, and Subcutaneous Tissue)

Chapter 15 in the Tabular List in volume 3 of ICD-9-CM includes codes for the following procedures:

- 85, Operations on the breast
- 86, Operations on skin and subcutaneous tissue

Operations on the Breast

Procedures such as mastectomy, mammoplasty, and insertion of breast tissue expanders and breast implants are subdivisions of category 85. Diagnostic procedures such as biopsies of the breast are also subdivisions of category 85.

Code 85.0, Mastotomy, is used for incision and drainage of a breast abscess. A mastotomy is also performed for the insertion of a Mammosite catheter after a lumpectomy has been performed for carcinoma of the breast. If the catheter is inserted during a session when the radiation seeds were not implanted at the same time, code 85.0 is used for the catheter placement. If the catheter is placed and radioactive seeds are delivered through the catheter for internal radiation to tissue near the lumpectomy site during the same session, only code 92.27, Implantation or insertion of radioactive elements, is assigned. This code assignment includes all the components of the procedure. Subcategory 85.1 includes diagnostic procedures performed on the breast, such as closed [percutaneous] [needle] biopsy (85.11) or an open biopsy of the breast (85.12).

A lumpectomy of the breast, performed for a benign or malignant breast mass, can be one of three possible procedures. Code 85.21, Local excision of lesion of breast, is the most likely procedure and is the code assignment when the term *lumpectomy* is referenced in the Alphabetic Index to Procedures, volume 3. If physicians perform a more extensive procedure to remove a breast lump, documentation may reveal that a resection of a breast quadrant (85.22) or a partial mastectomy (85.23) was performed. Careful reading of the operative description is recommended.

Code 85.3, Reduction mammoplasty, and subcutaneous mammectomy codes are subdivided to identify the types of procedures performed for breast reductions.

Code 85.4, Mastectomy, is subdivided to identify the extent of the procedure and the side(s) involved (unilateral or bilateral).

Code 85.5, Augmentation mammoplasty, includes unilateral and bilateral breast enlargements, including injection of saline into breast tissue expanders.

A variety of breast reconstruction surgeries are described with a wide range of codes from 85.6, Total breast reconstruction, to other repair and plastic operations on the breast identified by codes 85.81 through 85.99.

Operations on Skin and Subcutaneous Tissue

Category 86, Operations on skin and subcutaneous tissue, includes subdivisions with procedures such as insertion of infusion pumps and totally implantable vascular access devices, excision of skin, and subcutaneous lesions and skin grafting.

Debridement

Debridement is the removal of foreign material and contaminated or devitalized tissue from, or adjacent to, a traumatic or infected lesion until the surrounding healthy tissue is exposed. ICD-9-CM classifies debridement to the following two codes: 86.22, Excisional debridement of wound, infection, or burn; and 86.28, Nonexcisional debridement of wound, infection, or burn.

The following guidelines apply to coding debridement:

- For coding purposes, excisional debridement, code 86.22, is assigned when it is performed by any healthcare provider. Prior to advice given in the Second Quarter 2000 *Coding Clinic* newsletter, this code had been reserved for physician use only. Today, it can be used by other healthcare providers, such as nurses, therapists, or physician assistants who perform excisional debridement. Excisional debridement is the surgical removal, or cutting away, of necrotic tissue or slough, usually performed with a scalpel. Excisional debridement can be performed in the operating room, the emergency department, or at bedside, depending on the extent of the area to be debrided.

- For coding purposes, nonexcisional debridement performed by a physician or nonphysician healthcare professional is assigned code 86.28. Nonexcisional debridement can include the use of forceps (tweezers), scissors, hydrogen peroxide, wet dressings of water, or whirlpool baths. Nonexcisional debridement often includes the clipping away of loose necrotic tissue fragments.

The term *sharp debridement* may be found in documentation of wound debridements performed by physical therapists. The use of a sharp instrument does not always mean it is an excisional debridement. Generally debridement performed by a physical therapist is nonexcisional debridement, code 86.28. Only if the documentation describes the sharp debridement as a definite cutting away of tissue, such as cutting outside and beyond the wound margin, should this be coded with 86.22. This code does not include the minor removal of loose fragments with scissors or scraping away tissue with a sharp instrument, as both of these procedures would be coded to 86.28. Pulsed or pulsatile lavage, mechanical lavage, mechanical irrigation, or high-pressure irrigation are also examples of nonexcisional debridement.

Review Exercise: Chapter 15

Assign ICD-9-CM diagnosis and procedure codes to the following:

1. Decubitus ulcer of sacrum with excisional debridement by the physician in the operating room

   707.3   86.22

2. Blue nevus of foot; excision of nevus, foot

   216.7   86.3

3. Dermatitis due to detergent

   692.0

4. Chronic ulcer of left ankle; full-thickness skin graft, left lower leg

   707.13   86.63

5. History of breast cancer; status post mastectomy, right breast; insertion of unilateral breast implant

   V10.3   V51

6. Adenocarcinoma of right breast, lower inner quadrant; quadrant resection of breast, lower inner quadrant

   174.3   85.22

7. Benign breast cyst, left; percutaneous needle breast biopsy

   610.0   85.11

8. Idiopathic urticaria

   708.1

9. Hypertensive kidney disease with chronic kidney disease, stage V; insertion of totally implantable vascular access device

   403.91   585.5   86.07

10. Cellulitis of the upper arm with nonexcisional debridement performed by the physical therapist

    682.3   86.28

Chapter 16

Diseases of the Musculoskeletal System and Connective Tissue

Chapter 13, Diseases of the Musculoskeletal System and Connective Tissue (710–739)

Chapter 13, Diseases of the Musculoskeletal System and Connective Tissue, in the Tabular List in volume 1 of ICD-9-CM is divided into the following categories and section titles:

Categories	Section Titles
710–719	Arthropathies and Related Disorders
720–724	Dorsopathies
725–729	Rheumatism, Excluding the Back
730–739	Osteopathies, Chondropathies, and Acquired Musculoskeletal Deformities

Fifth-Digit Subclassification

At the beginning of chapter 13, information on using the fifth-digit subclassification with the following categories is given: 711–712, 715–716, 718–719, and 730. The fifth-digit subclassification is repeated at the beginning of each of those series of codes.

Systemic Lupus Erythematosus

Systemic lupus erythematosus (SLE) is a chronic generalized connective tissue disorder ranging from mild to fulminating and marked by skin eruptions, arthralgia, fever, leukopenia, visceral lesions, and other constitutional symptoms, as well as many autoimmune phenomena, including hypergammaglobulinemia with the presence of antinuclear antibodies and LE cells.

ICD-9-CM classifies SLE to code 710.0. At the beginning of this code, a note advises use of an additional code to identify manifestations such as nephritis or endocarditis. In addition, at the beginning of category 710, Diffuse diseases of connective tissue, a note advises use of an additional code if there is lung involvement or the presence of myopathy.

Arthritis

ICD-9-CM classifies arthritic conditions to categories 711 through 716. It should be noted that many codes in these categories are set in italic type to indicate that they are not intended to be the first-listed code.

Rheumatoid Arthritis

Rheumatoid arthritis, a chronic, crippling condition, affects the joints of the hands, wrists, elbows, feet, and ankles. Periods of remission and exacerbation occur in afflicted patients. Although the exact etiology is unknown, immunologic changes and tissue hypersensitivity, complicated by a cold and damp climate, may have a contributory effect. The synovial membranes are primarily affected. The joints become inflamed, swollen, and painful, as well as stiff and tender. A characteristic sign of rheumatoid arthritis is the formation of nodules over body surfaces. During an active period of rheumatoid arthritis, the patient suffers from malaise, fever, and sweating.

ICD-9-CM classifies rheumatoid arthritis to category 714. Again, a note advises coders to use additional codes to identify any manifestations, such as myopathy and polyneuropathy. Rheumatoid arthritis that affects children is coded to subcategory 714.3, Juvenile chronic polyarthritis.

Dorsopathies (720–724)

The section "Dorsopathies" (720–724) contains codes describing intervertebral disc disorders and spondylosis, in addition to other back disorders. It should be noted that categories 721 (spondylosis and allied disorders) and 722 (intervertebral disc disorders) have fourth-digit subcategories that designate the presence or absence of myelopathy, which refers to a functional disorder of the spinal cord.

Osteopathies, Chondropathies, and Acquired Musculoskeletal Deformities (730–739)

The section "Osteopathies, Chondropathies, and Acquired Musculoskeletal Deformities" (730–739) includes codes describing osteomyelitis, bone cysts, malunion and nonunion of fractures, pathological fractures, acquired deformities of the limbs, and curvature of the spine.

Osteomyelitis

Category 730, Osteomyelitis, periostitis, and other infections involving bone, is further subdivided to fourth-digit subcategories that describe acute or chronic osteomyelitis, as well as osteopathy or bone infections resulting from other diseases such as poliomyelitis. The fifth-digit subclassification identifies the site involved. An additional code should be assigned that describes the organism involved.

Pathologic Fractures

Pathologic fractures are classified to subcategory 733.1, with the fifth-digit subclassification identifying the specific site. These types of fractures occur in existing diseases such as osteoporosis or bone metastasis, both of which are capable of weakening the bone. Often pathologic fractures are spontaneous in nature; however, minor injuries can result in a fracture because the bone is already weakened. Stress fractures (733.93–733.95) are excluded from the codes for pathologic fracture.

Malunion and Nonunion Fractures

Malunion of a fracture (733.81) refers to a fracture that was reduced, but the bone ends did not align properly during the healing process. Malunions are often diagnosed during the healing stages and require surgical intervention.

Nonunion of a fracture (733.82) is the failure of the bone ends to align or heal. This usually requires a reopening of the fracture site, with some type of internal fixation and bone grafting performed. Nonunion fractures are often more difficult to treat than malunions. An additional diagnosis code for late effect of fracture (905.0–905.5) is also assigned.

Stress Fractures

Bones may develop "fatigue" or stress fractures from repetitive forces applied before the bone and its supporting structures have time to accommodate such force. When a stress fracture is first suspected, x-rays are often negative. Days or weeks may pass before the fracture line is visible. However, a presumptive diagnosis is necessary to begin prompt treatment. The term *stress reaction* is synonymous with stress fracture.

Previously, ICD-9-CM grouped pathologic and stress fractures together. As of October 2001, three new codes were created for stress fractures or stress reaction of the tibia and fibula (733.93), metatarsals (733.94), and other bones (733.95).

Arthroscopic Surgery

An arthroscope is a small, tubular instrument containing magnifying lenses, a light source, and a video camera. Very small instruments are used with the arthroscope to perform surgical procedures on a joint, such as repair or removal of tissue or to take a biopsy. Arthroscopic surgery is commonly performed today on most joints, including the knee, shoulder, wrist, and ankle. Arthroscopic surgery is often performed on an outpatient basis, and these procedures cause less damage to the body, minimize pain and scarring, and allow a faster recovery than open joint procedures involving an arthrotomy.

Arthroscopy of a joint is coded with ICD-9-CM volume 3 codes in the range of 80.20–80.29. However, the use of an arthroscope is often the "approach" during a therapeutic or diagnostic joint procedure. When a more definitive procedure is performed through an arthroscope, only the definitive procedure code is assigned. An additional code for the arthroscopy is not needed. For example, if a patient had an arthroscopic arthroplasty of the knee with a chondroplasty and debridement of meniscus performed, only the code 81.47, Other repair of knee, would be assigned. The arthroscopic approach code, 80.26, is not assigned.

Review Exercise: Chapter 16

Assign ICD-9-CM codes to the following:

1. Displacement of thoracic intervertebral disc and laminectomy with excision of disc

    722.11   80.51

2. Primary localized osteoarthrosis of the hip

    715.15

3. Acute juvenile rheumatoid arthritis

    714.31

4. Lumbar spondylosis with myelopathy

    721.42

(Continued on next page)

Review Exercise: Chapter 16 (Continued)

5. Chondromalacia of the patella

   717.7

6. Systemic lupus erythematosus

   710.0

7. Acute osteomyelitis of ankle due to staphylococcus aureus

   730.07   041.11

8. Pathologic fracture of the vertebra due to metastatic carcinoma of the bone from the lung

   733.13   198.5   162.9

9. Acquired talipes equinovarus

   736.71

10. Pyogenic arthritis of hand due to streptococcus Group B

    711.04   041.02

11. Postlaminectomy syndrome of the thoracic region

    722.82

12. Kyphosis due to osteoporosis

    733.00   737.41

13. Left knee internal derangement with old medial meniscal tear; arthroscopy of left knee with partial medial meniscectomy   717.82

    717.9   80.26   80.6

14. Nonpyogenic arthritis of the hip due to staphylococcal infection

    716.95   041.10

15. Ankylosing spondylitis

    720.0

16. Baker's cyst of knee with excision

    727.51   83.39

17. Pathologic fracture of the humerus due to postmenopausal osteoporosis; closed reduction, fracture of humerus

    733.11   733.01   79.01

18. Paget's disease of the bone (no bone tumor noted)

    731.0

19. Aneurysmal bone cyst, left tibia; excision of cyst

    733.22   77.67

20. Slipped upper femoral epiphysis (nontraumatic)

    732.2

1st 2.

7.

1st 2.

Chapter 17

Congenital Anomalies and Certain Conditions Originating in the Perinatal Period

Newborns often suffer from congenital anomalies and certain other conditions that originate in the perinatal period. This chapter addresses the coding of the congenital and perinatal conditions.

When coding the birth of an infant, a code from categories V30–V39 is used according to the type of birth. This code is assigned once only to a newborn as a principal diagnosis at the time of birth. Instructions on the assignment of the V30–V39 series codes can be found in chapter 23 of this text.

Official Newborn Coding Guidelines

The ICD-9-CM Official Guidelines for Coding and Reporting contain directions regarding chapter 14 of ICD-9-CM, Congenital Anomalies, and chapter 15 of ICD-9-CM, Certain Conditions Originating in the Perinatal Period. The guidelines can be found in appendix I of this textbook.

The newborn, or perinatal, period is defined as before birth through the first 28 days after birth. All clinically significant conditions noted on routine newborn examinations should be coded. A condition is significant if it requires one or more of the following:

- Clinical evaluation

- Therapeutic treatment

- Diagnostic procedures

- Extended length of hospital stay

- Increased nursing care and/or monitoring

- Implications for future healthcare needs

The perinatal guidelines are identical to the general coding guidelines for the selection of additional diagnoses, with the exception of the final item—implications for future healthcare needs. Codes should be assigned for conditions that have been specified by the provider as having implications for future healthcare needs. Codes from the perinatal chapter should not be assigned unless the provider has established a definitive diagnosis. The physician determines whether a condition is clinically significant.

Chapter 14, Congenital Anomalies (740–759)

A congenital anomaly is an irregularity or abnormality that is present at, and existing from, the time of birth. Chapter 14 in the Tabular List in volume 1 of ICD-9-CM classifies congenital anomalies. The chapter is organized by body system, beginning with the central nervous system. Because many conditions can be either congenital in origin or acquired, coders must carefully review the subterms in the Alphabetic Index to select the appropriate code to describe congenital conditions.

When a specific abnormality is diagnosed at the time of birth, the congenital anomaly is listed as an additional diagnosis, with the V30–V39 series used to indicate the newborn status. Congenital anomalies may also be the principal or first-listed diagnosis for admissions or encounters subsequent to the newborn admission. Codes for congenital anomalies may be used throughout the life of the patient. For example, a forty-year old patient with Down's syndrome would be assigned code 758.0 at the time of a healthcare visit. If a congenital anomaly has been corrected, a personal history code should be used to identify the history of the anomaly.

Infant Coding Guidelines

When a specific abnormality is diagnosed for an infant, assign an appropriate code from categories 740 through 759, Congenital anomalies. Such abnormalities may occur as a set of symptoms or as multiple malformations. A code should be assigned for each presenting manifestation of the syndrome when the syndrome is not indexed specifically in ICD-9-CM.

> **EXAMPLE:** A child was diagnosed with Sticker's Syndrome. *Coding Clinic* (1999, 3Q, pp. 16–17) advised coders to assign code 756.89 for other specified anomalies of muscle, tendon, fascia, and connective tissue. Each manifestation of the syndrome is coded separately because this syndrome is not specifically indexed in ICD-9-CM. The patient may have myopia (367.1), retinal detachment (361.9), sensorneural hearing loss (389.10), and cleft palate (749.00), among other hereditary eye and joint disorders. Each documented condition would be coded separately in addition to 756.89.

Principal versus Additional Diagnosis

If a congenital anomaly is noted during the hospital admission when the infant was born, the code describing the anomaly is assigned as an additional diagnosis. The principal diagnosis is a code from the section "Liveborn Infants According to Type of Birth" (V30–V39).

> **EXAMPLE:** Liveborn male infant born in the hospital with Tetralogy of Fallot: V30.00, Single liveborn, delivered in hospital without mention of cesarean delivery; 745.2, Tetralogy of Fallot

However, if the patient was transferred on the day of birth to another hospital for care of the congenital anomaly, the principal diagnosis at the second hospital would be the congenital anomaly.

> **EXAMPLE:** Liveborn male infant transferred for care of thoracic spina bifida with hydrocephalus: 741.02, Spina bifida of dorsal [thoracic] region with hydrocephalus

Common Congenital Anomalies

Congenital anomalies, also known as birth defects, have been the leading cause of infant mortality in the United States over the past several years. Birth defects substantially contribute to childhood morbidity and long-term disability. More than 4,500 different birth defects have been identified. Congenital anomalies can affect almost every body system.

There are three major categories of known causes:

- Chromosomal disorders (either hereditary or arising during conception)

- Exposure to an environmental chemical (for example, medications, alcohol, cigarettes, solvents)

- Mother's illness during pregnancy, exposing the infant to viral or bacterial infections

The stage of fetal development at the time of exposure to one of the two latter causes is critical. Fetal development is particularly vulnerable in the first trimester of pregnancy. The life expectancy and quality of life for individuals with many birth defects has improved greatly over the past forty years. This is a result of pioneering surgery that can correct certain defects before the infant is born, as well as neonatal intensive care units that provide specialized care and advanced technology to treat the infant.

Central Nervous System Defects

Central nervous system (CNS) defects involve the brain, spinal cord, and associated tissue. These include neural tube defects (anencephaly, spina bifida, and encephalocele), microcephalus, and hydrocephalus.

One of the more common CNS defects is spina bifida. Spina bifida is a defective closure of the vertebral column. It ranges in severity from the occult type revealing few signs to a completely open spine (rachischisis). In spina bifida cystica, the protruding sac contains meninges (meningocele), the spinal cord (myelocele), or both (myelomeningocele). Commonly seen in the lumbar, low thoracic, or sacral region, spina bifida extends for three to six vertebral segments. When the spinal cord or lumbosacral nerve roots are involved, as is usually the case, varying degrees of paralysis occur below the involved level. This may result in orthopedic conditions such as clubfoot, arthrogryposis, or dislocated hip. The paralysis also usually affects the sphincters of the bladder and rectum. In addition, an excessive accumulation of cerebrospinal fluid within the ventricles, called hydrocephalus, is associated with at least 80 percent of the lumbosacral type of spina bifida.

In ICD-9-CM, most types of spina bifida, excluding spina bifida occulta, are assigned to category 741. This category is further subdivided to fourth-digit subcategories that describe the presence or absence of hydrocephalus. The fifth-digit subclassification describes the site of the spina bifida. Spina bifida occulta (756.17), however, is classified to category 756, Other congenital musculoskeletal anomalies.

If surgical repair is deemed necessary, the opening in the vertebral column is closed. If hydrocephalus exists, a shunt (most often a ventriculo-peritoneal shunt) also may be necessary.

ICD-9-CM classifies repairs of spina bifida to code 03.5, Plastic operations on spinal cord and structures. Code 03.51 is assigned for spinal meningocele; code 03.52, for spinal myelomeningocele; and code 03.59, when the type is unspecified.

Cardiovascular System Defects

Cardiovascular system defects involve the heart and circulatory systems. They are the most common group of birth defects in infants. Surgical procedures repair defects and restore circulation to as normal as possible. Some defects can be repaired before birth, while others may require multiple surgical procedures after birth. Smaller defects may be repaired in a cardiac catheterization laboratory instead of an operating room. Some of the more commonly occurring cardiovascular defects are patent ductus arteriosus, atrial septal defect, ventricular septal defect, and pulmonary artery anomalies.

Descriptions of cardiovascular system defects are as follows:

- Hypoplastic left heart syndrome (746.7) is a condition in which the entire left half of the heart is underdeveloped. This condition may be repaired in a series of three procedures over one year. If not treated, the condition can be fatal within a month.

- Common truncus or persistent truncus arteriosus (PTA) (745.0) is a failure of the fetal truncus arteriosus to divide into the aorta and pulmonary artery. It can be corrected surgically.

- Pulmonary valve atresia (746.01) and stenosis (746.02) is an obstruction or narrowing of the pulmonary heart valve. Mild forms are relatively well tolerated and require no intervention. More severe forms are surgically corrected.

- Tetralogy of Fallot (TOF) (745.2) is a defect characterized by four anatomical abnormalities within the heart that results in poorly oxygenated blood being pumped to the body. It can be corrected surgically.

- Total anomalous pulmonary venous return (TAPVR) (747.41) is a malformation of all of the pulmonary veins. In this condition, the pulmonary veins empty into the right atrium, or a systemic vein, instead of into the left atrium.

- Transposition of great vessels or great arteries (TGV) (745.10–745.19) is a defect in which the positions of the aorta and the pulmonary artery are transposed. Immediate surgical correction is required.

- Tricuspid valve atresia and stenosis (746.1) is the absence or narrowing of the valve between the right atrium and ventricle. Severe cases are surgically corrected.

- Aortic valve stenosis (AS) (746.3) is the narrowing or obstruction of the aortic heart valve. This can be surgically repaired in some cases.

- Atrial septal defect (ASD) (745.5) is a hole in the wall between the upper chambers of the heart (the atriums). The openings may resolve without treatment or require surgical intervention. This condition may also be referred to as patent foramen ovale.

- Coarctation of the aorta (747.10) is a defect in which the aorta is narrowed somewhere along its length. Surgical correction is recommended even for mild defects.

- Endocardial cushion defect is a spectrum of septal defects arising from imperfect fusion of the endocardial cushions in the fetal heart (745.60–745.69). These defects are repaired surgically.

- Patent ductus arteriosus (PDA) is a condition in which the channel between the pulmonary artery and the aorta fails to close at birth (747.0). Many of these close spontaneously and cause no consequences. The condition can also be surgically and medically repaired.

- Ventricular septal defect (VSD) (745.4) is a hole in the lower chambers of the heart, or the ventricles. The openings may resolve without treatment; however, the condition can be surgically corrected. Ebstein anomaly is a deformation or displacement of the tricuspid valve with the septal and posterior leaflets being attached to the wall of the right ventricle. Only severe cases are corrected surgically.

Respiratory System Defects

Respiratory system congenital anomalies, mainly in the lungs, trachea, and nose, are life-threatening, but less common than those involving other major organs. The major defect is lung atresia or hypoplasia—the failure to develop or underdevelopment of one or both lungs (748.5).

Digestive System Defects

Digestive system defects include orofacial defects (e.g., choanal atresia, or cleft palate and lip) and gastrointestinal defects (for example, esophageal atresia, rectal and intestinal atresia and stenosis, and pyloric stenosis).

Cleft Lip and Cleft Palate

Cleft lip, cleft palate, and combinations of the two are the most common congenital anomalies of the head and neck. A cleft is a fissure or elongated opening of a specified site, usually occurring during the embryonic stage. A cleft palate is a split in the roof of the mouth (the palate) and a cleft lip is the presence of one or two splits in the upper lip. Cleft lips and palates are classified as partial or complete, and can occur either bilaterally or unilaterally. The most common clefts are left unilateral complete clefts of the primary and secondary palate, and partial midline clefts of the secondary palate involving the soft palate and part of the hard palate. The incisive foramen serves as the dividing point between the primary and the secondary palate.

In ICD-9-CM, cleft palate and cleft lip are classified to category 749. This category is subdivided to describe cleft palate (749.0), cleft lip (749.1), and a combination of the two (749.2). These subcategories are further subdivided to identify unilateral or bilateral and complete or incomplete cleft palate or cleft lip. Documentation in the record should be reviewed to determine whether the cleft is complete or incomplete (partial). The physician should be queried when the documentation is unclear.

Surgical repair of cleft lips and/or palates is not conducted until after the twelfth week of life. Sometimes secondary revisions are required to correct any tissue deformities or scars. ICD-9-CM assigns code 27.54 for repair of cleft lip, code 27.62 for correction of cleft palate, and code 27.63 for revision of cleft palate repair.

Pyloric Stenosis

Pyloric stenosis is a narrowing of the outlet between the stomach and small intestine. It results from hypertrophy of the circular and longitudinal muscularis of the pylorus and distal antrum of the stomach. Typically, the infant feeds well from birth until two or three weeks after birth, at which time occasional regurgitation of food, or spitting up, occurs, followed several days later by projectile vomiting. Dehydration due to the vomiting is common. Surgery is the treatment of choice. Fredet-Ramstedt pyloromyotomy is performed following management of the dehydration.

ICD-9-CM assigns code 750.5 for pyloric stenosis. Code 43.3 describes the pyloromyotomy.

Genitourinary Tract Defects

Both male and female infants may be afflicted with defects of the reproductive organs and the urinary tract. Some are relatively minor and fairly common defects that can be repaired by surgery. Some of the GU tract defects are as follows:

- Bladder exstrophy (753.5) is a condition in which the bladder is turned inside out with portions of the abdominal and bladder walls missing. This must be surgically repaired.

- Epispadias (752.62) is a relatively rare defect in which the urethra opens on the top surface of the penis and surgical correction is needed.

- Hypospadias (752.61) is a relatively common defect that appears as an abnormal penile opening on the underside of the penis rather than at the end. Surgical correction may be needed for cosmetic, urologic, and reproductive reasons.

- Obstructive genitourinary defect is an obstruction of the ureter, renal pelvis, urethra, or bladder neck (753.20–753.29, 753.6). Severity of the condition depends on the level of the obstruction. Urine accumulates behind the obstruction and produces organ damage. This condition can be corrected surgically while the fetus is in the uterus or after birth.

- Renal atresia or hypoplasia (753.3) is the absence or underdevelopment of the kidneys and may be unilateral or bilateral. Newborns with bilateral renal atresia often expire due to respiratory failure within a few hours of birth. Unilateral renal atresia may not be detected for years.

- Polycystic kidney disease is an inherited disorder characterized by multiple, bilateral, grapelike clusters of fluid-filled cysts that grossly enlarge the kidneys, compressing and eventually replacing functioning renal tissue. The infantile form of this condition reveals an infant with pronounced epicanthal folds, a pointed nose, a small chin, and floppy, low-set ears. Signs of respiratory distress and congestive heart failure also may be present. This condition eventually deteriorates into uremia and renal failure.

ICD-9-CM classifies cystic kidney disease to subcategory 753.1, with the following fifth-digit subclassifications:

753.10   **Cystic kidney disease, unspecified**
753.11   **Congenital single renal cyst**
753.12   **Polycystic kidney, unspecified type**
753.13   **Polycystic kidney, autosomal dominant**
753.14   **Polycystic kidney, autosomal recessive**
753.15   **Renal dysplasia**
753.16   **Medullary cystic kidney**
753.17   **Medullary sponge kidney**
753.19   **Other specified cystic kidney disease**

When there is no further specification as to type of polycystic kidney disease, assign code 753.12. In addition, assign other complications that may be present, such as chronic kidney disease (585.1–585.9).

Musculoskeletal Defects

Musculoskeletal defects are relatively common disorders and range from minor problems to more serious conditions. Clubfoot is the most common musculoskeletal congenital anomaly.

Clubfoot

Clubfoot is a general term that is used to describe a variety of congenital structural foot deformities involving the lower leg, ankle, and foot joints, ligaments, and tendons. Clubfoot deformities include:

- Varus deformities, which are characterized by a turning inward of the feet (codes 754.50–754.59)

- Valgus deformities, which are characterized by a turning outward of the feet (codes 754.60–754.69)

- Talipes cavus, which is recognized by increased arch of the foot (code 754.71)

- Talipes calcaneus or equines, in which the entire foot exhibits an abnormal upward or downward misalignment (code 754.79)

The generic term *clubfoot* is classified as talipes, unspecified (code 754.70).

Chromosomal Defects

Chromosomal abnormalities are disorders that arise from abnormal numbers of chromosomes or from defects in specific fragments of the chromosomes. Each disorder is associated with a characteristic pattern of defects that arises as a consequence of the underlying chromosomal abnormality. Congenital heart defects, especially septal defects, are common among these infants and are a major cause of death. The more common chromosomal conditions include the following:

- Down's syndrome is associated with the presence of a third number 21 chromosome. It results in mental retardation, distinctive malformations of the face and head, and other abnormalities. The severity of these problems varies widely among the affected individuals. Down's syndrome is one of the more frequently occurring chromosomal abnormalities.

- Edward's syndrome is associated with the presence of a third number 18 chromosome. It causes major physical abnormalities and severe mental retardation. Many children with this disorder expire in the first year of life due to the abnormalities of the lungs and diaphragm, heart defects, and blood vessel malformations.

- Patau's syndrome is associated with the presence of a third number 13 chromosome. The infants have many internal and external abnormalities, including profound retardation. Death may occur in the first few days of life due to the respiratory difficulties, heart defects, and severe defects in other organ systems.

Exercise 17.1

Assign ICD-9-CM codes to the following (unless otherwise noted, assume this visit is subsequent to admission for birth):

1. Single liveborn male (born in the hospital via cesarean delivery) with congenital diaphragmatic hernia and repair of diaphragmatic hernia (abdominal approach)

   V30.01 756.6 53.7

2. Single liveborn male (born in the hospital) with polydactyly of fingers

   V30.00 755.01

3. Unilateral cleft lip and palate; repair of cleft lip

   749.22 27.54

4. Patent ductus arteriosus with repair

   747.0 38.85

5. Congenital talipes equinovalgus; Down's syndrome

6. Congenital hydrocephalus with insertion of ventriculo-peritoneal shunt

7. Hypoplasia of lung

8. Small omphalocele with repair

9. Childhood-type polycystic kidney

10. Thyroglossal duct cyst with excision

Chapter 15, Certain Conditions Originating in the Perinatal Period (760–779)

Chapter 15, Certain Conditions Originating in the Perinatal Period, in the Tabular List in volume 1 of ICD-9-CM includes the following categories and section titles:

Categories	Section Titles
760–763	Maternal Causes of Perinatal Morbidity and Mortality
764–779	Other Conditions Originating in the Perinatal Period

The perinatal period is defined as beginning before birth and lasting through twenty-eight days after birth.

Inclusion Notation

The following includes note appears at the beginning of chapter 15:

---

15. CERTAIN CONDITIONS ORIGINATING IN THE PERINATAL PERIOD (760–779)

Includes: conditions that have their origin in the perinatal period, before birth through the first 28 days after birth, even though death or morbidity occurs later

---

Although the perinatal period lasts through twenty-eight days following birth, the codes within chapter 15 may be assigned beyond that period when the condition still exists. However, the condition must have its origin in the perinatal period, even though it could continue to affect the patient beyond that time.

> **EXAMPLE:** Six-month-old was admitted to the hospital with acute respiratory failure due to bronchopulmonary dysplasia: 518.81, Acute respiratory failure; 770.7, Chronic respiratory disease arising in the perinatal period

In the above example, the patient developed bronchopulmonary dysplasia (BPD) during the perinatal period while receiving prolonged and high concentrations of inspired O_2. Although this patient is no longer in the perinatal period, the BPD is still present and, as such, should be coded. BPD occurs commonly in infants who had respiratory distress syndrome at birth, as well as those who have required endotracheal intubation and a respirator for many days.

Coding Guidelines

The following subsections offer guidelines that may be used when coding certain conditions originating in the perinatal period.

Categories 760–763

Codes from categories 760 through 763, Maternal causes of perinatal morbidity and mortality, are assigned only when the maternal condition has actually affected the fetus or newborn. The fact that the mother has an associated medical condition or experiences some complication of pregnancy, labor, or delivery does not justify the routine assignment of codes from these categories to the newborn's record.

A number of substances are known to have effects on the development of the fetus when the mother is exposed to the substance during pregnancy. Subcategory 760.7, Noxious influences affecting fetus or newborn via placenta or breast milk, identifies through the use of the fifth digit the substance found to have harmed the fetus or newborn. Some of the substances are legal and illegal drugs, such as narcotics and cocaine, but others include anti-infectives, anticonvulsants, and antimetabolic agents that must be continued through the pregnancy.

> **EXAMPLE:** Liveborn infant born (in hospital) with fetal alcohol syndrome to an alcohol-dependent mother: V30.00, Single liveborn, delivered in hospital without mention of cesarean delivery; 760.71, Alcohol affecting fetus via placenta or breast milk

> **EXAMPLE:** Delivery of a normal and healthy infant (in hospital) to a mother who occasionally uses cocaine: V30.00, Single liveborn, delivered in hospital without mention of cesarean delivery

In the first example, the use of alcohol by the mother was manifested in the infant; therefore, a code for fetal alcohol syndrome was assigned.

In the second example, however, the infant was healthy and normal despite the mother's occasional use of cocaine; therefore, the code to describe noxious influences of cocaine affecting the fetus (760.75) was not assigned.

Categories 764–765

Categories 764 and 765 are classified in the section "Other Conditions Originating in the Perinatal Period." Category 764 classifies slow fetal growth and fetal malnutrition. Category 765 classifies disorders related to short gestation and low birth weight.

Most physicians indicate a newborn's weight in grams. However, weight may also be recorded in pounds and ounces. One pound equals approximately 454 grams. A two-pound infant weighs about 907 grams, a five-pound infant weighs about 2,268 grams, and a ten-pound infant weighs about 4,536 grams. The ICD-9-CM system classifies an infant's weight in grams.

At the beginning of this section, the following fifth-digit subclassification that applies to categories 764, 765.0, and 765.1 is introduced:

0   unspecified [weight]
1   less than 500 grams
2   500–749 grams
3   750–999 grams
4   1,000–1,249 grams
5   1,250–1,499 grams
6   1,500–1,749 grams
7   1,750–1,999 grams
8   2,000–2,499 grams
9   2,500 grams and over

These fifth digits are used to identify the weight of the infant at birth, not the weight at subsequent visits.

The birth weight fifth digits are limited for use to category 764 and to codes 765.0, Extreme prematurity, and 765.1, Other preterm infants. The inclusion terms for these codes describe only birth weight with no reference to gestational age.

For the premature infant, the weeks of gestation are also valuable information. With codes from category 764 and subcategories 765.0 and 765.1, a code from subcategory code 765.2 is to be used as an additional code to specify weeks of gestation as documented by the physician. More than one code in the 765 category should be used to describe the preterm infant; that is, one to describe the birth weight, and a second code to indicate the completed weeks of gestation. Weeks of gestation may allow the physician to predict the probability of developmental problems later.

Codes from category 764 and subcategories 765.0 and 765.1 should not be assigned based solely on recorded birth weight or estimated gestational age, but on the attending physician's assessment of maturity of the infant. Because physicians may use different criteria in determining prematurity, the coder should not record a diagnosis of prematurity unless the physician documents this condition.

Meconium Staining

Meconium is a newborn's first stool, consisting of a combination of swallowed amniotic fluid and mucus from the baby.

The passage of meconium before birth is an indication of fetal distress. It is seen in infants small for gestational age, post dates, or those with cord complications or other factors compromising placental circulation. Meconium aspiration is defined as the presence of meconium below the vocal cords and occurs in up to 35 percent of live births with meconium staining. Meconium aspiration syndrome occurs in about 4 percent of deliveries complicated by meconium-stained fluid. Meconium aspiration syndrome occurs when meconium from amniotic fluid in the upper airway is inhaled into the lungs by the newborn with his or her first breath. This invokes an inflammatory reaction in the lungs, which can be fatal. Meconium staining is not meconium aspiration. Meconium aspiration is not meconium aspiration syndrome. ICD-9-CM provides distinct codes for the different conditions involving meconium:

763.84   Meconium passage during delivery
770.11   Meconium aspiration without respiratory symptoms
770.12   Meconium aspiration with respiratory symptoms
779.84   Meconium staining

Respiratory Problems in Infants after Birth

Conditions classified to subcategory 770.8, Other respiratory problems after birth, are frequently present in infants. Subcategory 770.8, along with its fifth digits, includes different newborn respiratory conditions that vary in type and severity. Many infants suffer from more than one condition listed under 770.8, for example, code 770.84, Respiratory failure of newborn, which may exist with other respiratory problems. Subcategory 770.8 does not include conditions related to lack of oxygen at birth, which are properly indexed to codes within subcategory 768, Intrauterine hypoxia and birth asphyxia.

Code 770.6, Transient tachypnea of newborn (TNN), is a different, more serious respiratory condition that occurs in infants.

Infections

ICD-9-CM classifies perinatal infections to category 771, Infections specific to the perinatal period. Although the perinatal period extends through the twenty-eighth day of life, the following inclusion note appears at the beginning of category 771:

Includes: infections acquired before or during birth
          or via the umbilicus

Therefore, an infant who develops a urinary tract infection at the age of twenty days would be assigned code 771.82, Urinary tract infection of newborn. Newborn, neonatal, and perinatal refer to the time period of birth through twenty-eight days of life. If the infection is acquired within the first twenty-eight days of life, the perinatal code is used.

Subcategory 771.8, Other infections specific to the perinatal period, is another series of codes used frequently with newborns. It includes infections ranging from urinary tract infection to septicemia. Unique codes exist for septicemia or sepsis of newborn (771.81) and bacteremia of newborn (771.83.) There is direction under 771.8 to "use additional code to identify organism" (041).

Neonatal Cardiac Dysrhythmia

Infants may have either brachycardia or tachycardia after birth that is unrelated to the stress of labor or delivery or other intrauterine complications. These symptoms are almost always a symptom of an underlying condition, but the cause may not be immediately known. Neonatal bradycardia is coded to 779.81, and neonatal tachycardia is coded to 779.82.

Review Exercise: Chapter 17

Assign ICD-9-CM codes to the following (assume this visit is subsequent to the admission for birth, unless otherwise noted, and in the perinatal period):

1. Live newborn (born in hospital) with fetal distress with onset before labor

   _V30.00   768.2_

2. Erythroblastosis fetalis

   _773.2_

3. Hyperbilirubinemia of prematurity; prematurity (birth weight of 2,000 gm with 35 completed weeks of gestation); phototherapy

   _774.2   765.18   765.28   99.83_

4. Erb's palsy

   _767.6_

5. Hypoglycemia in infant with diabetic mother

   _775.0_

6. Necrotizing enterocolitis discovered in a newborn at birth

   _777.5_

7. Premature "crack" baby born in hospital to a mother dependent on cocaine; birth weight of 1,247 gm, 32 completed weeks of gestation

   _765.14 760.75   765.26_

8. Newborn readmitted on day 10 of life with pneumonia

   _770.89   779.89   486_

9. Newborn transferred to University Hospital for treatment of septicemia of newborn

   _771.81_

10. Disseminated intravascular coagulation in a 15-day-old infant

    _776.2_

11. Single newborn delivered via cesarean section; large for gestational age (mother is diabetic)

    _V30.01   766.0   760.+   775.0_

12. Transferred from hospital A to hospital B with spina bifida involving the dorsal region with hydrocephalus; repair of myelomeningocele with insertion of ventriculoperitoneal shunt (assign codes for hospital B)

    _741.02   03.52   02.34_

13. Newborn (born in hospital) via normal spontaneous vaginal delivery with respiratory failure of newborn; 50 hours of mechanical ventilation with endotracheal intubation

    _V30.00   770.84   96.71_

14. Newborn transferred to hospital B with Tetralogy of Fallot; Blalock-Taussig procedure with cardiopulmonary bypass (assign codes for hospital B)

    _745.2   39.0   39.61_

15. Newborn male, born in hospital, via repeat cesarean section with hypospadias

    _V30.01   752.61_

Chapter 18

Symptoms, Signs, and Ill-Defined Conditions

Chapter 16, Symptoms, Signs, and Ill-Defined Conditions (780–799)

Chapter 16, Symptoms, Signs, and Ill-Defined Conditions, in the Tabular List in volume 1 of ICD-9-CM contains the following categories and section titles:

Categories	Section Titles
780–789	Symptoms
790–796	Nonspecific Abnormal Findings
797–799	Ill-Defined and Unknown Causes of Morbidity and Mortality

Definitions

A sign is objective evidence of a disease observed by the physician. A symptom is any subjective evidence of disease reported by the patient to the physician.

Some symptoms, such as hives (708.9), gastrointestinal hemorrhage (578.9), menstrual pain (625.3), and dehydration (276.51), have been classified elsewhere in ICD-9-CM. Such symptoms are associated with a given organ system and thus are assigned to the chapter in ICD-9-CM that deals with the corresponding organ system.

Other symptoms are associated with many systems or are of unknown cause; they are classified to chapter 16. Examples of these types of symptoms include coma, convulsions, fever, jaundice, chest pain, cough, nausea, vomiting, respiratory arrest, and anorexia.

When to Use a Code from Chapter 16

Carefully read the long note that appears at the beginning of chapter 16. It outlines the uses of codes included in this chapter. The conditions, signs, and symptoms included in categories 780 through 796 consist of:

- Cases for which no more specific diagnosis can be made even after all facts bearing on them have been investigated

- Signs or symptoms existing at the time of initial encounter that proved to be transient and whose causes could not be determined

- Provisional diagnosis in a patient who failed to return for further investigation or care

- Cases referred elsewhere for investigation or treatment before the diagnosis was made

- Cases in which a more precise diagnosis was not available for any other reason

- Certain symptoms that represent important problems in medical care and might be classified in addition to a known cause

- A symptom that was treated in an outpatient setting and did not have the workup necessary to determine a definitive diagnosis

Symptoms (780–789)

The first section of chapter 16 includes a variety of symptoms. In some cases, symptoms may be assigned as additional diagnoses. The following guidelines should be of assistance in determining when to assign a symptom as an additional diagnosis:

- **Conditions that are an integral part of a disease process:** Signs and symptoms that are integral to the disease process should not be assigned as additional codes.

  > EXAMPLE: Nausea and vomiting with gastroenteritis: 558.9, Other and unspecified noninfectious gastroenteritis and colitis
  >
  > Only the code for gastroenteritis (558.9) is assigned. The code for nausea and vomiting (787.01) is not assigned because these are symptoms of gastroenteritis.

- **Conditions that are not an integral part of a disease process:** Additional signs and symptoms that may not be routinely associated with a disease process should be coded when present.

  > EXAMPLE: Patient with metastases to brain admitted in comatose state: 198.3, Secondary malignant neoplasm of brain and spinal cord; 780.01, Coma

  The code for coma (780.01) should be added as an additional diagnosis; coma is a significant condition that is not routinely associated with brain metastases.

Symptoms and signs are used frequently to describe reasons for service in outpatient settings. Outpatient visits do not always allow for the type of study that is needed to determine a diagnosis. Often the purpose of the outpatient visit is to relieve the symptom rather than to determine or treat the underlying condition. Coders must code the outpatient's condition to the highest level of certainty. The highest level of certainty is often an abnormal sign or symptom code that is assigned as the reason for the outpatient visit.

Most subcategories in the "Symptoms (780–789)" section are grouped by body systems, such as category 781, Symptoms involving nervous and musculoskeletal systems, and category 785, Symptoms involving cardiovascular system.

Category 780, however, classifies general symptoms that are not related to one specific body system. Subcategory 780.9 has been further divided to include code 780.91, Fussy infant (baby), and codes 780.92, Excessive crying of infant (baby), 780.93, Memory loss, 780.94,

Early satiety, and 780.95, Other excessive crying (for child, adolescent, or adult.) Code 780.99, Other general symptoms, describes conditions for which no specific cause can be determined.

Nonspecific Abnormal Findings (790–796)

Categories 790–796 contain codes for nonspecific abnormal findings from laboratory, x-ray, pathologic, and other diagnostic tests. The following guidelines apply when coding nonspecific abnormal findings in the inpatient setting:

- Abnormal findings from laboratory, x-ray, pathologic, and other diagnostic results are not coded and reported unless the physician indicates their clinical significance. If the findings are outside the normal range and the physician has ordered other tests to evaluate the condition or has prescribed treatment, it is appropriate to ask the physician whether the diagnosis code(s) for the abnormal findings should be added.

- Exclusion notes in this section direct coders to search elsewhere in ICD-9-CM when documentation in the health record states the presence of a specific condition. Codes for these specific conditions are located in the Alphabetic Index under the main term "Findings, abnormal, without diagnosis."

Often abnormal findings are the reason for additional testing to be performed on patients in the outpatient setting. For example, elevated prostate specific antigen (PSA) (code 790.93) may be a reason for continued testing or monitoring of a patient. The code does not provide a specific diagnosis, but indicates an abnormal finding for a specific organ. Abnormal findings recorded in the record may or may not be appropriate to code. If the coder notes an abnormal laboratory finding that appears to have triggered additional testing or therapy, the coder should ask the physician whether the abnormal finding is a clinically significant condition.

On other occasions, the coder will notice abnormal findings on radiological studies that may well be incidental to the patient's current condition. For example, an elderly patient with congestive heart failure is given a chest x-ray. A finding of degenerative arthritis is noted in the radiologist's conclusion, but no apparent treatment or further evaluation has occurred. It is unlikely that the arthritis should be coded.

The radiologist's findings can be used to identify the specific site of a fracture when the physician's diagnosis statement is nonspecific. For example, the attending physician writes "Fracture, left tibia." However, the radiologist describes the injury as a fracture of the shaft of the tibia. The coder may code 823.20, Fracture, tibia, shaft, based on the specific findings of the radiologist (*Coding Clinic* 1999).

The radiologist's findings may also be used to clarify an outpatient's diagnosis or reason for services. For example, a patient comes to the hospital for an outpatient x-ray. The physician's order for the x-ray is "possible kidney stones." The radiologist's statement on the radiology report is "bilateral nephrolithiasis." Based on the fact that the radiologist is a physician, it is appropriate to code the calculus of the kidney, 592.0, as the patient's diagnosis (*Coding Clinic* 2000).

Coding of Pap Smears

The coding of Pap smears often involves the coding of nonspecific abnormal findings. Because the classification of abnormal Pap smears has become more specific in recent years, ICD-9-CM now includes more code options under subcategory 795.0.

The Bethesda System of Cytologic Examination is used by 90 percent of the laboratories in the United States and has been endorsed by national and international societies as the preferred method of reporting the results of abnormal Papanicolaou (Pap) smears. The Bethesda System was first published in 1989, then revised in 1991 and again in 2001. The ICD-9-CM classification has been updated to reflect the 2001 version, including revising code titles and inclusion terms, as well as adding new codes. In the most recent revision of ICD-9-CM, several codes that were formerly classified as a dysplasia of the cervix (622.1) have been reclassified to codes 795.03 and 795.04 as Pap smear of cervix with low-grade squamous intraepithelial lesion and with high-grade squamous intraepithelial lesion. Other new codes describe a Pap smear with cervical high-risk human papillomavirus (HPV) DNA test positive (795.05) and with cervical low-risk human papillomavirus (HPV) DNA test positive (795.09). Another new code describes an unsatisfactory smear or an inadequate sample (795.08).

The excludes note for subcategory 795.0 refers the coder to other subcategories for confirmed dysplasia or carcinoma in situ conditions.

Coding of Anthrax Exposure

Another category of nonspecific abnormal findings has emerged as a result of possible bioterrorist activities and the existence of confirmed cases of anthrax. Different degrees of exposure to anthrax may be coded as follows:

- Code 795.31 is used for the asymptomatic patient who tests positive for anthrax by nasal swab.

- Code V01.81 would be used when the individual has been actually exposed to anthrax or has come in contact with anthrax spores but has not tested positive.

- Code V71.82 is used for the individual who seeks medical evaluation with concerns about anthrax exposure but is found not to have been exposed.

Chapter 21 of this book includes a listing of E codes approved by the National Center for Health Statistics to classify, report, and analyze injuries, sequelae of injuries, and deaths associated with different kinds of terrorist events.

Codes for nonspecific abnormal test results or findings may be found under the Alphabetic Index entries of "abnormal, abnormality, abnormalities," "findings, abnormal, without diagnosis," "elevation," or "positive."

Ill-Defined and Unknown Causes of Morbidity and Mortality (797–799)

The "Ill-Defined and Unknown Causes of Morbidity and Mortality" section of chapter 16 includes conditions for which further specification is not provided in the health record or for which the underlying cause is unknown. These codes should not be used when a more definitive diagnosis is available.

Asphyxia once meant the stopping of the pulse, but the term has more recently been associated with hypoxia and hypercapnia. Hypoxia refers to a deficiency of oxygen reaching the tissues of the body, usually due to low inspired oxygen. Hypoxemia is deficient oxygenation of the blood. Hypercapnia refers to elevated levels of carbon dioxide in the arterial blood. Low oxygen levels can be present without asphyxiation. These different conditions have distinct codes in ICD-9-CM:

786.09	Hypercapnia
799.01	Asphyxia
799.02	Hypoxemia

Inpatient Coding Guidelines

The ICD-9-CM Official Guidelines for Coding and Reporting address the use of sign and symptom codes as a principal diagnosis and when a sign or symptom code should not be used. The guidelines also address the correct use of sign and symptom codes as additional diagnoses.

Using Signs and Symptoms as Principal Diagnosis for Inpatient Encounters

According to guideline II.A. of the Official Guidelines for Coding and Reporting, codes for symptoms, signs, and ill-defined conditions from chapter 16 are not to be used as principal diagnoses when a related definitive diagnosis has been established. For example, with abdominal pain due to acute gastric ulcer, only the gastric ulcer is coded. However, the symptom can be designated as principal diagnosis when the patient is admitted for the purpose of treating the symptom and there is no treatment or evaluation of the underlying disease. For example, a patient is admitted for dehydration due to gastroenteritis for the purpose of rehydration. The gastroenteritis alone could have been treated on an outpatient basis. In this case, the code for the dehydration can be designated as principal diagnosis even though the cause of the condition is known.

Another reference is made to signs and symptoms in the official coding guidelines in item II.E.: When a symptom(s) is followed by contrasting/comparative diagnoses, the symptom code is sequenced first.

All the contrasting/comparative diagnoses should be coded as suspected conditions, for example, abdominal pain due to either pancreatitis or cholecystitis.

Using Signs and Symptoms as Additional Diagnoses

Codes for signs and symptoms are assigned as additional codes only when the sign or symptom is not integral to the underlying condition. It also may be appropriate to code a sign or symptom when its presence is significant in relationship to the patient's condition and/or the care given. When ascites is present in a patient with liver cirrhosis, for example, the ascites often must be treated separately from the cirrhosis.

Signs and symptoms are not coded when they are implicit in the diagnosis or when the symptoms are included in the condition code. For example, with chest pain due to myocardial infarction (MI), no symptom code is assigned for the chest pain because it is implicit in the MI. Another example is the diagnosis of atherosclerosis of the extremities with gangrene. The gangrene is not coded separately because it is included in code 440.24, Atherosclerosis of the extremities with gangrene.

Note: The coding guideline for symptoms followed by contrasting/comparative diagnosis applies only to the selection of the principal diagnosis. For example, if the physician lists a secondary diagnosis statement of vertigo due to Meniere's syndrome versus labyrinthitis, only the vertigo is coded (*Coding Clinic* 1998).

Outpatient Coding Guidelines

Many outpatient visits are coded with ICD-9-CM codes for signs and symptoms when a definitive diagnosis has not been established. Coders of outpatient visits must follow Section IV: Diagnostic Coding and Reporting Guidelines for Outpatient Services, within the ICD-9-CM Official Guidelines for Coding and Reporting.

Signs, symptoms, abnormal test results, or other reasons for the outpatient visit are used when a physician qualifies a diagnostic statement as "probable," "suspected," "questionable," "rule out," or "working diagnosis." The condition qualified in that statement should not be coded as if it existed. Rather, the condition should be coded to the highest degree of certainty, such as the signs or symptoms the patient exhibits.

These guidelines differ from acute care, short-term, long-term, and psychiatric hospital inpatient rules, where a qualified condition is coded as if it exists, because the evaluation and management of the suspected condition in these settings is often equal to the treatment of the same condition that has been confirmed.

The term *ruled out* designates the fact that the condition stated to be ruled out *does not* exist. This condition, therefore, cannot be coded and the preceding signs, symptoms, or abnormal test results are coded instead.

Review Exercise: Chapter 18

Assign ICD-9-CM codes to the following outpatient encounters:

1. Abnormal pap smear of the cervix, atypical squamous cell changes of undetermined significance (ASC-US)

   795.01

2. Sudden infant death syndrome

   798.0

3. Sleep apnea with insomnia

   780.51

4. Shortness of breath, cause undetermined

   786.05

5. Abnormal mammogram

   793.80

6. Urgency of urination

   788.63

7. Pneumonia with cough

   486

8. Elevated blood pressure reading; hypertension not confirmed

   796.2

9. Stress urinary incontinence in male patient

   788.32

10. Laennec's cirrhosis of liver with ascites

    571.2 , 789.5   571.5

Review Exercise: Chapter 18 (Continued)

11. Seizures; epilepsy, ruled out

    780.39

12. Right upper quadrant abdominal pain

    789.01

13. Chronic fatigue syndrome

    780.71

14. Abdominal mass with jaundice

    789.30, 782.4

15. Chest pain, noncardiac in origin

    786.59

16. Abnormal glucose tolerance test

    790.22

17. Elevated PSA

    790.93

18. Respiratory arrest of unknown origin

    799.1

19. Failure to thrive in 2-year-old child

    783.41

20. Rule out diabetes; patient complains of polydipsia and polyuria for several weeks prior to the office visit

    783.5   788.42

Chapter 19

Injury and Poisoning I

Chapter 17, Injury and Poisoning (800–999)

Chapter 17, Injury and Poisoning, in the Tabular List in volume 1 of ICD-9-CM includes the following categories and section titles:

Categories	Section Titles
800–829	Fractures
830–839	Dislocation
840–848	Sprains and Strains of Joints and Adjacent Muscles
850–854	Intracranial Injury, Excluding Those with Skull Fracture
860–869	Internal Injury of Thorax, Abdomen, and Pelvis
870–897	Open Wound
900–904	Injury to Blood Vessels
905–909	Late Effects of Injuries, Poisonings, Toxic Effects, and Other External Causes
910–919	Superficial Injury
920–924	Contusion with Intact Skin Surface
925–929	Crushing Injury
930–939	Effects of Foreign Body Entering through Orifice
940–949	Burns
950–957	Injury to Nerves and Spinal Cord
958–959	Certain Traumatic Complications and Unspecified Injuries
960–979	Poisoning by Drugs, Medicinal and Biological Substances
980–989	Toxic Effects of Substances Chiefly Nonmedicinal as to Source
990–995	Other and Unspecified Effects of External Causes
996–999	Complications of Surgical and Medical Care, Not Elsewhere Classified

Clearly, chapter 17 of ICD-9-CM encompasses a wide variety of injuries, as well as poisonings and surgical and medical complications. This chapter addresses injuries, and the next chapter addresses poisonings, adverse effects, and complications of surgical and medical care.

Injuries are traumatic in nature, resulting in damage to a body part. The damage may occur to such an extent that the tissues are destroyed. Various external causes such as blows, falls, guns, knives, industrial equipment, or household items may be responsible for injuries.

ICD-9-CM classifies injuries into well-defined categories such as fractures, dislocations, sprains, and open wounds, which are easier to understand than some disease processes. Traumatic injuries, however, may predispose a person to a nontraumatic disease. For example, bacteria may settle at the site of a bone fracture and cause acute osteomyelitis.

Main Terms for Injuries

The Alphabetic Index to Diseases in ICD-9-CM classifies injuries according to their general type, such as a wound, fracture, or dislocation. The subterms under the general type of injury identify the anatomical site.

Wound, open . . .
    abdomen, abdominal . . . 879.2
       complicated 879.3
       wall (anterior) 879.2
         complicated 879.3
         lateral 879.4
           complicated 879.5
     alveolar (process) 873.62
       complicated 873.72

Instructions for Coding Injuries

ICD-9-CM uses fifth digits in the injury section to provide data on level of consciousness, specific anatomical site, and severity of injury. Fifth digits must be used as indicated in the ICD-9-CM system.

Exercise 19.1

Describe the data the fifth digit provides for each of the following codes:

1. 800.06

_____

2. 811.12

_____

3. 832.04

_____

4. 866.01

_____

5. 942.14

_____

Fractures (800–829)

A fracture is a break in the bone due to either a traumatic injury or a disease process. Tenderness and swelling develop at the site of the break, with a visible or palpable deformity, pain, and weakness. X rays show a partial or an incomplete break at the site of the fracture.

In ICD-9-CM, traumatic fractures are classified to categories 800 through 829. At the fourth-digit level, fractures are identified as closed or open. In closed fractures, the skin remains intact; in open fractures, a break in the skin occurs. At the beginning of the section "Fractures" (800–829), the following list of terms synonymous with *open and closed* appears:

The descriptions "closed" and "open" used in the fourth-digit subdivisions include the following terms:

closed (with or without delayed healing):

comminuted	impacted
depressed	linear
elevated	simple
fissured	slipped epiphysis
fracture NOS	spiral
greenstick	

open (with or without delayed healing):

compound	puncture
infected	with foreign body
missile	

When there is no indication as to whether the fracture is open or closed, the code describing a closed fracture is assigned.

Coders are permitted to use an x-ray report to assign a more specific fracture diagnosis code. The physician may not list the specific site of the fracture, but an x-ray report in the health record shows the precise site. It is appropriate for the coder to assign the more specific code from the x-ray report without consulting the physician. However, if there is any question as to the appropriate diagnosis, the coder must contact the physician.

A fifth-digit subclassification often is used in fracture coding to identify the specific site involved.

---

816   Fracture of one or more phalanges of hand

Includes: finger(s)   thumb

The following fifth-digit subclassification is for use with category 816:

0   phalanx or phalanges, unspecified
1   middle or proximal phalanx or phalanges
2   distal phalanx or phalanges
3   multiple sites

816.0   Closed

816.1   Open

In the preceding example, the fourth digit describes a closed or open fracture of the phalanges, with the fifth digit identifying the specific site of the fracture.

Remember that pathologic fractures are not considered traumatic and, as such, are not classified to chapter 17 of ICD-9-CM with the traumatic fracture codes. Pathologic fractures, codes 733.10–733.19, are discussed in chapter 13 of ICD-9-CM.

Exercise 19.2

Assign ICD-9-CM codes to the following:

1. Simple greenstick fracture, shafts of tibia and fibula

2. Comminuted fracture of humerus

3. Fracture of femur due to gunshot

4. Compound fracture of lower end of ulna

5. Fracture of right fibula due to osteogenesis imperfecta

Multiple Fractures

Whenever possible, separate codes should be assigned for multiple fractures unless the Alphabetic Index or Tabular List provides instructions to the contrary.

> **EXAMPLE:** Closed fracture of the distal radius: 813.42, Other fractures of distal end of radius (alone)

> **EXAMPLE:** Closed fracture of the metacarpal bone: 815.00, Closed fracture of unspecified metacarpal bone(s)

Combination categories for multiple fractures are provided for use in the following situations:

- When the health record contains insufficient detail

> **EXAMPLE:** "Multiple fractures of right upper limb" is the only information provided in the health record: 818.0, Ill-defined fractures of upper limb

In this example, no additional information is provided in the health record as to the specific sites of the upper limb involved; therefore, code 818.0 is assigned.

- When the reporting form limits the number of codes that can be assigned

> **EXAMPLE:** Patient had many traumatic injuries, including several fractures of the hand bones, which were identified in the health record. Because of all the other more critical injuries, space was not available on the form to code each metacarpal fracture separately: 817.0, Closed multiple fractures of hand bones

In this example, the single code 817.0 would be assigned for the multiple fractures of the hand bones.

Exercise 19.3

Assign ICD-9-CM codes to the following:

1. Open frontal fracture with subarachnoid hemorrhage with brief loss of consciousness

   _____

2. Supracondylar fracture of the right humerus and fracture of the olecranon process of the right ulna

   _____

3. Open fracture of the patella

   _____

4. Multiple fractures of the right lower extremity

   _____

5. Infected shaft of the tibia fracture

   _____

Dislocation (830–839)

Dislocation is the displacement of a bone from its joint. The joints most commonly affected are in the fingers, thumbs, and shoulders. Pain and swelling occur, as well as the loss of use of the injured part. To promote healing, the dislocation can be reduced and the joint immobilized by applying a cast.

A dislocation that occurs with a fracture is included in the fracture code. The reduction of the dislocation is included in the code for the fracture reduction.

ICD-9-CM classifies the dislocation of a joint without associated fracture to categories 830 through 839. These categories also include subluxations, that is, an incomplete or a partial dislocation. The fourth-digit classification differentiates between open and closed dislocations. At the beginning of the section "Dislocation" (830–839), the following list of terms synonymous with *open and closed* appears:

> The descriptions "closed" and "open," used in the fourth-digit subdivisions, include the following terms:
>
> | closed: | open: |
> |---------|-------|
> | complete | compound |
> | dislocation NOS | infected |
> | partial | with foreign body |
> | simple | |
> | uncomplicated | |

When a dislocation is not indicated as closed or open, it should be classified as closed. As with fractures, ICD-9-CM uses the fifth digit to identify the specific site.

> **832   Dislocation of elbow**
>
> The following fifth-digit subclassification is for use with category 832:
>
> > **0   elbow unspecified**
> > **1   anterior dislocation of elbow**
> > **2   posterior dislocation of elbow**
> > **3   medial dislocation of elbow**
> > **4   lateral dislocation of elbow**
> > **9   other**
>
> **832.0   Closed dislocation**
>
> **832.1   Open dislocation**

Sprains and Strains (840–848)

A sprain is an injury of the supporting ligaments of a joint resulting from a turning or twisting of a body part. Sprains are extremely painful and are accompanied by swelling and discoloration. They require rest for the injury to heal. Whiplash is a specific type of sprain, usually due to a sudden throwing of the head forward and then backward. It results in a compression of the cervical spine that involves the bones, joints, and intervertebral disks.

A strain is simply an overstretching or overexertion of some part of the musculature that usually responds to rest.

Codes within the categories 840 through 848 are current injuries. Patients also may suffer from chronic strains of the neck or back or derangements of different joints. The physician may describe these conditions as chronic, old, or recurrent. Using terms such as *sprain/strain* or *derangement,* the coder should refer to the subterm for the site and use another subterm to describe the chronic, old, or recurrent condition. The coder will be referred to codes within the "Diseases of the Musculoskeletal System" section, categories 710–739.

Exercise 19.4

Assign ICD-9-CM codes to the following:

1.   Anterior dislocation of the elbow

_____

2.   Dislocation of the first and second cervical vertebrae

_____

3.   Compound dislocation of hip

_____

4.   Sprain of lateral collateral ligament of knee

_____

5.   Acute lumbosacral strain

_____

Intracranial Injury, Excluding Those with Skull Fracture (850–854)

At the beginning of this section on intracranial injury, the following note appears: "The description 'with open intracranial wound,' used in the fourth-digit subdivisions, includes those specified as open or with mention of infection or foreign body." As mentioned in chapter 1 of this publication, the notes in ICD-9-CM often provide a definition that must be applied to that section, category, or subcategory. The purpose of the note in this section is to offer information that when a diagnostic statement includes the terms *open, infected,* or *foreign body,* the fourth-digit code describing an open intracranial wound should be assigned.

In addition to this section note, a fifth-digit subclassification for categories 851–854 is provided.

Cerebral Concussion

A cerebral concussion is a transient loss of consciousness for less than 24 hours (usually far less) after a traumatic head injury. Although no intracranial damage occurs, the patient may experience bradycardia, hypotension, and respiratory arrest for a few seconds, as well as retrograde and posttraumatic amnesia. The patient is put under 48-hour observation to check for the development of complications. A computerized axial tomography (CAT) scan may be performed to rule out any intracranial injury. Codes for cerebral concussion range from 850.0 to 850.9, based on the exact injury that occurred.

Cerebral Contusion

Often caused by a blow to the head, a cerebral contusion is a more severe injury involving a bruise of the brain with bleeding into brain tissue, but without disruption of the brain's continuity. The loss of consciousness that occurs often lasts longer than that of a concussion. A laceration or fracture often accompanies the contusion. Any type of laceration of the brain results in some destruction of brain tissue and a subsequent scarring that may cause posttraumatic epilepsy. Codes for cerebral laceration and contusion range from 851.0 through 851.9, with fifth digits added to indicate whether a loss of consciousness or concussion occurred.

Subdural Hematoma

A subdural hematoma is the formation of a hematoma between the dura and the leptomeninges. Often resulting from a tear in the arachnoid, the acute form of subdural hematoma is associated with a laceration or contusion. Chronic subdural hematomas may result from closed head injuries such as falls. Symptoms include headache, increasing drowsiness, hemiparesis, and seizures.

Internal Injury of Thorax, Abdomen, and Pelvis (860–869)

Internal injuries of the thorax, abdomen, and pelvis are classified to categories 860 through 869. The fourth-digit subcategories describe the presence or absence of an open wound. The fifth-digit subclassification identifies the specific site, the specific type of injury, or the severity of the injury.

861.0   **Heart, without mention of open wound into thorax**

     861.00   **Unspecified injury**

     861.01   **Contusion**

         Cardiac contusion

         Myocardial contusion

     861.02   **Laceration without penetration of heart chambers**

     861.03   **Laceration with penetration of heart chambers**

861.1   **Heart, with open wound in thorax**

     861.10   **Unspecified injury**

     861.11   **Contusion**

     861.12   **Laceration without penetration of heart chambers**

     861.13   **Laceration with penetration of heart chambers**

---

864   **Injury to liver**

The following fifth-digit subclassification is for use with category 864:

     0   **unspecified injury**

     1   **hematoma and contusion**

     2   **laceration, minor**

         Laceration involving capsule only or without significant
involvement of hepatic parenchyma [i.e., less than 1 cm deep]

     3   **laceration, moderate**

         Laceration involving parenchyma, but without major disruption
of parenchyma [i.e., less than 10 cm long and less than
3 cm deep]

     4   **laceration, major**

         Laceration with significant disruption of hepatic
parenchyma [i.e., 10 cm long and 3 cm deep]

         Multiple moderate lacerations, with or without hematoma

         Stellate lacerations of liver

     5   **laceration, unspecified**

     9   **other**

864.0   **Without mention of open wound into cavity**

864.1   **With open wound in cavity**

Exercise 19.5

Assign ICD-9-CM codes to the following:

1. Traumatic subdural hemorrhage with open intracranial wound; loss of consciousness, unknown time

   _____

2. Cerebral contusion with brief loss of consciousness

   _____

3. Traumatic laceration of the liver, moderate

   _____

4. Traumatic hemothorax with open wound into thorax and concussion with loss of consciousness

   _____

5. Traumatic duodenal injury

   _____

Open Wound (870–897)

ICD-9-CM classifies open wounds to categories 870 through 897. An open wound is an injury of the soft tissue parts associated with rupture of the skin. Open wounds may be animal bites, avulsions, cuts, lacerations, puncture wounds, and traumatic amputation. In addition, an open wound may be a penetrating wound, which involves the passage of an object through tissue that leaves an entrance and exit, as in the case of a knife or gunshot wound.

The seriousness of an open wound depends on its site and extent. If a major vessel or organ is involved, a wound may be life-threatening. For example, the rupture of a large artery or vein may cause blood to accumulate in one of the body cavities, which is referred to as hemothorax, hemopericardium, hemoperitoneum, or hemarthrosis, depending on the body cavity involved. The significance of the hemorrhage rests on the volume of the blood loss, the rate of loss, and the site of hemorrhage. Large losses may induce hemorrhagic shock. Crushing wounds are excluded from these categories and, instead, are classified to categories 925 through 929.

Instructional Notes

Three instructional notes appear at the beginning of the section "Open Wound" (870–897).

OPEN WOUND (870–897)

Includes: animal bite   laceration
             avulsion   puncture wound
             cut   traumatic amputation

Excludes: *burn (940.0–949.5)*
             crushing (925–929.9)
             puncture of internal organs (860.0–869.1)
             superficial injury (910.0–919.9)
             that incidental to:
                 dislocation (830.0–839.9)
                 fracture (800.0–829.1)
                 internal injury (860.0–869.1)
                 intracranial injury (851.0–854.1)

Note: The description "complicated" used in the fourth-digit sub-
         divisions includes those with mention of delayed healing,
         delayed treatment, foreign body, or infection.

         ▶ Use additional code to identify infection. ◀

In the preceding example, the includes note identifies wounds that are classified to categories 870 through 897 and the excludes note identifies wounds that are classified elsewhere in ICD-9-CM. The third note defines the term *complicated*. The definition contains specific criteria that must be documented in the health record before a code is selected to describe a complicated wound.

> **EXAMPLE:**   Delayed healing of open wound of foot: 892.1, Complicated open wound of foot except (toes) alone

In this example, the wound was considered complicated because the diagnostic statement included the terminology "delayed healing"; therefore, code 892.1 was assigned.

The description "complicated" used in the fourth-digit subdivisions includes those with mention of delayed healing, delayed treatment, foreign body, or infection. Following the note is an ICD-9-CM instruction, "Use additional code to identify infection."

Fourth- and Fifth-Digit Subdivisions

ICD-9-CM uses the fourth-digit subcategories and the fifth-digit subclassification to identify the type of open wound, the site of the wound, complicated or uncomplicated wounds, and involvement of tendon.

---

874   Open wound of neck

    874.0   Larynx and trachea, without mention of complication

        874.00   Larynx with trachea
        874.01   Larynx
        874.02   Trachea

    874.1   Larynx and trachea, complicated

        874.10   Larynx with trachea
        874.11   Larynx
        874.12   Trachea

---

880   Open wound of shoulder and upper arm

The following fifth-digit subclassification is for use with category 880:

      0   **shoulder region**
      1   **scapular region**
      2   **axillary region**
      3   **upper arm**
      9   **multiple sites**

880.0   **Without mention of complication**
880.1   **Complicated**
880.2   **With tendon involvement**

Repair of Open Wounds

Open wounds, such as laceration of skin, are typically repaired by the suturing of skin and subcutaneous tissue or by the use of the newer tissue adhesives. Procedure code 86.59 includes the repair of open wound by suturing, as well as the application of Dermabond, a tissue adhesive.

Exercise 19.6

Assign ICD-9-CM codes to the following:

1. Avulsion of eye

    _____

2. Traumatic below-the-knee amputation with delayed healing

    _____

3. Open wound of buttock

    _____

4. Open wound of wrist involving tendons

    _____

5. Laceration of external ear

    _____

Burns (940–949)

Burns are assigned to categories 940 through 949 in ICD-9-CM and include burns due to electricity, flames, hot objects, lightning, radiation, chemicals, and scalding.

Burns also are classified by depth, extent, and, where needed, agent (E code). By depth, burns are classified as first degree (erythema), second degree (blistering), and third degree (full-thickness involvement), as described below:

*   A first-degree burn is the least severe and includes damage to the epidermis or outer layer of skin alone.

- A second-degree burn involves the epidermis and dermis. There is edema and blistering of the skin, which is red and moist.

- A third-degree burn is the most severe and includes all three layers of skin: epidermis, dermis, and subcutaneous. The skin appears charred, white, and dry.

Guidelines for Coding Burns and Encounters for Late Effects of Burns

The following official guidelines apply when coding burns and encounters for the late effects of burns:

- Code all burns with the highest degree of burn sequenced first.

- Classify burns of the same local site (a three-digit category level [940–947]), but of different degrees, to the subcategory identifying the highest degree recorded in the diagnosis.

- Code nonhealing burns as acute burns. Code necrosis of burned skin as a nonhealed burn.

- Assign code 958.3, Posttraumatic wound infection, not elsewhere classified, as an additional code for any documented infected burn site.

- When coding multiple burns, assign separate codes for each burn site. Category 946, Burns of multiple specified sites, should be used only if the locations of the burns are not documented.

- Category 949, Burn, unspecified, is extremely vague and should seldom be used.

- Assign codes from category 948, Burns classified according to extent of body surface involved, when the site of the burns is not specified or when there is a need for additional data. Use category 948 as additional coding when it is necessary to provide data for evaluating burn mortality, such as that needed by burn units. Also, use category 948 as an additional code for reporting purposes when there is mention of a third-degree burn involving 20 percent or more of body surface. In assigning a code from category 948, observe the following criteria:

  —Fourth-digit codes are used to identify the percentage of total body surface involved in a burn (all degrees).

  —Fifth digits are assigned to identify the percentage of body surface involved in a third-degree burn.

  —The fifth digit 0 is assigned when less than 10 percent of body surface or no body surface is involved in a third-degree burn.

- Category 948 is based on the classic "rule of nines" in estimating body surface involved: head and neck are assigned 9 percent; each arm, 9 percent; each leg, 18 percent; the anterior trunk, 18 percent; the posterior trunk, 18 percent; and the genitalia, 1 percent. Physicians may change these percentage assignments, where necessary, to accommodate infants and children who have proportionately larger heads than adults, as well as patients whose buttocks, thighs, or abdomens are proportionately larger than normal.

- Code encounters for the treatment of the late effects of burns (for example, scars or joint contractures) to the residual condition (sequela), followed by the appropriate late effect code (906.5–906.9). A late effect E code also may be used, if desired.

- When appropriate, both a sequela with a late effect code and a current burn code may be assigned on the same record.

Sunburn is caused by overexposure to the ultraviolet rays from sunlight. Sunburns can be described as first, second, or third degree, depending on the depth of the burn. Sunburns are not classified in the range of 940–949 with traumatic burns due to flames or other sources of heat. Instead, sunburns are classified to codes 692.70–692.79, contact dermatitis due to solar radiation.

Coding Debridements of Wounds, Infections, or Burns

Excisional debridement, 86.22, is assigned when the procedure is performed by physicians, nurses, therapists, or physician assistants. Nonexcisional debridement performed by a physician or other healthcare professional is assigned to 86.28.

Exercise 19.7

Assign ICD-9-CM codes to the following:

1. Second-degree burn of chest wall and first-degree burn of face

   _____

2. Deep third-degree burn of forearm

   _____

3. Third-degree burns of back involving 20 percent of body surface

   _____

4. Thirty percent body burns with 10 percent third degree

   _____

5. First- and second-degree burns of palm

   _____

6. Nonhealing second-degree burns of right upper arm and right hand

   _____

7. Infected second-degree burn of left thigh

   _____

8. First- and second-degree burns on multiple sites of legs

   _____

9. Full-thickness burns of back

   _____

10. First- and second-degree burns of scalp with third-degree burns of shoulder

   _____

Superficial Injury and Contusion with Intact Skin (910–924)

Superficial injuries such as abrasions or contusions are not coded when associated with more severe injuries (for example, fractures, open wounds) of the same site. The following subsections describe the conditions for coding superficial injury, contusion with intact skin surface, and crushing injury.

Superficial Injury (910–919)

Superficial injuries are classified to categories 910 through 919. This section includes a variety of superficial injuries, from abrasions to superficial foreign bodies. The fourth-digit subcategories specify type of injury and presence or absence of infection.

910	**Superficial injury of face, neck, and scalp, except eye**
910.0	Abrasion or friction burn without mention of infection
910.1	Abrasion or friction burn, infected
910.2	Blister without mention of infection
910.3	Blister, infected
910.4	Insect bite, nonvenomous, without mention of infection
910.5	Insect bite, nonvenomous, infected
910.6	Superficial foreign body (splinter) without major open wound and without mention of infection
910.7	Superficial foreign body (splinter) without major open wound, infected
910.8	Other and unspecified superficial injury of face, neck, and scalp without mention of infection
910.9	Other and unspecified superficial injury of face, neck, and scalp, infected

Contusion with Intact Skin Surface (920–924)

Contusions are injuries of the soft tissue. Although the skin is not broken, the small vessels or capillaries are ruptured and the result is bleeding into the tissue. When the blood becomes trapped in the interstitial spaces, the result is a hematoma.

ICD-9-CM classifies these types of contusions to categories 920 through 924. The fourth-digit subcategories are subdivided to identify the specific site involved.

Crushing Injury (925–929)

Crushing injuries usually occur when part or all of an extremity is pulled into, and compressed by, rollers in a machine, such as those found in industrial plants. A crushing injury also may occur in a nonindustrial setting. Avulsion of skin and fat or a friction burn of the tissues may result. Abrasion burns are often severe, including third degree. Vessels, nerves, and muscles may be avulsed, and bones may be dislocated or fractured. A common complication is secondary congestion, which can lead to paralysis and to severe muscle fibrosis and joint stiffness. Muscle compartments may need decompression, and muscles and ligaments may need to be sectioned. Often the overall circulation of the extremity is of greater concern than definitive management of specific structures. These types of injuries may be called wringer, compression, crush, crushed, or crushing injuries.

Injury to Blood Vessels (900–904), Nerves and Spinal Cord (950–957)

This subsection describes the conditions for coding injury to blood vessels and the nerves and spinal cord.

A point to remember: When a primary injury results in minor damage to peripheral nerves or blood vessels, list the primary injury first, with additional code(s) from categories 950 through 957, Injury to nerves and spinal cord, and/or from categories 900 through 904, Injury to blood vessels. Also, when the primary injury is to the blood vessels or nerves, list the primary injury first.

Injury to Blood Vessels (900–904)

The codes for injuries to blood vessels include arterial hematomas, avulsions, cuts, lacerations, ruptures, and traumatic aneurysms or fistulas that are secondary to other injuries such as fractures or open wounds. Codes from categories 900–904 are usually assigned as additional diagnoses, with the underlying injury listed first.

> **EXAMPLE:** Open wound of the forearm with injury to the ulnar blood vessel:
> 881.00, Open wound of forearm without mention of complication;
> 903.3, Injury to ulnar blood vessels

Injury to Nerves and Spinal Cord (950–957)

The codes for injury to nerves and the spinal cord include injuries with or without the presence of an open wound. Category 952, Spinal cord injury without evidence of spinal bone injury, is subdivided at the fourth- and fifth-digit levels to identify the specific sites involved.

Exercise 19.8

Assign ICD-9-CM codes to the following:

1. Open wound of the lower leg with tendon involvement and injury to the anterior tibial artery

    _____

2. Nonvenomous insect bite, elbow, infected

    _____

3. Contusion of the lower leg and knee

    _____

4. Spinal cord injury, C_1–C_4

    _____

5. Crushing injury of left hand and wrist

    _____

Effects of Foreign Body Entering through Orifice (930–939)

Foreign objects often are found in various body openings in the pediatric population. Children sometimes put small items in their noses or ears or swallow coins or marbles.

Foreign bodies also can lodge in the larynx, bronchi, or esophagus, usually during eating. Foreign bodies in the larynx may produce hoarseness, coughing, and gagging, and partially obstruct the airway, causing stridor. A grasping forceps through a direct laryngoscope can remove foreign bodies from the larynx.

Foreign bodies in the bronchi usually produce an initial episode of coughing, followed by an asymptomatic period before obstructive and inflammatory symptoms occur. Foreign bodies are removed from the bronchi through a bronchoscope.

Foreign bodies in the esophagus produce immediate symptoms of coughing and gagging, with the sensation of something being "stuck in the throat," as well as causing difficulty in swallowing. Foreign bodies in the esophagus can be removed through an esophagoscope. Intraocular foreign bodies require removal by an ophthalmic surgeon.

ICD-9-CM classifies foreign bodies in orifices to categories 930 through 939. These categories are further subdivided to fourth-digit subcategories that identify the specific site or orifice. These codes can be found in the Alphabetic Index by referencing the main term "Foreign body" and the subterm "entering through orifice." When the foreign body is associated with an open wound, it is coded as an open wound, complicated by site. A foreign body inadvertently left in an operative wound is considered to be a complication of a procedure and is coded 998.4.

Exercise 19.9

Assign ICD-9-CM codes to the following:

1. Removal of coin from bronchus

   _____

2. Foreign body in eye

   _____

3. Marble in colon

   _____

4. Bean in nose

   _____

5. Q-Tip stuck in ear

   _____

Chapter 20

Injury and Poisoning II

Chapter 17, Injury and Poisoning (800–999)

Chapter 20 provides further explanation of chapter 17, Injury and Poisoning, in ICD-9-CM.

Alphabetic Index

ICD-9-CM provides two different sets of code numbers to differentiate between poisonings and adverse effects or adverse reactions to substances. Codes 960–979 are used to identify poisoning by drugs and medicinal and biological substances. These codes are found through a separate index known as the Table of Drugs and Chemicals. This table also is used to classify the appropriate E code for the drug or chemical involved with an adverse reaction, while the actual condition identified as the adverse effect is coded with disease codes. The Table of Drugs and Chemicals follows the Alphabetic Index to Diseases.

Table of Drugs and Chemicals

The Table of Drugs and Chemicals provides an alphabetic listing of drugs and other agents. The first column identifies the specific substance. The second column, titled "Poisoning," is used when a particular case meets the criteria for poisoning (criteria follow). The remaining five columns describe the circumstance under which the adverse reaction or poisoning occurred.

Adverse Effects of Drugs

Adverse effects can occur in situations in which medication is administered properly and prescribed correctly in both therapeutic and diagnostic procedures. A brief discussion of common causes of adverse effects follows:

- Cumulative effects result when the inactivation and/or excretion of the drug is slower than the rate at which the drug is being administered. This is often documented as drug toxicity in the health record.

- Hypersensitivity or allergic reaction is a qualitatively different response to a drug acquired only after reexposure to the drug.

- Synergistic reaction is enhancing the effect of a prior or concurrent administration of another drug.

- The effectiveness of a drug may change as the result of interaction with another prescribed medication.

- Side effects are the unwanted, predictable pharmacologic effects that occur within therapeutic code ranges.

Instructions for Coding Adverse Effects

The following instructions apply when coding adverse effects:

1. Code the manifestation or the nature of the adverse effects, such as urticaria, vertigo, gastritis, and so forth.

2. Locate the drug in the "Substance" column of the Table of Drugs and Chemicals in the Alphabetic Index to Diseases.

3. Select the E code for the drug from the "Therapeutic Use" column of the Table of Drugs and Chemicals. Use of the E code is mandatory when coding adverse effects.

   EXAMPLE: Atrial tachycardia due to digitalis glycosides intoxication: 427.89, Other specified cardiac dysrhythmias (atrial tachycardia); E942.1, Cardiotonic glycosides and drugs of similar action causing adverse effects in therapeutic use (adverse effect of digitalis)

4. If the adverse effect is the result of the interaction between two or more prescription drugs, assign E codes for both drugs.

   EXAMPLE: Premature supraventricular beats due to the interaction of digitalis glycosides and Valium, both correctly prescribed and administered: 427.61, Supraventricular premature beats; E942.1, Cardiotonic glycosides and drugs of similar action causing adverse effects in therapeutic use (adverse effect of digitalis); E939.4, Benzodiazepine-based tranquilizers causing adverse effects in therapeutic use (adverse effect of Valium)

5. Late effect of an adverse effect of a correct substance properly administered is coded as follows:

   - First code the residual or late effect, such as blindness or deafness.

   - Assign code 909.5, Late effect of adverse effect of drug, medicinal or biological substance, to identify a late effect of an adverse reaction. Use the Alphabetic Index to Diseases and see "Late, effect(s) (of), adverse effect of drug, medicinal or biological substance" to locate code 909.5.

   - No specific E code is provided to identify the external cause of a late effect of an adverse reaction to a correct substance properly administered. The residual effect will differ from the immediate reaction. However, the E code is the same as the original code selected from the "Therapeutic Use" column of the Table of Drugs and Chemicals.

     EXAMPLE: Hearing loss occurring as a result of previously administered streptomycin therapy: 389.9, Unspecified hearing loss; 909.5, Late effect of adverse effect of drug, medicinal or biological substance; E930.6, Antimycobacterial antibiotics causing adverse effects in therapeutic use

See figure 20.1 for assistance in coding adverse reactions to correct substances properly administered.

Figure 20.1.   Coding adverse reactions to correct substances properly administered

Current Condition		Late Effect
Code effect: Coma, vertigo, etc.	←Principal Diagnosis→	Code effect: Deafness, blindness, etc.
		Plus
		Late effect 909.5
And		**And**
E code from "Therapeutic Use" column of Table of Drugs and Chemicals (E930–949)	←Other Diagnosis→	E code from "Therapeutic Use" column of Table of Drugs and Chemicals (E930–949)

Use of codes E930–E949 is mandatory when coding adverse effects.

Exercise 20.1

Assign ICD-9-CM diagnosis codes to the following:

1. Ataxia due to the interaction of carbamazepine and erythromycin

2. Vertigo from dye administered for intravenous pyelogram

3. Constipation from Oncovin injected for Hodgkin's disease

4. Excessive drowsiness due to side effects of Periactin

5. Hemiplegia resulting from previous adverse reaction to Enovid

Unspecified Adverse Effects of Drugs

Sometimes an adverse effect of a drug is unknown or, more often, not documented in the health record. Normally, unspecified adverse effects of drugs are indicated by diagnostic statements such as:

- Toxic effect of
- Drug toxicity
- Drug intoxication
- Drug allergy/hypersensitivity

Instructions for Coding Unspecified Adverse Effects of Drugs

Certain coding instructions apply when coding unspecified adverse effects. These include:

- In the inpatient setting, the health record documentation should provide enough information to determine the specific adverse effect or reaction of a particular medication. In such circumstances, the information previously discussed for coding adverse reactions applies.

- In the event this information is unavailable and the documentation states toxicity, intoxication, or allergy to a particular drug with no specific reaction identified, assign code 796.0, Nonspecific abnormal toxicological findings. First, the physician should be queried to determine whether the toxicity, allergy, or intoxication is truly an adverse effect or a poisoning. Then, an E code from the "Therapeutic Use" column of the Table of Drugs and Chemicals is assigned to describe the drug or medicinal substance causing the adverse effect.

    EXAMPLE: While hospitalized, patient developed paroxysmal supraventricular tachycardia secondary to digitalis intoxication: 427.0, Paroxysmal supraventricular tachycardia; E942.1, Cardiotonic glycosides and drugs of similar action causing adverse effects in therapeutic use (adverse effect of digitalis)

    EXAMPLE: Documentation in the health record of an inpatient states aminophylline toxicity: 796.0, Nonspecific abnormal toxicological findings

    In this example, the coder should query the physician as to whether the toxicity is a poisoning or an adverse reaction (effect), as well as whether there are any associated reactions or manifestations. For this example, if the physician confirms that the toxicity is an adverse effect, E945.7, Anti-asthmatics causing adverse effects in therapeutic use (adverse effect of aminophylline), would be added. However, if the physician declares the toxicity to be a poisoning, an E code would be used to reflect the external cause of the poisoning by aminophylline.

- In the outpatient setting, unspecified adverse effects or reactions may be reported with code 995.2, Unspecified adverse effect of drug, medicinal and biological substance. However, the coder should read the note in the Tabular List under code 995.2, which states: "This code is not for use in the inpatient setting and only for limited use in the outpatient setting when no signs or symptoms of the drug are documented." Code 995.2 is found in the Alphabetic Index to Diseases under "Effect, adverse, NEC, drugs and medicinals NEC." In addition, an E code from the "Therapeutic Use" column of the Table of Drugs and Chemicals is assigned to describe the drug or medicinal substance causing the adverse effect.

    EXAMPLE: Drug reaction to penicillin: 995.2, Unspecified adverse effect of drug, medicinal and biological substance; E930.0, Penicillin causing adverse effects in therapeutic use (adverse effect of penicillin)

Note: Code 995.2 is permissible in the outpatient setting in rare circumstances, when no further documentation is available (*Coding Clinic* 1997). If the drug reaction was described as penicillin toxicity with no specific reaction identified, it would be assigned code 796.0. If the drug causing the unspecified adverse reaction was unknown, code E947.9, Unspecified drug or medicinal substance, would be assigned. This code is indexed under the main term "Drug" in the Table of Drugs and Chemicals.

- Late effect of an unspecified adverse effect is coded in the same manner as late effects of specified adverse effects.

    —First code the residual or late effect, such as blindness or deafness.

    —Code 909.5, Late effect of adverse effect of drug, medicinal or biological substance, is assigned to identify a late effect of an unspecified adverse reaction. Code 909.5 is found in the Alphabetic Index to Diseases under "Late effect(s) (of), adverse effect of drug, medicinal or biological substance."

    —If the specific residual is not identified, first code 909.5.

    —Select the appropriate code from the "Therapeutic Use" column of the Table of Drugs and Chemicals to identify the drug involved.

    > EXAMPLE: Residuals of previous severe allergic reaction to chemotherapy (fluorouracil), which was discontinued six months ago: 909.5, Late effect of adverse effect of drug, medicinal or biological substance; E933.1, Antineoplastic and immunosuppressive drugs causing adverse effects in therapeutic use (adverse effect of fluorouracil)

Exercise 20.2

Assign ICD-9-CM codes to the following:

1. Emergency department patient with allergic reaction to unspecified drug

2. Residuals from previous episode of acute hypersensitivity to sulfonamide

3. Inpatient with asymptomatic Dilantin toxicity

4. Rash due to unspecified drug

Poisonings

Poisoning refers to conditions caused by drugs, medicinal substances, and other biological substances only when the substance involved is not used according to a physician's instructions. Poisonings can occur in the following ways:

- The wrong dosage of medication given in error during a diagnostic or therapeutic procedure, or during the course of medical care

- The wrong dosage of medication given in error by nonmedical personnel, such as a mother to an infant or a child to an elderly parent

- Medication given to the wrong person by medical or nonmedical personnel

- Medication taken by the wrong person

- The wrong dosage of medication self-administered

- Intoxication (other than cumulative effect)

- Overdose

- Medications (prescription or nonprescription) taken in combination with alcoholic beverages

- Over-the-counter medications taken in combination with prescribed medications without consulting a physician

Instructions for Coding Poisonings

The following instructions apply when coding poisonings:

1. Use the Table of Drugs and Chemicals in the Alphabetic Index to Diseases to locate the drug or other agent.

2. Assign the code from the "Poisoning" column.

3. Code the specified effect of the poisoning, such as coma, vertigo, drowsiness, and so forth.

4. Identify the external cause of poisoning from the appropriate column of the Table of Drugs and Chemicals. If the intent (accident, self-harm, or assault) of the cause of an injury or poisoning is unknown or unspecified, code the intent as undetermined, E980–E989. If the intent (accident, self-harm, or assault) of the cause of an injury or poisoning is questionable, probable, or suspected, code the intent as undetermined, E980–E989 (Official Coding Guidelines). Use of the E codes is optional for many facilities; however, some states mandate the coding of external causes (E codes).

   > **EXAMPLE:** Overdosed on aspirin, suicide attempt: 965.1, Poisoning by salicylates (overdose on aspirin); E950.0, Suicide and self-inflicted poisoning by analgesics, antipyretics, and antirheumatics (suicide attempt)

5. Late effect of a poisoning is coded as follows:

   - First code the residual (specified effect), such as deafness or blindness.

   - Assign a code to identify a late effect of poisoning by drugs: 909.0, Late effect of poisoning due to drug, medicinal or biological substance; or 909.1, Late effect of toxic effects of nonmedical substances.

     —Code 909.0 is found in the Alphabetic Index to Diseases under "Late, effect(s) (of), poisoning due to drug, medicinal or biological substance."

     —Code 909.1 is found in the Alphabetic Index to Diseases under "Late effect(s) (of), toxic effect of, nonmedical substance."

   - Use the Alphabetic Index to External Causes to assign one of the following E codes to describe the late effect of an external cause:

     —E929.2, Late effects of accidental poisoning: Found in the Index to External Causes under "Late effect of, poisoning, accidental"

     —E959, Late effects of self-inflicted injury: Found in the Index to External Causes under "Late effect of, suicide, attempt (any means)"

     —E969, Late effects of injury purposely inflicted by other person: Found in the Index to External Causes under "Late effect of, assault"

     —E977, Late effects of injuries due to legal intervention: Found in the Index to External Causes under "Late effect of, legal intervention"

—E989, Late effects of injury, undetermined whether accidentally or purposely inflicted: Found in the Index to External Causes under "Late effect of, injury undetermined whether accidentally or purposely inflicted"

Note: Although E codes are usually optional, it is best to double-check the requirements of the particular state or facility where the coding is being done.

See figure 20.2 for assistance in coding poisonings.

Codes 960–979 are never used in combination with codes E930–E949 because codes 960–979 identify poisonings and codes E930–E949 identify the external cause of adverse reactions to correct substances properly administered.

Figure 20.2.   Coding poisonings

Current Injury		Late Effect
Code from 960–979	←Principal Diagnosis→	Specified effect—deafness, blindness, etc.
Plus		*Plus*
Specified effect—tachycardia, coma	←Other Diagnosis→	Late effect 909.0 or 909.1
And		**And**
E code from one of the following "External Cause" columns of Table of Drugs and Chemicals: accident suicide attempt assault undetermined	←Other Diagnosis→	E929.2 or E959 or E969 or E977 or E989

In general, E codes for poisonings are optional, although many healthcare facilities and some states mandate their use.

Exercise 20.3

Assign ICD-9-CM codes to the following:

1. Accidental ingestion of mother's oral contraceptives

2. Stricture of esophagus due to accidental lye ingestion three years ago

3. Listlessness from prescribed Valium and six pack of beer (grain alcohol). The intent is undetermined.

4. Lead poisoning from eating paint, accidental injury by a child

5. Carbon monoxide poisoning from car exhaust in a suicide attempt, victim found in car parked in garage

Complications of Surgical and Medical Care, Not Elsewhere Classified (996–999)

When a causal relationship is stated between a condition and the surgical or medical care, a code from categories 996 through 999 may be assigned. A time limit has not been identified because some complications may occur during or directly following surgery, while others may occur later during the same hospitalization or even days, weeks, or months after discharge. In some cases, documentation in the record will clearly state a complication, such as colitis due to radiation therapy. In other cases, documentation in the record will identify symptoms that may refer to a complication.

The section "Complications of Surgical and Medical Care, Not Elsewhere Classified" is subdivided into the following categories:

996 **Complications peculiar to certain specified procedures**
997 **Complications affecting specified body systems, not elsewhere classified**
998 **Other complications of procedures, not elsewhere classified**
999 **Complications of medical care, not elsewhere classified**

Classification of Complications

Complications specific to one anatomical site are classified in the chapter of ICD-9-CM for that anatomical site. All other complications are included in codes 996 through 999.

The following large exclusion note appears at the beginning of the complications section:

Complications of Surgical and Medical Care,
Not Elsewhere Classified (996–999)

Excludes: *adverse effects of medicinal agents (001.0–799.9, 995.0–995.8)*
burns from local applications and irradiation (940.0–949.5)
complications of:
  conditions for which the procedure was performed
  surgical procedures during abortion,
    labor, and delivery (630–676.9)
poisoning and toxic effects of drugs and chemicals (960.0–989.9)
postoperative conditions in which no complications
    are present, such as:
    artificial opening status (V44.0–V44.9)
    closure of external stoma (V55.0–V55.9)
    fitting of prosthetic device (V52.0–V52.9)
specified complications classified elsewhere
    anesthetic shock (995.4)
    electrolyte imbalance (276.0–276.9)
    postlaminectomy syndrome (722.80–722.83)
    postmastectomy lymphedema syndrome (457.0)
    postoperative psychosis (293.0–293.9)
    any other condition classified elsewhere in the Alphabetic
      Index when described as due to a procedure

The excludes note lists many complications/conditions that are not classified to this section. For example, adverse effects of medicinal agents are assigned to codes 001.0 through 799.9 and 995.0 through 995.89.

Category 996

Category 996 includes codes that identify complications in the use of artificial substitutes or natural sources. The large inclusion note at the beginning of this category describes procedures in which artificial substitutes or natural sources are used.

Codes 996.00–996.59 identify mechanical complications of prosthetic devices, implants, and grafts. Complications include the mechanical breakdown, displacement, leakage, mechanical obstruction, perforation, or protrusion of the device, implant, or graft.

Total joint replacement (TJR) is one of the most commonly performed and successful operations in orthopedic surgery. Success rates of greater than 90 percent in terms of implant survivorship, reduction in joint pain, and improvement in function have been reported at ten- to fifteen-year follow-up. As the population in the United States ages, and advances in technology lead to the expansion of the indications for TJR to include younger and more active patients, the prevalence of TJR is expected to increase over the next decade. While the vast majority of hip and knee replacements last for fifteen to twenty years or more, some hip and knee replacements can fail, necessitating revision surgery. Common reasons for revision joint replacement surgery include mechanical loosening of the prosthesis, dislocation of the prosthetic joint, fracture of the bone around the implant, and implant fracture or failure. To classify the mechanical reasons for revision joint replacement, ICD-9-CM diagnosis codes 996.40 through 996.49 are provided. In addition to one of these codes, the patient should also be assigned a code from the V43.60–V43.69 range to identify the joint previously replaced by prothesis.

Other reasons for revision joint replacement surgery are infection or inflammatory reactions due to internal joint prosthesis (996.66) or other complications, such as pain due to the presence of the internal joint prosthesis (996.77.)

996.4 **Mechanical complication of internal orthopedic device, implant, and graft**

Mechanical complications involving:

external (fixation) device utilizing internal screw(s),
   pin(s), or other methods of fixation
grafts of bone, cartilage, muscle, or tendon
internal (fixation) device such as nail, plate, rod, etc.

Use additional code to identify joint replaced by prosthesis (V43.60–V43.69)

Excludes:	*complications of external orthopedic device, such as:*
	pressure ulcer due to cast (707.0)

Subcategory 996.6 identifies infection and inflammatory reaction due to an internal prosthetic device, implant, and graft. The fifth-digit subclassification identifies the type of device, implant, or graft, or the organ system involved. Included under this subcategory heading is a directional note: Use additional code to identify joint (V43.60–V43.69)

996.61 **Due to cardiac device, implant, and graft**

Cardiac pacemaker or defibrillator:

electrode(s), lead(s)
pulse generator
subcutaneous pocket
Coronary artery bypass graft
Heart valve prosthesis

Subcategory 996.7 classifies other complications of internal prosthetic devices, implants, and grafts, such as embolism, fibrosis, hemorrhage, pain, stenosis, and thrombus, as well as complications not otherwise specified. Again, the fifth-digit subclassification identifies the specific device or organ system involved.

996.73   Due to renal dialysis device, implant, and graft

Code 996.8 classifies complications of transplanted organs, including failure or rejection of the transplanted organ. The specific organ is identified at the fifth-digit subclassification. An additional code should be assigned to identify the nature of the complication, such as cytomegalovirus infection.

> **EXAMPLE:**   **996.81, Complications of transplanted kidney**
> **078.5, Cytomegaloviral disease**

Code 996.9 classifies complications of a reattached extremity or body part. The fifth-digit subclassification identifies the specific extremity or body part.

996.92   Complications of reattached hand

Category 997

Category 997 includes complications of specified body systems not classified elsewhere in ICD-9-CM. The subcategories and subclassifications identify the organ system involved or the specific complication, such as hepatic failure resulting from a surgical procedure (997.4).

997.4   Gastrointestinal complications
　　　Complications of:
　　　　intestinal (internal) anastomosis and bypass, not elsewhere classified,
　　　　　except that involving urinary tract
　　Hepatic failure
　　Hepatorenal syndrome　　　} specified as due to a
　　Intestinal obstruction NOS　} procedure

　　| *Excludes:* | *gastrostomy complications (536.9–536.49)* |

*specified gastrointestinal complications
　classified elsewhere, such as:
　　blind loop syndrome (579.2)
　　colostomy and enterostomy complications (569.60–569.69)
　　gastrojejunal ulcer (534.0–534.9)
　　infection of external stoma (569.61)
　　pelvic peritoneal adhesions, female (614.6)
　　peritoneal adhesions (568.0)
　　peritoneal adhesions with obstruction (560.81)
　　postcholecystectomy syndrome (576.0)
　　postgastric surgery syndromes (564.2)*

A note at the beginning of category 997 states "Use additional code to identify complications." It serves as a reminder that an additional code should be assigned to further identify the specific complication.

EXAMPLE: **997.1, Cardiac complications**
427.31, Atrial fibrillation

Category 998

Category 998 includes other complications of procedures not classified elsewhere in ICD-9-CM. The subcategories identify the type of complication, such as postoperative shock, hemorrhage or hematoma, accidental puncture or laceration, foreign body accidentally left in operation wound or body cavity, postoperative infection, postoperative fistula, and reaction to foreign body accidentally left in operation wound or body cavity. Disruption of operation wound is classified according to whether it is an internal or external operation wound. The unspecified disruption is coded to the external operation wound code.

Category 999

Category 999 includes complications of medical care not elsewhere classified. The inclusion note at the beginning of this category identifies the types of complications included in this category. Similarly, it identifies complications classified elsewhere in ICD-9-CM.

999   Complications of medical care, not elsewhere classified
Includes: complications, not elsewhere classified, of:
dialysis (hemodialysis) (peritoneal) (renal)
extracorporeal circulation
hyperalimentation therapy
immunization
infusion
inhalation therapy
injection
inoculation
perfusion
transfusion
vaccination
ventilation therapy
 	
Excludes: *specified complications classified elsewhere*
    such as:
complications of implanted device (996.0–996.9)
contact dermatitis due to drugs (692.3)
dementia dialysis (294.8)
    transient (293.9)
dialysis disequilibrium syndrome (276.0–276.9)
poisoning and toxic effects of drugs
    and chemicals (960.0–989.9)
postvaccinal encephalitis (323.5)
water and electrolyte imbalance (276.0–276.9)

Instructions for Coding Complications

The following instructions apply when coding complications:

1. Locate the main term for the complication in the Alphabetic Index to Diseases (for example, malabsorption).

2. Check for a subterm indicating that the condition is a result of a complication of medical or surgical care.

> **Malabsorption**   579.9
> postsurgical   579.3

3. If a specific code is not identified, consult the main term "Complications" to locate an appropriate code by condition or system.

> **Complications**
> aortocoronary (bypass) graft   996.03

4. When no appropriate code can be found, assign the following nonspecific complication codes only if documentation in the health record supports their assignment:

> **Complications**
> medical care NEC   999.9
> surgical procedures   998.9

5. A second code may be assigned for more specificity if the complication code is too general.

> **997.1   Cardiac complications**
> Cardiac
>   arrest
>   insufficiency   during or resulting from
> Cardiorespiratory failure   a procedure
> Heart failure
>
> *Excludes:* *the listed conditions as long-term effects of cardiac surgery or due to the presence of cardiac prosthetic device (429.4)*

In the preceding example, a second code would be assigned to further describe the cardiac complication, such as cardiac arrest or heart failure.

Exercise 20.4

Assign ICD-9-CM codes to the following:

1. Infection from ventriculoperitoneal shunt

    _____

2. Displaced breast prosthesis

    _____

3. Leakage of mitral valve prosthesis

    _____

4. Postoperative superficial thrombophlebitis of the right leg

    _____

5. Postmastoidectomy complication

    _____

Review Exercise: Chapters 19 and 20

Assign the appropriate ICD-9-CM codes to the following:

1. Urticaria due to Tetracycline, prescribed by physician

   708.0   E946.0

2. Operative wound dehiscence

   998.32

3. Methadone overdose, suicide attempt

   965.02   E950.0

4. Air embolism

   958.0

5. Compound fracture of the tibia with open reduction and internal fixation

   823.90   79.36

6. Contusion of the cheek and forearm

   920   923.10

7. Left Colles' fracture with closed reduction

   813.41   79.02

8. Open wound of the forearm with tendon involvement

   881.20

9. Patient mixed Diuril and alcoholic beverage, which resulted in syncope, described as an accident   980.0

   974.3   E858.5   780.2

10. Severe vomiting due to Cytoxan, which is being administered for bone metastasis with unknown primary site

    535.4   E933.1

11. Dislocated hip prosthesis with closed reduction

    79.75

12. Postoperative wound infection with cellulitis, lower leg; cellulitis due to staphylococcus aureus infection

    998.59   682.6   04.11

13. Chronic cholecystitis with cholelithiasis with postoperative atelectasis; cholecystectomy with intraoperative cholangiogram

    574.10   518.0   51.22   87.53

14. Concussion with no loss of consciousness, with abrasion of the elbow and foot

    850.0   913.0   917.0

15. Attempted suicide with 15 Tylenol (acetaminophen) and 10 ampicillin; depression

    965.4   E950.0   960.0   E950.4   311

Chapter 21

Supplementary Classifications— E Codes

External Causes of Injury and Poisoning (E800–E999)

E codes classify environmental events, circumstances, and other conditions as the cause of injuries and other adverse effects. Coding external causes of injuries and poisonings provides data for research and evaluation of injury prevention strategies. E codes capture how the injury or poisoning happened (cause), the intent (intentional, such as an assault; or unintentional, such as an accident), and the place where the event occurred.

The E Codes Supplementary Classification in the Tabular List in volume 1 of ICD-9-CM includes the following categories and section titles:

Categories	Section Titles
E800–E848	Transport Accidents
E849	Place of Occurrence
E850–E858	Accidental Poisoning by Drugs, Medicinal Substances, and Biologicals
E860–E869	Accidental Poisoning by Other Solid and Liquid Substances, Gases, and Vapors
E870–E876	Misadventures to Patients during Surgical and Medical Care
E878–E879	Surgical and Other Medical Procedures as the Cause of Abnormal Reaction of Patient, or Later Complication, without Mention of Misadventure at the Time of Procedure
E880–E888	Accidental Falls
E890–E899	Accident Caused by Fire and Flames
E900–E909	Accidents Due to Natural and Environmental Factors
E910–E915	Accidents Caused by Submersion, Suffocation, and Foreign Bodies
E916–E928	Other Accidents
E929	Late Effects of Accidental Injury
E930–E949	Drugs, Medicinal and Biological Substances Causing Adverse Effects in Therapeutic Use
E950–E959	Suicide and Self-Inflicted Injury
E960–E969	Homicide and Injury Purposely Inflicted by Other Persons
E970–E979	Legal Intervention
E980–E989	Injury Undetermined Whether Accidentally or Purposely Inflicted
E990–E999	Injury Resulting from Operations of War

E Codes as Additional Codes Only

E codes from the supplementary classification are used in addition to a code from the main chapters of ICD-9-CM classification. An E code cannot be assigned as the principal, first-listed, or the only listed diagnosis code. E codes provide additional information that may be extremely useful to public health agencies and may assist healthcare planners to determine the kinds of accidents a particular facility treats. They can identify patients who were injured in transportation accidents, fires, or national disasters, as well as in a wide variety of other situations.

Alphabetic Index

The Alphabetic Index to External Causes of Injury and Poisoning (E Code) is a separate index that follows the Table of Drugs and Chemicals in volume 2 of ICD-9-CM. The E code index is organized by main terms describing the accident, circumstance, event, or specific agent that caused the injury or other adverse effect, such as a collision, earthquake, or dog bite.

> **Fall, falling** (accidental) E888.9
>   building E916
>   burning E891.8
>   private E890.8
>   down
>   escalator E880.0
>   ladder E881.0
>   in boat, ship, watercraft E833
>   staircase E880.9
>   stairs, steps—*see* Fall, from, stairs
>   earth (with asphyxia or suffocation (by pressure)
>   (*see also* Earth, falling) E913.3

Exercise 21.1

Identify the external event that caused the following injuries and assign E codes only:

1. Fractured radius resulting from accidental fall into hole

   E883.9

2. Fracture of humerus due to fall from cliff

   E884.1

3. Firecracker injury with second-degree burn of face

   E923.0

4. Burn of left palm from splashing grease

   E924.0

5. Hematoma of buttocks from tackle during football game

   E886.0

Use of E Codes

The use of E codes in many healthcare facilities is optional, except for categories E930 through E949, Drugs, Medicinal and Biological Substances Causing Adverse Effects in Therapeutic Use. (Refer to chapter 20 for the use of these E codes.) Each healthcare facility must decide whether it needs the information the E codes provide. Today, information on industrial accidents may be of great value to hospitals planning to market healthcare plans to employers in their market area.

A point to remember: Some states mandate the use of some or all E codes. Always check with the policy of the facility or state mandate where the coding is being done to confirm the use of E codes.

An E code may be used as an additional code in any category if documentation in the health record supports that use. However, an E code cannot be assigned as a principal or first-listed diagnosis.

Guidelines for Coding External Causes of Injuries, Poisonings, and Adverse Effects of Drugs (E Codes)

The guidelines discussed in the following subsections apply when coding and collecting E codes from health records in hospitals, outpatient clinics, emergency departments, other ambulatory care settings, and physicians' offices, except when other specific guidelines apply.

General E Code Guidelines

An E code may be used with any code in the range of 001 through V85.4 that indicates an injury, poisoning, or adverse effect due to an external cause. General guidelines include:

- Assign the appropriate E code for all initial encounters or treatments of an injury, poisoning, or adverse effect of drugs—but not for subsequent treatment.

- Use a late effect E code for subsequent visits when a late effect of the initial injury or poisoning is being treated. There is no late effect E code for adverse effects of drugs.

- Do not use a late effect E code for subsequent visits for follow-up care (for example, to assess healing, to receive rehabilitative treatment) of the injury or poisoning when no late effect of the injury has been documented.

- Use the full range of E codes to completely describe the cause, intent, and place of occurrence, if applicable, for all injuries, poisonings, and adverse effects of drugs.

- Assign as many E codes as necessary to fully explain each external cause. If only one E code can be recorded, assign the one most related to the principal diagnosis.

- Select appropriate E codes by referring to the Index to External Causes and by reading inclusion and exclusion notes in the Tabular List.

Multiple-Cause Coding Guidelines for E Codes

If two or more events cause separate injuries, an E code should be assigned for each cause. The E code to be listed first will be selected on the following basis:

1. E codes for child and adult abuse take priority over all other E codes, except as described in the child and adult abuse guidelines below.

2. E codes for terrorism events take priority over all other E codes except child and adult abuse.

3. E codes for cataclysmic events take priority over all other E codes, except for child and adult abuse and terrorism.

4. E codes for transport accidents take priority over all other E codes, except for cataclysmic events and for child and adult abuse and terrorism.

The first E code listed should correspond to the cause of the most serious diagnosis due to an assault, accident, or self-harm, following the order of the hierarchy just listed.

Child and Adult Abuse Guidelines for E Codes

When the cause of an injury or neglect is intentional child or adult abuse (995.5–995.59, 995.80–995.85), the first E code listed should be assigned from categories E960 through E968, Homicide and Injury Purposely Inflicted by Other Persons (except category E967). An E code from category E967, Child and adult battering and other maltreatment, should be added as an additional E code to identify the perpetrator, if known. The title of category E967 was recently changed to "Perpetrator of Child and Adult Abuse." Additionally, inclusion terms for codes E967.0 and E967.2 include the partner of the child's parent or guardian. An inclusion term for code E967.3 was added to better explain the relationship between perpetrator and victim. E967.3 is used when the perpetrator is the spouse, ex-spouse, partner, or ex-partner of the victim.

In cases of neglect when the intent is determined to be accidental, the first E code listed should be E904.0, Abandonment or neglect of infants and helpless persons.

Guidelines for Unknown or Suspected Intent

If the intent (accident, self-harm, assault) of the cause of an injury or poisoning is unknown or unspecified, assign codes from categories E980 through E989, Injury Undetermined Whether Accidentally or Purposely Inflicted.

If the intent (accident, self-harm, assault) of the cause of an injury or poisoning is questionable, probable, or suspected, also assign codes from categories E980 through E989.

Undetermined Cause

When the intent of an injury or poisoning is known, but the cause is unknown, use code E928.9, Unspecified accident; E958.9, Suicide and self-inflicted injury by unspecified means; or E968.9, Assault by unspecified means. These E codes should be used only rarely because documentation in the health record, in both inpatient and outpatient settings, should normally provide sufficient detail to determine the cause of the injury.

Definitions and Instructions Related to Transport Accidents

At the beginning of the E code supplementary classification in the Tabular List, definitions and examples related to transport accidents are given. Carefully review this material to ensure accurate E code assignment.

Exercise 21.2

Using the definitions and instructions in the E code supplementary classification related to transport accidents, classify the following:

1. Snowmobile
    E820.9

2. Person changing a tire on a vehicle
    E818.2 ?

3. Parachute
    E843.7

4. Tractor accident on the highway
    E816.9 ?

5. Baby carriage
    E829.9

Place of Occurrence E Codes

Category E849, Place of occurrence, is provided to note the place where an injury or poisoning occurred. This category describes only the place where the event occurred, not the patient's activity at the time of the event.

Code E849 and its subdivisions are italicized in the Tabular List to indicate that this code is not to be used for primary coding. The E code identifying the cause of the accident, event, or adverse effect must be assigned first, followed by the place of occurrence E code, where applicable.

Do not use E849.9 if the place of occurrence is not stated. Only code the specific place of occurrence as documented in the patient's record.

Place of occurrence E codes can be located in the Index to External Causes under the main term "Accident occurring (at) (in)."

Exercise 21.3

Assign all the appropriate E codes to the following:

1. Choked on food at riding school
    E911, E849.4

2. Hit by baseball on baseball field
    E917.0, E849.4

3. Slipped on slippery surface at store
    E885.9, E849.6

4. Hit by falling tree in forest
    E916, E849.8

5. Developed swimmer's cramp in swimming pool of private home
    E910.2, E849.0

Classification of Death and Injury Resulting from Terrorism

After the September 11, 2001 terrorist events, an urgent need was recognized for a classification that can be used to characterize and statistically classify, report, and analyze injuries, sequelae of injuries, and deaths associated with such events. The following E codes went into effect October 1, 2002.

The use of these E codes is described in the terrorism guidelines added to the ICD-9-CM Official Guidelines for Coding and Reporting, effective October 1, 2002.

When the cause of an injury is identified by the Federal Bureau of Investigation (FBI) as terrorism, the first-listed E code should be a code from category E979, Terrorism. The definition of terrorism employed by the FBI is found in the inclusion note at E979 in the Tabular List. The terrorism E code is the only E code that should be assigned. Additional E codes from the assault categories should not be assigned.

An E code for terrorism should not be assigned if the cause of an injury is only suspected to be the result of terrorism. Instead, a code in the range of E codes should be assigned based on the circumstances as documented.

Code E979.9 is assigned for the secondary effects of terrorism for conditions occurring subsequent to the terrorist event. This code should not be assigned for conditions that are due to the initial terrorist act.

The terrorism subclassification went into effect October 1, 2002, and includes the following E codes:

E979.0   **Terrorism involving explosion of marine weapons**
E979.1   **Terrorism involving destruction of aircraft**
E979.2   **Terrorism involving other explosions and fragments**
E979.3   **Terrorism involving fires, conflagration, and hot substances**
E979.4   **Terrorism involving firearms**
E979.5   **Terrorism involving nuclear weapons**
E979.6   **Terrorism involving biological weapons**
E979.7   **Terrorism involving chemical weapons**
E979.8   **Terrorism involving other means**
E979.9   **Terrorism, secondary effects**

Codes E999.0, Late effect of injury due to war operations, and E999.1, Late effect of injury due to terrorism, can also be used as applicable.

Fourth-Digit Subdivisions

Fourth digits are provided in many E code categories to identify the injured person. Those categories requiring fourth digits are preceded by a section mark to refer to a footnote at the bottom of the page. Fourth-digit subdivisions for the external cause (E) code appear immediately after the Alphabetic Index to External Causes. The fourth-digit subdivisions also appear in the Tabular List of E codes.

The fourth-digit subdivisions are specific to each of the following E code category groups:

Railway Accidents (E800–E807)
Motor Vehicle Traffic and Nontraffic Accidents (E810–E825)
Other Road Vehicle Accidents (E826–E829)
Water Transport Accidents (E830–E838)
Air and Space Transport Accidents (E840–E845)

For example, the fourth digit for a pedestrian is 2 in E800 through E807 and 0 in E826 through E829.

Exercise 21.4

Assign all appropriate E codes to the following:

1. Fall from train by railway passenger

   E804.1

   29.33

2. Pedestrian knocked down by an animal-drawn vehicle

   E827.7   ? E827.0

3. Passenger fell from ship gangplank onto dock

   E835.3   ? E834.3

4. Rider thrown from horse

   E828.5   E828.2

5. Passenger hit by boat while waterskiing

   E838.5   E838.4

E Codes for Late Effects

When the condition being coded is a late effect of an illness or injury, the E code for the late effect must be assigned rather than a current E code, if the healthcare facility assigns E codes. The E codes for external causes of late effects include:

E929   **Late effects of accidental injury**
E959   **Late effects of self-inflicted injury**
E969   **Late effects of injury purposely inflicted by other person**
E977   **Late effects of injury due to legal intervention**
E989   **Late effects of injury, undetermined whether accidentally or purposely inflicted**
E999   **Late effect of injury due to war operations**

Coding Guidelines for Late Effects of External Causes

The following guidelines apply when coding late effects of external causes:

- Late effect E codes exist for injuries and poisonings, but not for adverse effects of drugs, misadventures, and surgical complications.

- A late effect E code (E929, E959, E977, E969, E977, E989, or E999.1) should be used with any report of a late effect or sequela resulting from a previous injury or poisoning (905–909).

- A late effect E code should never be used with a related current nature of injury code.

- Use a late effect E code for subsequent visits when a late effect of the initial injury or poisoning is being treated. There is no late effect E code for adverse effect of drugs. Do not use a late effect E code for subsequent visits for follow-up care (for example, to assess healing, to receive rehabilitative therapy) of the injury or poisoning when no late effect of the injury has been documented.

Coding of Late Effects

Typically, patients with late effects are coded according to the following criteria:

- Residual effect or the condition the patient has at present, found in the Alphabetic Index to Diseases

- Late effect or the condition the patient originally had that produced the residual, found in the Alphabetic Index to Diseases under the term "Late effect"

- E code for late effect of original accident or event, found in the Index to External Causes under the term "Late effect"

A detailed discussion of the coding of late effects is presented in chapter 22 of this book.

Exercise 21.5

Assign all appropriate ICD-9-CM codes, including E codes, to the following:

1. Osteomyelitis of femur due to an old compound fracture resulting from an automobile accident six months ago in which patient was the driver

   730.25, 821.10, E929.0

2. Convulsions due to an old skull fracture sustained when patient fell from a ladder two years ago

   780.39, 803.00, E929.3

3. Deviated nasal septum due to an old nasal fracture; patient hit with a ball while playing baseball

   470, 802.0, E917.0

4. Scars of arm due to an old burn sustained in a house fire three years ago

   709.2, E929.4

5. Anoxic brain damage due to gunshot wound of the head sustained four years ago; reported as a homicide attempt

   348.1   E965.4

Chapter 22

Late Effects

Definition of Late Effects

A late effect is the residual effect, or condition produced and present today, that remains after the acute phase of an illness or injury has terminated. A residual is the temporary or permanent healthcare problem that follows the acute phase of an illness or injury. The code for the acute phase of an illness or injury that led to the late effect condition is never used with a code for the late effect.

Coding of late effects generally requires two codes sequenced in the following order: The code for the condition or nature of the late effect that is present today, known as the residual, is sequenced first. The code for the late effect or the cause of the residual is sequenced second.

> **EXAMPLE:** Hemiplegia following old cerebral thrombosis
> Scarring following third-degree burn
> Traumatic arthritis following fracture
>
> The hemiplegia, scarring, and traumatic arthritis represent residuals of a previous illness or injury. The cerebral thrombosis, third-degree burn, and fracture represent the causes of the residuals, or what is referred to as the late effect.

An exception to the above guideline would apply in those instances where the code for late effect is followed by a manifestation code identified in the Tabular List and title or the late effect code has been expanded (at the fourth and fifth-digit levels) to include the manifestation(s). The code for the acute phase of an illness or injury that led to the late effect is never used with a code for the late effect.

Late Effects of Cerebrovascular Disease

Coding of late effects of cerebrovascular disease is an example of an exception to the general rule that late effects require two codes as listed above. This includes cerebrovascular accident (CVA), such as cerebral thrombosis or intracranial hemorrhage. Category 438, Late effects of cerebrovascular disease, provides combination codes that identify both the residual (cognitive deficits, aphasia, hemiplegia) and the cause (the cerebrovascular accident), which was previously coded to categories 430–437 when the acute episode occurred. To locate the combination codes for late effects following CVAs, the main term to be used in the Alphabetic Index to Diseases is "Late, effects, (of) cerebrovascular disease," with numerous subterms that identify the current residual condition. More than one code in category 438 may be used to describe a patient with multiple residual conditions present after the acute phase of the CVA is treated.

Late Effect Terminology

The following are examples of terminology found in diagnostic statements that indicate late effects:

- Residuals of
- Old
- Sequela of
- Late
- Due to or following previous illness or injury

Passage of Time and Residual Effects

Sometimes the diagnosis will indicate that sufficient time has passed from the occurrence of the acute illness or injury to the development of the residual effect. For example, a fracture in a young person should heal in four to six weeks; in an older person, in six to twelve weeks. When healing does not occur, the physician may indicate the patient has a nonunion fracture that requires a late effect code.

There is no time limit or set period during which a condition may be designated a residual effect. It may be apparent early, as in a cerebrovascular accident, or it may occur months or years later, as with a previous injury, such as a fracture.

Exercise 22.1

Circle the residual and write in the cause on the following blank for each of the following diagnoses:

1. (Contracture left heel tendons) due to poliomyelitis

   _____ poliomyelitis _____

2. (Mild mental retardation) following viral encephalitis

   _____ viral encephalitis _____

3. (Seizure disorder) secondary to intracranial abscess

   _____ intracranial abscess _____

4. (Aphasia) due to old cerebrovascular accident

   _____ cerebrovascular accident _____

5. (Paralysis of arm) due to old radial nerve injury

   _____ radial nerve injury _____

Coding of Late Effects

ICD-9-CM contains the following limited number of late effect codes to identify the cause of the late effect:

137	Late effects of tuberculosis
138	Late effects of acute poliomyelitis
139	Late effects of other infectious and parasitic diseases
268.1	Rickets, late effects
326	Late effects of intracranial abscess or pyogenic infection
438	Late effects of cerebrovascular disease
677	Late effect of complication of pregnancy, childbirth, and the puerperium
905	Late effects of musculoskeletal and connective tissue injuries
906	Late effects of injuries to skin and subcutaneous tissues
907	Late effects of injuries to the nervous system
908	Late effects of other and unspecified injuries
909	Late effects of other and unspecified external causes
997.6	Amputation stump complication

Late effects of specific diseases may be found in chapters in ICD-9-CM on specific diseases. For example, late effects of cerebrovascular disease, category 438, is included in the chapter on diseases of the circulatory system.

Alphabetic Index Entry

The code for the cause of the late effect can be located in the Alphabetic Index to Diseases under the main term "Late" and the subterm "effect(s) (of)."

Late—*see also* condition
    effect(s) (of)—*see also* condition
    cerebrovascular disease (conditions classifiable to
    430–437) 438.9
        with
            alterations of sensations 438.6
            aphasia 438.11
            apraxia 438.81
            ataxia 438.84
            cognitive deficits 438.0
            disturbances of vision 438.7
            dysphagia 438.82
            dysphasia 438.12
            facial droop 438.83
            facial weakness 438.83
            hemiplegia/hemiparesis
                affecting
                    dominant side 438.21
                    nondominant side 438.22
                    unspecified side 438.20

Coding Guideline

The residual condition or nature of the late effect is sequenced first, followed by the cause of the late effect. However, in a few instances the code for the late effect is followed by a manifestation code identified in the Tabular List. In these instances, the title or the late effect code has been expanded at the fourth- and fifth-digit levels to include the manifestations.

> **EXAMPLE:** Scar of the right hand secondary to a laceration sustained two years ago: 709.2, Scar conditions and fibrosis of skin; 906.1, Late effect of open wound of extremities, without mention of tendon injury

> **EXAMPLE:** Dysphasia secondary to old cerebrovascular accident sustained one year ago: 438.12, Late effect of cerebrovascular disease, speech and language deficits, dysphasia

Coding Guideline Exceptions

Exceptions to the preceding coding guideline are as follows:

1. If the health record does not identify the specific residual effect, code only the late effect code.

    > **EXAMPLE:** Documentation in the health record states "late effect of polio": 138, Late effects of acute poliomyelitis

2. If the Alphabetic Index to Diseases indicates a different sequence, follow the directions of the index.

    > **EXAMPLE:** Scoliosis due to poliomyelitis during childhood
    > The following entries appear in the Alphabetic Index to Diseases:

    > **Scoliosis** (acquired) (postural) 737.30
    >   congenital 754.2
    >   due to or associated with . . .
    >   poliomyelitis 138 *[737.43]*

    > The Alphabetic Index directs the coder to sequence first the late effect code (138), followed by the residual *[747.43]*, which is in italicized print and, therefore, should not be reported as the principal diagnosis or first-listed code.

    > 138   **Late effects of acute poliomyelitis**
    > *737.43* *Scoliosis associated with other conditions*

3. If ICD-9-CM does not provide a code to describe the cause of the late effect, assign a code only for the residual. Conditions that are stated to be due to previous surgery are not considered late effects. Depending on the circumstances, a history-of code or surgical complication code may be reported.

Residual Effect Not Stated

The late effect code can be assigned by itself when the diagnostic statement indicating a late effect does not include the residual condition.

> EXAMPLE: Late effect of rickets (Rickets developed in childhood, patient is now an adult.)
>
> Only code 268.1, Rickets, late effect, is assigned because the specific effect(s) is (are) not identified.

Residual Effect Directed by Alphabetic Index

In some cases, when the residual is referenced in the Alphabetic Index to Diseases, the code for a late effect is listed first, followed by a manifestation code in italics and within slanted brackets. In such an instance, the Alphabetic Index takes precedence, with the code for the late effect sequenced first, followed by the code for the residual.

> EXAMPLE: Kyphosis due to poliomyelitis during childhood
>
> Codes 138, Late effects of acute poliomyelitis, and 737.41, *Kyphosis associated with other conditions,* are assigned. The code for the residual (kyphosis) is sequenced after the late effect code as indicated in the Alphabetic Index:

Kyphosis (acquired) (postural) 737.10
   due to or associated with . . .
      poliomyelitis 138 *[737.41]*

Exercise 22.2

Assign ICD-9-CM codes to the following residuals and late effects. It is not necessary to assign E codes in these exercises.

1. Epileptic seizures due to previous encephalitis

    _345.90 , +39.0 326_

2. Malunion fracture of humerus due to old fracture

    _733.81 , 905.2_

3. Residuals of old gunshot wound of leg

    _891.0 909.4 906.1_

4. Paraplegia from previous laceration of spinal cord

    _344.1 , 907.2_

5. Keloid of arm due to old crushing injury

    _701.4 , 906.4_

6. Aphasia due to cerebrovascular accident one year ago

    _438.11_

7. Traumatic arthritis following fracture of left ankle

    _716.17 , 905.4_

8. Scarring due to third-degree burn of left leg

    _709.2 , 906.7_

9. Contracture of right wrist due to poliomyelitis

    _718.43 138_

10. Irradiation hypothyroidism following previous radiation therapy for carcinoma of the head and neck [Do not code the carcinoma in this example.]

    _244.1 , 909.2_

Chapter 23

Supplementary Classifications— V Codes

Factors Influencing Health Status and Contact with Health Services (V01–V84)

Commonly referred to as V codes, categories V01 through V85 of ICD-9-CM are included in "Supplementary Classification of Factors Influencing Health Status and Contact with Health Services," in the Tabular List in volume 1.

V code classifications are available for the following situations:

- When a person who is currently not sick uses health services for some purpose, such as acting as a donor, receiving prophylactic care such as an inoculation or vaccination, or receiving counseling on health-related issues.

  EXAMPLE: Physician office visit for prophylactic flu shot: V04.81, Need for prophylactic vaccination and inoculation against influenza

- When a person with a resolving disease or injury or one with a chronic, long-term condition requiring continuous care encounters the healthcare system for specific aftercare of that disease or injury (for example, dialysis for renal disease, chemotherapy for malignancy, or cast change). A diagnosis or symptoms code should be used whenever a current, acute diagnosis is being treated or a sign or symptom is being studied.

  EXAMPLE: Patient is admitted for chemotherapy for acute lymphocytic leukemia: V58.1, Encounter for chemotherapy; 204.00, Acute lymphocytic leukemia; 99.25, Chemotherapy

- When circumstances or problems influence a person's health status but are not in themselves a current illness or injury.

  EXAMPLE: Patient visits physician's office with a complaint of chest pain with an undetermined cause; patient is status post open-heart surgery for mitral valve replacement, six months ago: 786.50, Chest pain, unspecified; V43.3, Heart valve replaced by other means

- For newborns, to indicate birth status.

  EXAMPLE: Single newborn delivered via cesarean section: V30.01, Single live-born delivered by cesarean delivery

V codes are assigned more frequently in hospital ambulatory care departments and other primary care sites, such as physicians' offices, than in acute, inpatient facilities. V codes may be used as either a first-listed (principal diagnosis code in the inpatient setting) or secondary code depending on the circumstances of the encounter. Certain V codes may only be used as first listed, others only as secondary codes.

V codes are diagnosis codes and indicate a reason for a healthcare encounter. They are not procedure codes. A procedure code must be assigned in addition to the diagnosis V code to indicate a procedure was performed.

The ICD-9-CM Official Guidelines for Coding and Reporting include an extensive section addressing the use of V codes and their intended purposes.

V Code Categories and Section Titles

The V code supplementary classification contains the following categories and section titles:

Categories	Section Titles
V01–V06	Persons with Potential Health Hazards Related to Communicable Diseases
V07–V09	Persons with Need for Isolation, Other Potential Health Hazards and Prophylactic Measures
V10–V19	Persons with Potential Health Hazards Related to Personal and Family History
V20–V29	Persons Encountering Health Services in Circumstances Related to Reproduction and Development
V30–V39	Liveborn Infants According to Type of Birth
V40–V49	Persons with a Condition Influencing Their Health Status
V50–V59	Persons Encountering Health Services for Specific Procedures and Aftercare
V60–V69	Persons Encountering Health Services in Other Circumstances
V70–V84	Persons without Reported Diagnosis Encountered during Examination and Investigation of Individuals and Populations
V85	Body Mass Index

Coders should review the multiple guidelines in ICD-9-CM Official Guidelines for Coding and Reporting, which was updated April 1, 2005. Within Section I, ICD-9-CM Conventions, General Coding Guidelines, and Chapter-Specific Guidelines, specific guidelines appear for V codes. Detailed information about the intent and appropriate use of V codes is provided in Section I, C-18, Supplemental Classification of Factors Influencing Health Status and Contact with Health Services (V Codes).

Main Terms

V codes are indexed in the Alphabetic Index to Diseases along with codes for diseases, conditions, and symptoms. It is necessary, however, to become familiar with the main terms in the Alphabetic Index to Diseases that are related to V codes. First, look for terms that describe the reason for the encounter or admission. (The terms documented in the health record will often not lead to the appropriate code.)

Then ask: Why is the patient receiving services?

EXAMPLE: The health record states closure of colostomy: V55.3, Attention to colostomy; 46.52, Closure of stoma of large intestine

The statement in the preceding example requires a V code (V55.3) because the patient was admitted for attention to an artificial opening. In addition, a procedure code (46.52) should be assigned for the closure.

Figure 23.1 shows how the main terms in the Alphabetic Index to Diseases lead to V codes.

Figure 23.1.   Main terms leading to V codes

Admission (encounter)	Donor	Pregnancy
Aftercare	Encounter for	Problem
Attention to	Examination	Prophylactic
Boarder	Exposure	Replacement by artificial or
Care (of)	Fitting (of)	mechanical device or prosthesis of
Carrier (suspected) of	Follow up	Resistance, resistant
Checking	Health	Screening
Chemotherapy	Healthy	Status (post)
Contact	History (personal) of	Supervision (of)
Contraception, contraceptives	Maintenance	Test(s)
Convalescence	Maladjustment	Therapy
Counseling	Newborn	Transplant(ed)
Dependence	Observation	Unavailability of medical facilities
Dialysis	Outcome of delivery	Vaccination

Persons with Potential Health Hazards Related to Communicable Diseases (V01–V06) and Persons with Need for Isolation, Other Potential Health Hazards and Prophylactic Measures (V07–V09)

Categories V01 through V06 of the V code supplementary classification are assigned when a patient has come in contact with, or has been exposed to, a communicable disease and is in need of prophylactic vaccination and inoculation against a disease. The person does not show any signs or symptoms of the disease he or she was exposed to or came in contact with.

Category V01, Contact with or Exposure to Communicable Diseases

The V01 category codes for contact and exposure to communicable disease may be used as the first-listed code to explain an encounter for testing. However, these codes may be used more commonly as a secondary code to identify a potential health risk.

The status codes in category V02 indicate that the patient is either a carrier or suspected carrier of an infectious disease but currently does not exhibit the symptoms of the disease. Status codes in the V code classification are informational because the conditions they describe may affect the course of treatment. Remember, "status" is different from "history" in ICD-9-CM. The history codes in the V code classification indicate the patient no longer has the disease.

Categories V03–V06, Need for Prophylactic Vaccination and Inoculation

Categories V03–V06 are typically used to describe outpatient encounters for inoculations and vaccinations. The patient is being seen to receive a prophylactic inoculation against a disease.

A procedure code must also be used to show the inoculation occurred. Vaccinations and inoculation codes may be used as secondary codes during well-baby or well-child care visits if the service was given as part of routine preventive healthcare.

These codes are located in the Alphabetic Index under the main terms "Contact," "Exposure," "Prophylactic," and "Vaccination."

> **EXAMPLE:** Exposure to rubella: V01.4, Contact with or exposure to rubella

> **EXAMPLE:** Vaccination against diphtheria: V03.5, Need for prophylactic vaccination and inoculation against diphtheria alone

Category V08, Asymptomatic Human Immunodeficiency Virus (HIV) Infection Status

Category V08, Asymptomatic human immunodeficiency virus [HIV] infection status, is also discussed in chapter 4 of this book. The V08 code indicates the patient has tested positive for the HIV but has not manifested symptoms of the human immunodeficiency disease or AIDS.

Category V09, Infection with Drug-Resistant Microorganisms

The category V09, Infection with drug-resistant microorganisms, should be used as an additional code to indicate the presence of drug resistance of an infectious organism for infectious conditions classified elsewhere. Sequence the infection code first and then the V09 code. V09 codes are to be used when the documentation in the health record indicates that a patient's infection has a known causative bacteria or other organism that is resistant to the medication therapy administered. Documentation may exist that the patient has methicillin-resistant staphylococcus aureus (MRSA) as the causative organism of an infection. This is coded with ICD-9-CM subcategory code V09.0. MRSA, unfortunately, is a rather common hospital-acquired infection. Subcategory code V09.8 is used frequently to identify patients with an infection with microorganisms resistant to other specified drugs, such as Vancomycin-resistant organisms. Examples of this are Vancomycin (glycopeptide) intermediate staphylococcus aureus (VISA/GISA), Vancomycin-resistant enterococcus (VRE), or Vancomycin-resistant staphylococcus aureus (VRSA/GRSA). The infection resistance codes are indexed under the main term "Resistance, resistant (to) followed by the drug name."

> **EXAMPLE:** Staphylococcus aureus infection resistant to penicillin medication: 041.11, Staphylococcus aureus; V09.0, Infection with microorganisms resistant to penicillins

Persons with Potential Health Hazards Related to Personal and Family History (V10–V19)

The word *history* as used with all V codes may not be consistent with the intent of the word *history* when used by a physician to describe a patient's condition.

Personal history in ICD-9-CM means the patient's past medical condition no longer exists and the patient is not receiving any treatment for the condition. However, the information is important because the condition has the potential for recurrence and the patient may require continued monitoring. A physician may use the word *history* to describe a current condition the patient is being treated for, such as history of diabetes mellitus or history of hypertension.

If the patient is receiving treatment for the condition, it would not be classified as a "history" code in ICD-9-CM.

Family history codes in ICD-9-CM, categories V16–V19, are used when a patient's family member(s) has a particular disease that puts the patient at higher risk of contracting the same condition. Physicians generally mean the same thing when using the term *family history.*

Personal history codes are frequently used in conjunction with follow-up V codes and family history V codes, as well as screening V codes, to explain the reason for the visit or diagnostic testing. These codes are important information as their presence may alter the type of treatment the patient receives.

Categories V10 through V19 include codes for personal and family histories of malignant neoplasms and other health problems. The personal history of malignant neoplasm (V10) category includes primary cancer sites only. **Note:** There are no personal history of secondary neoplasm sites or carcinoma in situ sites. The instructional notes listed under each subcategory refer to specific code ranges for primary malignancies categories (categories 140–195.) Secondary and CA in situ malignancies are excluded from this range of codes.

A patient with leukemia or lymphoma in remission should be classified to the 200–208 categories instead of the V codes in this range. The history of leukemia or lymphatic or hematopoietic neoplasms codes in the V10.6 and V10.7 subcategories means the patient is completely cured of the disease.

Category V12, Personal history of certain other diseases has been expanded over the past several years to include specific conditions that have the potential to affect future healthcare services. History of infections of the central nervous system (V12.42), history of circulatory disorders (V12.50–V12.59), and history of pneumonia (V12.61) codes enable the tracking of specific conditions over the lifetime of the patient.

History of urinary (tract) infections (V13.02) and history of nephrotic syndrome (V13.03) can be relevant when similar conditions are currently present. Codes within the V13.1 and V13.2 subcategories describe a woman who has had a problem during previous pregnancies but currently is not pregnant. Other codes in the V13 category should be used cautiously because the word *history* may be misinterpreted. For example, rarely does a person have a history of arthritis (V13.4) or a history of a congenital anomaly (V13.6). Instead, these are lifelong conditions that the physician may document as "history" while actually intending to describe the patient's current health status.

Category V14 and code V15.0 are exceptions to the general rule that history codes mean the condition is no longer present. A person who has had an allergic reaction to food or a substance is always considered allergic to that substance. These V codes indicate that the person is not currently exhibiting an allergic reaction but, instead, has the potential for a reaction if exposed to the substance in the future.

A patient with a history of fall(s) or identified as at risk for falling can be classified with code V15.88. This code is used to identify patients at risk for falling or who have a history of falls with or without subsequent injuries. The code is not limited to a specific age group of patients. However, falls are an important public health problem affecting about one third of adults age 65 and older each year. About 20 to 30 percent of those who fall will suffer moderate to severe injuries, including hip and other fractures and head trauma. Adults aged 75 or older who fall are more likely to be admitted to a long-term care facility for a year or longer. In this same population, over 60 percent of deaths are from falls. The code V15.88 can be used to identify patients who require closer monitoring to prevent falls, to justify specific diagnostic or therapeutic services to identify causes of falling, or to order preventive evaluation or services.

These V codes are indexed under "History (personal) of" in the Alphabetic Index. Note the subterm "family" is indented under "history (personal) of" and is the point of reference for familial conditions.

EXAMPLE: Personal history of breast carcinoma: V10.3 (describes a condition coded to 174 or 175 when present and treated)

EXAMPLE: Personal history of allergy to penicillin: V14.0, Personal history of allergy to penicillin

EXAMPLE: Family history of diabetes: V18.0, Family history of diabetes mellitus

EXAMPLE: Personal history of noncompliance with medical treatment: V15.81, Personal history of noncompliance with medical treatment

Persons Encountering Health Services in Circumstances Related to Reproduction and Development (V20–V29)

Categories V20–V29 include codes for health supervision of infant or child (V20), constitutional states in development (V21), supervision of normal and high-risk pregnancies (V22 and V23), postpartum care (V24), contraceptive management (V25) and surveillance (V25.4), sterilization (V25.2), procreative management (V26), outcome of delivery (V27), antenatal screening (V28), and observation and evaluation of newborn for suspected condition not found (V29).

Category V22, Normal Pregnancy

Category V22 is assigned for supervision of a pregnancy. Codes V22.0, Supervision of normal first pregnancy, and V22.1, Supervision of normal subsequent pregnancies, are generally used in outpatient settings and for routine prenatal visits. When a complication of the pregnancy is present, the code for that condition is assigned rather than a code from category V22. These codes are not used with any other pregnancy code in chapter 11 of ICD-9-CM because the V22 code indicates the patient is pregnant and healthy, while the chapter 11 codes indicate an obstetrical problem or condition exists. Codes V22.0 and V22.1 are indexed under "Pregnancy, supervision (of) (for)" in the Alphabetic Index to Diseases.

Code V22.2, Pregnant state, incidental, would be assigned as an additional code only if a pregnant patient was seen for a reason unrelated to the pregnancy. It is the physician's responsibility to document that the pregnancy is in no way complicating the reason for the visit or the nonobstetrical condition currently being treated. Otherwise, a code from chapter 11 in ICD-9-CM is used. Code V22.2 is indexed under the main term "Pregnancy" in the Alphabetic Index.

EXAMPLE: Patient seen in the emergency room with a sprained wrist; doctor states the patient is also 30 weeks pregnant, but the pregnancy is not affected: 842.00, Sprains and strains of unspecified site of wrist; V22.2, Pregnant state, incidental

Category V23, Supervision of High-Risk Pregnancy

Category V23 provides information on conditions that may add risk to a present pregnancy. A code from V23 can be assigned as a principal or first-listed diagnosis or as an additional code. A code from chapter 11 in ICD-9-CM can be assigned with a code from category V23. Typically these codes are used for prenatal outpatient visits. Code V23.7, Insufficient prenatal care, may be assigned to patients who had little or no prenatal care. Healthcare providers must define "insufficient" prenatal care and consistently capture this code for the information to be valuable. Codes within the V23.8 subcategories identify elderly (35 years or older) or very young (less than 16 years) pregnant females whose age and current pregnancy make them high risk for problems and thus worthy of close monitoring. The V23 category codes are indexed under the main terms "Pregnancy, supervision (of) (for)" and "Pregnancy, management affected by" in the Alphabetic Index.

EXAMPLE:	Pregnancy, 19-week gestation with history of infertility: V23.0, Pregnancy with history of infertility
EXAMPLE:	Full term with intrauterine death, spontaneous delivery; no prenatal care received during pregnancy: 656.41, Intrauterine death; V23.7, Insufficient prenatal care; V27.1, Single stillborn; 73.59, Other manually assisted delivery

Category V24, Postpartum Care and Examination

Category V24 is used primarily in the outpatient setting for uncomplicated follow-up during the postpartum period. Code V24.0 is the principal diagnosis when the mother delivers outside the hospital prior to admission and is admitted for routine postpartum care and no complications are noted. If a postpartum complication is found, however, the appropriate pregnancy diagnosis code is assigned rather than a code from category V24. Category V24 codes are indexed under "Postpartum, observation" in the Alphabetic Index.

EXAMPLE:	Visit to physician for routine postpartum exam; no complications were noted: V24.2, Routine postpartum follow-up
EXAMPLE:	Patient delivered at home and admitted to hospital with postpartum hemorrhage: 666.14, Other immediate postpartum hemorrhage

Category V25, Encounter for Contraceptive Management

Category V25 includes codes for contraceptive management, such as general contraceptive counseling and advice, insertion of an intrauterine contraceptive device, menstrual extraction, and surveillance of previously prescribed contraceptive methods. Codes from this category are indexed under "Contraception, contraceptive" in the Alphabetic Index.

EXAMPLE:	Visit to physician for prescription of birth control pills: V25.01, Prescription of oral contraceptives

Code V25.2, Sterilization, is often assigned as an additional diagnosis when a sterilization procedure is performed during the same admission as a delivery. It may also be assigned as a principal diagnosis when the admission is solely for sterilization.

EXAMPLE:	Spontaneous delivery of full-term live infant with tubal ligation performed the day after delivery: 650, Normal delivery; V27.0, Outcome of delivery, single liveborn; V25.2, Sterilization; 73.59, Other manually assisted delivery; 66.39, Other bilateral destruction or occlusion of fallopian tube
EXAMPLE:	Patient desires sterilization; tubal ligation performed: V25.2, Sterilization; 66.39, Other bilateral destruction or occlusion of fallopian tube

Category V26, Procreative Management

Procreative management describes healthcare services related to producing an offspring. Services related to genetic testing and infertility services can be described with these codes. Screening for genetic carrier status is becoming more commonplace to identify individuals for certain serious genetic disease. For example, a couple may be screened either preconception or early in pregnancy to determine carrier status. If both partners are carriers, different pregnancy management may be instituted. Carrier status screening has become the professional standard of care for cystic fibrosis, Canavan disease, hemoglobinopathies, and Tay-Sachs disease. As most of the individuals are noncarriers, it is inappropriate to use disease codes to describe the screening encounter; instead, code V26.31 is appropriate. Other codes within subcategory V26.3 identify encounters for genetic counseling and other genetic testing.

Healthcare encounters for reversal of a previous tubal ligation or vasectomy, artificial insemination, investigation and testing, and genetic counseling are included here. Codes V26.51 and V26.52 describe sterilization status for both men and women and are frequently confused with code V25.2. The "status" codes, V26.51 and V26.52, describe past treatment to acquire sterilization, whereas a person who desires sterilization during the current episode of care is coded with V25.2, Admission for sterilization. The Alphabetic Index to Diseases should be followed closely so as not to confuse these different episodes of healthcare.

> **EXAMPLE:** A female patient undergoes fertility testing by fallopian insufflation, V26.21

> **EXAMPLE:** A male patient is admitted for a vasoplasty after previous sterilization 2 years ago, V26.0

Category V27, Outcome of Delivery

A code from Category V27, Outcome of delivery, should be included on every maternal record when a delivery has occurred. These codes are not to be used on subsequent postpartum records or on the newborn record. They are always secondary codes on the maternal record at the time of delivery. The V27 code indicates whether the delivery produced a single or multiple birth and whether the infants were liveborn or stillborn. The unspecified code, V27.9, should not be used because the maternal health record will identify the details of the delivery. Codes in category V27 are indexed under "Outcome of delivery" in the Alphabetic Index.

> **EXAMPLE:** Spontaneous delivery of full-term live infant: 650, Normal delivery; V27.0, Outcome of delivery, single liveborn; 73.59, Other manually assisted delivery

A point to remember: Category V27 codes are only assigned to the mother's health record. These codes should not appear on the baby's health record. Do not confuse the V27 maternal codes with the V30 newborn codes that are used to describe the newborn's birth status.

Category V29, Observation and Evaluation of Newborn for Suspected Condition Not Found

Category V29 codes are available for situations where a newborn (the first twenty-eight days of life) is suspected of having a particular condition that is ruled out after examination and observation. Do not assign a code from category V29 when the patient has identified signs or symptoms of a suspected problem; instead, in these cases code the sign or symptom. V29 codes are used only for healthy newborns and infants for which no condition after study is found to be present. V29.0 can be a principal or secondary diagnosis code when the newborn is an inpatient. At the time of birth, if a suspected condition is not found, category V29 is used as an additional code because the V30–V39 category code must be listed first to indicate the status of the birth. However, category V29 may be used as a principal code for readmissions or encounters when the V30 code no longer applies. Additional diagnosis codes may be used in addition to the observation code on the newborn record, but only if the additional codes describe a condition unrelated to the suspected condition being evaluated.

Codes for this category are located in the Alphabetic Index under the main term "Observation (for), suspected, condition, newborn."

EXAMPLE:	Five-day-old newborn is admitted to the hospital with suspected sepsis; following blood cultures, the sepsis was ruled out: V29.0, Observation for suspected infectious conditions
EXAMPLE:	Single liveborn infant delivered by cesarean delivery in the hospital; suspected of having a neurological condition that is ruled out after observation and study: V30.01, Single liveborn, born in hospital, delivered by cesarean delivery; V29.1, Observation for suspected neurological condition

Liveborn Infants According to Type of Birth (V30–V39)

A code from categories V30 through V39 is used to identify all types of births and is always the first code listed on the health record of the newborn. The V30–V39 code is used "once in a lifetime" when the infant is born. If the newborn is transferred to another institution, the V30 series is not used at the second institution or on the infant's subsequent admissions or outpatient visits to any healthcare provider. The V30–V39 categories describe single or multiple liveborns, and single or multiple stillborns. Codes for these categories are indexed under "Newborn" in the Alphabetic Index. Any disease or birth injury should also be coded as additional diagnoses, if applicable.

Fourth- and Fifth-Digit Subdivisions

At the beginning of categories V30 through V39, instructions for fourth and fifth digits are given.

.0 **Born in hospital (requires a fifth digit)**
.1 **Born before admission to hospital**
.2 **Born outside hospital and not hospitalized**

The fourth digit .0 is assigned when a baby is born in the hospital. The following fifth-digit subclassification is used with the fourth digit .0:

0 **delivered without mention of cesarean delivery**
1 **delivered by cesarean delivery**

EXAMPLE:	Exceptionally large liveborn male infant delivered in hospital via low cervical cesarean section: V30.01, Single liveborn, delivered in hospital by cesarean delivery; 766.0, Exceptionally large baby

The fourth digit .1 is assigned when a baby is admitted to the hospital immediately following birth. These codes are not assigned to newborns transferred from other hospitals.

EXAMPLE: Infant admitted to hospital following birth at home: V30.1, Single liveborn, delivered before admission to hospital

EXAMPLE: Infant transferred to hospital B from hospital A with a congenital heart defect—Tetralogy of Fallot. Hospital B would assign the following: 745.2, Tetralogy of Fallot

The fourth digit .2 is assigned when a baby is born outside the hospital and is not hospitalized. Therefore, this fourth digit should not be used in the acute care setting.

EXAMPLE: Single liveborn infant, examined at home after birth. Physical examination essentially normal. Infant will remain at home. Home visit is coded: V30.2, Single liveborn, born outside hospital and not hospitalized

Exercise 23.1

Assign ICD-9-CM diagnosis and procedure codes (when applicable) to the following:

1. Exposure to tuberculosis

   _____V01.1_____

2. Admission for sterilization; bilateral endoscopic ligation and division of fallopian tubes

   _____V25.2 , 66.22_____

3. Family history of colon carcinoma

   _____V16.0_____

4. Twin with stillborn mate delivered in the hospital via cesarean delivery

   _____V32.01_____

5. Antenatal screening for chromosomal anomalies by amniocentesis; amniocentesis

   _____V28.0 , 75.1 (+)_____

Persons with a Condition Influencing Their Health Status (V40–V49)

At the beginning of this section for categories V40–V49, a note states: "These categories are intended for use when these conditions are recorded as 'diagnoses' or 'problems.'" Typically, the codes in these categories are assigned as additional diagnoses. Categories V40–49 are "status" codes that describe the sequelae or residual of a past disease or condition. The codes may indicate a transplanted organ or tissue or the presence of an artificial opening such as a colostomy. Postsurgical states are described with these codes to indicate the presence of a mechanical or prosthetic device such as a cardiac pacemaker or an intrauterine contraceptive device. Other codes in this section describe postprocedural status to indicate a certain procedure has been performed in the past, such as a coronary bypass or angioplasty. A status code is informative because the patient's condition or status may influence the course of treatment he receives in the future.

Category V42, Organ or Tissue Replaced by Transplant

Category V42 is used for homologous or heterologous (animal or human) organ transplants. These codes are indexed under "Status (post), transplant" in the Alphabetic Index.

> **EXAMPLE:** Status post kidney transplant (human donor): V42. 0, Kidney replaced by transplant

A code, V49.83, Awaiting heart transplant status, is included in another category of ICD-9-CM. Some patients who are on a waiting list for a heart transplant may be hospitalized due to the severity of their illness. V49.83 is a status code to distinguish patients who are hospitalized while awaiting a new heart from patients who are hospitalized for direct treatment of their heart disease. This code could be also used to indicate that the patient is on the heart transplant waiting list.

Category V43, Organ or Tissue Replaced by Other Means

Category V43 is used when coding replacement of an organ with an artificial device, mechanical device, or prosthesis. Codes in this category are indexed under "Status (post), organ replacement, by artificial or mechanical device or prosthesis of" in the Alphabetic Index.

> **EXAMPLE:** Status post hip replacement with a prosthetic device: V43.64, Hip joint replaced by other means

Category V44, Artificial Opening Status

Category V44 is subdivided to identify the presence of an artificial opening, such as a tracheostomy (V44.0), ileostomy (V44.2), colostomy (V44.3), cystostomy (V44.5), and so forth. These codes are indexed under "Status (post)" in the Alphabetic Index.

> **EXAMPLE:** Status post colostomy: V44.3, Colostomy status

The exclusion note at the beginning of category V44 instructs coders to use a code from categories V55.0 through V55.9 when the encounter or admission is for attention to or management of that artificial opening.

Category V45, Other Postsurgical States

Category V45 includes codes for a variety of postsurgical states, such as cardiac pacemaker in situ (V45.01), renal dialysis status (V45.1), presence of cerebrospinal fluid drainage device (V45.2), aortocoronary bypass status (V45.81), and cataract extraction status (V45.61).

V45.7, Acquired absence of organ, was created to indicate the status of an acquired absence of an organ in contrast to a congenital absence. This status is useful in describing the reason for the visit when a patient is seen for reconstructive surgery. The code is intended to be used for patient care where the absence of an organ affects treatment. Subcategory V45.7 includes codes to describe the acquired absence, through surgery or other medical intervention, of breast, intestine, kidney, lung, stomach, urinary sites, genital organs, and other organs.

Codes from category V45 are indexed under "Status (post)" in the Alphabetic Index.

> **EXAMPLE:** Two-year-old admitted for hernia repair of right inguinal hernia; patient also has ventriculoperitoneal shunt: 550.90, Unilateral or unspecified (not specified as recurrent) inguinal hernia, without mention of obstruction or gangrene; V45.2, Presence of cerebrospinal fluid drainage device; 53.00, Unilateral repair of inguinal hernia, not otherwise specified

Category V46, Other Dependence on Machines

Codes from category V46 are assigned to cases when patients become dependent on machines, such as respirators, aspirators, and supplemental or long-term oxygen therapy. Patients who are dependent on ventilators may be admitted to a healthcare facility when their mechanical ventilator at home has equipment malfunctions or when a power outage causes their machine to fail. A specific code in this category, V46.12, indicates the encounter is associated with the patient's need for medical care due to the mechanical failure of his or her ventilator. Patients are often admitted to long-term care facilities specifically to be weaned from a ventilator. Code V46.13 is used to identify an encounter for weaning from a respirator or ventilator. These codes are indexed under "Dependence, on" in the Alphabetic Index.

> **EXAMPLE:** Patient in acute respiratory failure dependent on respirator:
> 518.81, Acute respiratory failure; V46.11, Dependence on respirator

Persons Encountering Health Services for Specific Procedures and Aftercare (V50–V59)

The following important note for categories V51–V58 appears at the beginning of this section:

> Categories V51–V58 are intended for use to indicate a reason for care in patients who may have already been treated for some disease or injury not now present, or who are receiving care to consolidate the treatment, to deal with residual states, or to prevent recurrence.

The word *aftercare* may not be used commonly by the physician to describe this particular episode of care for a patient. Instead, the physician may use terminology such as "follow-up" or "status post" or use an action word to describe the procedure to be performed, such as "closure" of a colostomy. Again, the language of physicians may not always coincide perfectly with the language of ICD-9-CM and the coder must identify that situation and make the necessary language adjustments in order to code the episode correctly. Aftercare visit codes describe the patient who has received the initial treatment for a disease or injury but requires continued care during the health or recovery phase. The aftercare may also describe the long-term consequences of the disease.

The aftercare V codes are not used if treatment is being given for a current or acute disease or injury. The diagnosis code should be used in this case.

Typically, aftercare codes are listed first to explain the specific reason for the visit or encounter. An aftercare code may also be used as an additional code when some type of aftercare is provided in addition to the reason for the admission or visit.

Categories V50 through V59 are subdivided to describe the type of service provided. Codes in categories V50 through V59 are indexed in the Alphabetic Index under "Admission (encounter), for," "Aftercare," and "Attention to." Typically, codes from these categories are assigned as a principal diagnosis.

Category V54, Other Orthopedic Aftercare

Category V54 is subdivided to describe particular orthopedic aftercare. Subcategory V54.0, Aftercare involving internal fixation device, identifies the reason for the encounter by describing the type of procedure to be performed: removal of a device or lengthening or adjusting a growth rod. Other codes describe the healing phase of fracture care. Coding guidelines for ICD-9-CM require that a fracture code be used only for the initial encounter for treatment. Subsequent encounters require the use of an aftercare code. Newer subcategories V54.1, Aftercare for healing traumatic fracture, and V54.2, Aftercare for healing pathologic fracture, exist to describe the services related to the healing process with the fracture site identified. A specific code, V54.81, describes aftercare following a joint replacement.

> **EXAMPLE:**   Removal of screw from healed fracture of arm: V54.01, Aftercare involving removal of fracture plate or other internal fixation device

> **EXAMPLE:**   A patient comes to the family physician's office for cast removal. The patient had suffered the fracture and received treatment while away at college, but healing has occurred and the cast needs to be removed. Code V54.89, Other orthopedic aftercare, describes the reason for the visit.

Category V55, Attention to Artificial Openings

Unlike category V44, Artificial opening status, category V55 describes attention to the artificial opening, which may include the following services:

- Adjustment or repositioning of catheter

- Closure

- Passage of sounds or bougies

- Reforming

- Removal or replacement of catheter

- Toilet or cleansing

Category V55 codes may be first-listed diagnoses or used as additional diagnoses codes. These codes identify encounters for catheter cleaning, fitting, and adjustment services, and other care that is distinct from actual treatment. These codes are not used when there is a complication of the device or catheter.

> **EXAMPLE:**   Emergency department visit for a patient who needs a replacement of a clogged gastrostomy tube: V55.1, Attention to gastrostomy

> **EXAMPLE:**   A patient is admitted for a scheduled closure of a colostomy: V55.3, Attention to colostomy

> **EXAMPLE:**   Encounter for replacement of cystostomy tube: V55.5, Attention to cystostomy

Category V56, Encounter for Dialysis and Dialysis Catheter Care

V56 codes are used to identify the main reason for the encounter, for example, extracorporeal or peritoneal dialysis and related services. The note "Use additional code to identify the associated condition" appears at the beginning of category V56. The associated condition, that is, the reason for the dialysis or dialysis catheter care, is listed second. Codes in category V56 are indexed under "Dialysis" in the Alphabetic Index.

> **EXAMPLE:** Visit for renal dialysis for patient with end-stage renal disease: V56.0, Encounter for extracorporeal dialysis; 585.6, End-stage renal disease

Category V57, Care Involving Use of Rehabilitation Procedures

Category V57 includes codes describing admissions or encounters for physical therapy, speech therapy, occupational therapy, and other rehabilitation procedures. When a patient is admitted for a rehabilitation procedure, the first code listed is the V code, followed by the codes for the disease or condition requiring rehabilitation. The fourth digit of the V57 code indicates the focus of treatment, for example, physical therapy or speech therapy.

Since the implementation of Medicare's rehabilitation prospective payment system in 2002, coders have been required to assign a code for the etiologic diagnosis to indicate the condition for which the patient is receiving rehabilitation. The etiologic diagnosis is required on the data collection instrument called the Inpatient Rehabilitation Facility–Patient Assessment Instrument (IRF-PAI). However, this does not change the official ICD-9-CM coding guidelines with regard to rehabilitation coding. The principal diagnosis for inpatient services or the first-listed diagnosis for outpatient services that must appear on the UB-92 claim form will still be a code from category V57, Care involving use of rehabilitation procedures, when the patient is receiving rehabilitation services.

Codes in category V57 are indexed under "Therapy" in the Alphabetic Index.

> **EXAMPLE:** Admission for physical therapy for hemiplegia due to CVA that occurred two weeks ago: V57.1, Care involving other physical therapy; 438.20, Late effect of cerebrovascular disease, hemiplegia

Category V58, Encounter for Other and Unspecified Procedures and Aftercare

Category V58 includes codes for admissions or encounters for radiotherapy, chemotherapy, attention to surgical dressings and sutures, other aftercare following surgery, and long-term (current) drug use, therapeutic drug monitoring, and so forth.

Aftercare codes describe patient encounters that take place after the initial treatment of a disease has been completed and the patient now requires continued care during the healing or recovery process. Patients may be admitted to skilled nursing facilities or long-term care hospitals for recovery or they may be receiving home care services. The aftercare codes describe services received during such a continuing phase of healthcare.

Aftercare codes are generally the first-listed code to describe the reason for the encounter. However, an aftercare code may be used as an additional code when the aftercare is provided during an admission for treatment of an unrelated condition. In addition, multiple aftercare codes can be used together to fully identify the reason for the aftercare services.

Aftercare codes are not used if treatment is directed at a current, acute disease or injury. The diagnosis code is used for these patients. Exceptions to this rule are code V58.0, Radiotherapy, and V58.1, Chemotherapy. These codes are always listed first, followed by the malignancy diagnosis code, when the patient's encounter is solely to receive radiation therapy or chemotherapy. Either code can be listed first if the patient is receiving both therapies during the same visit.

Subcategory V58.3 would be used for a surgical follow-up visit for change of surgical dressings, checking the wound for healing, or removal of sutures when there is no mention of any wound infection or other complications.

Broad categories exist for aftercare following surgery for neoplasms (V58.42), aftercare following surgery for injury and trauma (V58.43), and aftercare following surgery for specific body systems (V58.71–V58.78.) The aftercare codes are usually reported outside the acute care hospital setting to identify the postsurgical treatment after the initial treatment and surgery is completed. This postsurgical care may be received in a long-term care hospital or facility or through home care services. These codes should be used with other V codes for postoperative wound dressing care, ostomy care, or other similar V codes to completely describe the services. However, some codes should not be used together. For example, V58.43 should not be reported with one of the V54.1 codes when the surgical aftercare is for the treatment of a healing traumatic fracture because the fracture care code is more specific and there is an excludes note under V58.43. Inclusion terms appear under these aftercare codes to indicate the original disease or injury that was treated, for which aftercare is now being provided. For example:

V58.42, Aftercare following surgery for neoplasm
Conditions classifiable to 140–239.

Generally, one code from subcategories V54.1, V54.2, V54.4, and V54.7 is used per patient, unless the patient is recovering from multiple procedures and conditions.

Subcategory V58.6, Long-term (current) drug use, contains status codes that are intended to be used in addition to V58.83, Encounter for therapeutic drug monitoring, or other diagnosis codes. Subcategory V58.6 codes only state that a patient is on a prescribed drug for an extended period of time. There is no definition or time frame for long term. If a patient receives a drug on a regular basis and has multiple refills available for a prescription, it is appropriate to document long-term drug use. The code indicates a patient's continuous use of a prescribed drug for long-term treatment of a condition or for prophylactic use. It is not to be used to describe patients who have addictions to drugs.

Code V58.83, Encounter for therapeutic drug monitoring, is the correct code to use when a patient visit is for the purpose of undergoing a laboratory test to measure the drug level in the patient's blood or urine or to measure a specific function to assess the effectiveness of a drug. V58.83 may be used alone if the monitoring is for a drug that the patient is on for only a brief period, not long term. However, there is a "use additional code" note after code V58.83 to remind the coder to use an additional code for any associated long-term (current) drug use (V58.61–V58.69) to indicate what drug is being monitored.

EXAMPLE: Patient was seen in the physician's office for removal of sutures from healed open wound of the forearm: V58.3, Attention to surgical dressings and sutures

EXAMPLE: Admission for chemotherapy for patient with metastasis to bone; patient has history of breast carcinoma with mastectomy performed eight years ago: V58.1, Encounter for chemotherapy; 198.5, Secondary neoplasm of the bone; V10.3, Personal history of malignant neoplasm of breast; 99.25, Injection or infusion of cancer chemotherapeutic substance

EXAMPLE: Encounter for radiotherapy for patient with adenocarcinoma of the breast: V58.0, Encounter for radiotherapy; 174.9, Malignant neoplasm of breast

EXAMPLE: The patient is on anticoagulants and the physician orders a prothrombin time (PT) to be performed in the outpatient department: V58.83, Encounter for therapeutic drug monitoring; V58.61, Long-term (current) use of anticoagulants

Category V59, Donors

Codes from Category V59, Donors, are used for living individuals who are donating blood, tissue, or an organ to be transplanted into another individual. V59 codes are not used when a patient donates his or her own blood to possibly receive during an upcoming scheduled surgery; instead, the reason for the patient's surgery is coded. V59 codes are not used when the potential donor is examined (code V70.8). Also, these codes are not used for cadaveric donations, that is, when a patient's organ(s) are harvested at the time of death according to the patient's stated wishes.

Recently, the American College of Obstetricians and Gynecologists (ACOG) requested new codes for egg donors that identify the age of the donor and whether the eggs are intended to be used for anonymous donations or for a designated recipient. Codes V59.70–V59.74 identify the age of the egg or oocyte donor (either under age 35 or age 35 or over) and specify whether the intended recipient is anonymous or designated.

A sperm donor is indexed in ICD-9-CM to code V59.8, Donor, other specified organ or tissue.

Exercise 23.2

Assign ICD-9-CM diagnosis and procedure codes to the following:

1. Status post unilateral kidney transplant, human donor

   V42.0   ~~V59.4~~

2. Encounter for removal of cast; cast removal

   V54.89   97.88

3. Admitted to donate bone marrow; bone marrow aspiration

   V59.3   41.91

4. Encounter for chemotherapy for patient with Hodgkin's lymphoma; chemotherapy

   V58.11   201.90

5. Reprogramming of cardiac pacemaker

   V53.31

6. Routine circumcision of ten-year-old male; circumcision

   V50.2 , 64.0

7. Replacement of tracheostomy tube; trach tube replaced

   V55.0   97.23

8. Encounter for renal dialysis for patient in chronic renal failure; hemodialysis

   V56.0   586

9. Encounter for occupational therapy for patient with cognitive deficits secondary to an old CVA; occupational therapy

   V57.21   438.0

10. Encounter for fitting of artificial leg; fitting of prosthetic leg (below the knee)

    V52.1   84.46

(margin note: J47.81)

(margin note: Ch.)

Persons Encountering Health Services in Other Circumstances (V60–V69)

Categories V60 through V69 include a variety of codes that describe reasons for healthcare encounters and explain circumstances regarding healthcare services that do not fall into other categories. Certain V codes identify the reasons for the encounter, but others are used as additional codes to provide more details about the patient's healthcare services.

Category V60, Housing, Household, and Economic Circumstances

Codes in category V60, Housing, household, and economic circumstances, are used strictly as additional diagnosis codes to further explain the socioeconomic factors that may be influencing the patient's need for healthcare services.

Category V61, Other Family Circumstances

Category V61, Other family circumstances, is one of several categories in ICD-9-CM that may be used when a patient or family member receives counseling services after an illness or injury, or when support is required to cope with family and social problems. These codes are not used in conjunction with a diagnosis code when counseling is considered integral to the treatment for the condition. Subcategory codes V61.1, Counseling for marital and partner problems, and code V61.20, Parent–child problems, allow identification of counseling for family conflict and abuse-related issues, for both the victim and the perpetrator of parental child abuse. A different V code is used, V62.83, when counseling services are provided to the perpetrator of physical or sexual abuse. These counseling codes are used when only counseling services, not medical treatment, is rendered.

Category V62, Other Psychosocial Circumstances

Category V62 includes codes that classify those circumstances, or fear of them, affecting the person directly involved or others, mentioned as the reason for seeking or receiving medical advice or care. Rather than medical conditions, these are psychosocial conditions that often require counseling or other services to improve the individual's status or functioning. These codes may be listed as the only reason for an encounter or the codes may be used in addition to other diagnoses or reasons for visits to provide useful information on circumstances that may affect a patient's care or treatment. Examples of V62 codes include V62.0, Unemployment; V62.6, Refusal of treatment for reasons of religion or conscience; or V62.84, Suicidal ideation.

Category V63, Unavailability of Other Medical Facilities for Care

Category V63, Unavailability of other medical facilities for care, describes circumstances when a certain type of medical facility or service is not available and a patient has to be taken elsewhere or provided services in a facility that would not normally care for this type of patient. Code V63.1, Medical services in home not available, may be a first-listed or additional diagnosis code to explain the occasion when a home healthcare provider is not available and the patient may need to be admitted to an acute care hospital or long-term care facility.

Category V64, Persons Encountering Health Services for Specific Procedures, Not Carried Out

Category V64, Persons encountering health services for specific procedures, not carried out, was introduced in chapter 2 of this book as it further explains why a procedure or service was not performed. Codes in category V64 can only be used as additional diagnosis codes. The first four subcategory codes identify the circumstance when a particular procedure cannot be performed for different reasons.

Codes V64.00 through V64.09 describe specific reasons why an immunization or vaccination was not given. Tracking why an immunization was not given can be as important as tracking those that are given, according to the American Academy of Pediatrics. These codes identify the multiple reasons why a patient did not receive a routine immunization.

V64.1 and V64.2 state that a surgical or other procedure cannot be carried out because of a contraindication or a patient's decision. A contraindication is any medical condition that renders some form of treatment improper or undesirable. For example, the patient may have an infection, cardiac condition, or abnormal diagnostic test that would make performing the surgical procedure unsafe until the contraindication is resolved. The patient may also decide, sometimes at the last minute before surgery begins, that he does not want the surgery or procedure performed at this time and the procedure is cancelled. This code may also be used when a patient is recommended to have a procedure during the hospital stay and refuses. For example, the patient refuses coronary artery bypass surgery after a coronary arteriogram demonstrates significant coronary atherosclerosis. V64.2, Surgical or other procedure not carried out because of patient's decision, is used as an additional code to explain this event.

Code V64.3 is used when another circumstance causes the surgery or procedure to be cancelled. Such circumstances may be equipment failure in the surgery or procedure suite, unplanned absence of the surgeon or other necessary medical personnel, or lack of necessary medications or supplies.

Codes within subcategory V64.4, Closed surgical procedure converted to open procedure, are frequently used as additional diagnosis codes to explain when a planned endoscopic procedure cannot be completed and the physician must perform an open or invasive surgical procedure instead. Individual codes exist to explain the conversion of a laparoscopic, thoracoscopic, and arthroscopic procedure to a procedure using open surgical techniques. In each of these events, only the open surgical procedure is coded. An additional code is not required for the initially attempted endoscopic procedure.

Category V65, Other Persons Seeking Consultation

Codes from category V65, Other persons seeking consultation, are used to report services sought by one person on behalf of another person not in attendance, to describe an apparently healthy person who feigns illness to obtain medical care, or to classify a variety of counseling services not listed elsewhere. Codes within category V65 may be first-listed or additional diagnosis codes.

> **Example:** A patient frequently comes to the emergency department or a physician's office with a variety of vague complaints that usually include pain of some type. The doctor documents the patient as having "drug-seeking behavior." The patient's complaints or a code for unspecified drug abuse is listed first with an additional code of V65.2, Person feigning illness.

The counseling sessions that may be reported with a code for this category include dietary counseling, health education, counseling on substance use/abuse, HIV counseling (usually related to HIV testing), and training on the use of insulin pumps. Codes such as V65.49 and V65.8 may explain patient visits to physicians when the patient has no sign or symptom. For example, a patient may have a physician's office appointment to discuss her desire to have an elective bilateral removal of breast implants when there is no medical indication for the procedure. Code V65.8, Other reasons for seeking consultation, would be the principal or first-listed diagnosis because no abnormal symptoms or findings have prompted the surgery.

Category V66, Convalescence

Category V66 is used primarily for patients seeking convalescence, often in a long-term care facility or hospice, following surgery, radiotherapy, or chemotherapy. This category is subdivided to describe the reason for the convalescence. The convalescence codes are indexed in the Alphabetic Index under "Convalescence" and "Admission (encounter), for, convalescence following."

Code V66.7 describes an encounter for palliative care, that is, hospice care or end-of-life care. Code V66.7 is always a secondary code for the patient receiving palliative care for a terminal condition. The terminal condition, such as carcinoma, COPD, Alzheimer's disease, or AIDS, should be the principal diagnosis. Code V66.7 can also be used as a secondary diagnosis code during an inpatient admission or in any other healthcare setting when it is determined that palliative care should be initiated and no further treatment for the terminal illness is desired.

> **EXAMPLE:** Seventy-year-old patient admitted to a long-term care facility for convalescence following repair of hip fracture: V66.4, Convalescence following treatment of fracture

> **EXAMPLE:** Fifty-year-old patient is admitted to the hospital for management of pain that is caused by her widespread metastatic carcinoma of the liver, lungs, and bones, which spread from her breast carcinoma initially treated over 10 years ago. After consultation with her physicians and family, the patient elects to discontinue further treatment and receive hospice care with pain management services at home. The metastatic sites and history of breast cancer codes are listed first (according to the circumstances of the admission), with a secondary code, V66.7, Encounter for palliative care.

Category V67, Follow-up Examination

Carefully read the includes note under the category V67 title. It states "surveillance only following completed treatment." The term *follow-up* as it is intended in ICD-9-CM can be different from what a physician intends to describe when he uses the same phrase. The physician may be describing ongoing medical treatment or a recovery phase of the illness or recent surgery. Category V67, Follow-up examination, is to be used only to describe an encounter where the treatment of the condition is completed and the patient is undergoing surveillance or a "checkup" to determine if his or her disease-free status continues. When a physician states "follow-up" for hypertension that remains under treatment or "follow-up" after recent cardiac surgery, the V67 category is unlikely the appropriate set of codes to use. In these circumstances described by the physician, the hypertension under treatment is likely to be coded or a surgical aftercare code may be more appropriate to describe the healing/recovery phase after surgery.

Coding Guidelines

A code from category V67 is assigned as the principal diagnosis, or first-listed diagnosis code, to explain the reason for the encounter when the patient is admitted for the purpose of surveillance after the initial treatment for a disease or injury has been completed. The use of V67 means the condition has been fully treated and no longer exists. Following the V67 code, a second code can be used to indicate the reason for the follow-up, such as a personal history of a malignant neoplasm. If, during the follow-up examination, a recurrence, extension, or related condition is identified, the code for that condition is assigned as the principal diagnosis, or first-listed diagnosis code, rather than a code from category V67.

Category V67 is subdivided to describe the completed treatment, such as surgery, radiotherapy, or chemotherapy. Codes in this category are indexed under "Follow-up" and "Admission (encounter), for, follow-up examination" in the Alphabetic Index.

EXAMPLE: Patient admitted for follow-up cystoscopy to rule out recurrence of malignant neoplasm of the urinary bladder; patient had a transurethral resection of the bladder one year ago and has been cancer free to date; cystoscopy revealed no recurrence: V67.09, Follow-up examination following surgery; V10.51, History of malignant neoplasm of the urinary bladder; 57.32, Other cystoscopy

EXAMPLE: Patient admitted for follow-up colonoscopy to rule out recurrent adenoma of the colon; patient had removal of adenoma three years ago; colonoscopy was positive for recurrence and adenoma was removed: 211.3, Benign neoplasm of colon; 45.43, Endoscopic destruction of other lesion or tissue of large intestine

Persons without Reported Diagnosis Encountered during Examination and Investigation of Individuals and Populations (V70–V83)

The following note appears at the beginning of this section: Nonspecific abnormal findings disclosed at the time of these examinations are classifiable to categories 790 through 796.

Category V70, General Medical Examination

Like the codes in category V20.2, Routine infant or child health check, the codes in category V70 describe reasonably healthy children and adults who seek healthcare services for routine examinations, such as a general physical examination, or examinations for administrative purposes, such as a preschool examination. The codes are only used as first-listed diagnoses. These codes are not used if the examination is for the diagnosis of a suspected illness or for treatment of a disease. In these cases, the diagnosis code or possibly a category V71 code is used instead. If a diagnosis or condition is identified during the course of the general medical examination, it should be reported as an additional diagnosis code. Preexisting or chronic conditions, as well as history codes, may also be used as additional diagnoses as long as the examination was for the administrative purpose and not focused on treatment of the medical condition.

EXAMPLE: Fifty-five-year-old male has an appointment at this primary care physician's office for his annual physical examination. The patient has mild eczema that is treated with over-the-counter lotions, and he had an inguinal hernia repaired during the past year.

V70.0, Routine general medical examination at a healthcare facility; eczema, 692.9. The hernia is not coded because it no longer exists.

Category V71, Observation and Evaluation for Suspected Conditions Not Found

Codes from the category V71 are assigned as principal diagnoses for encounters or admissions to evaluate the patient's condition under the following circumstances:

- Some evidence suggests the existence of an abnormal condition.

- A health problem occurs following an accident or other incident that ordinarily results in such a problem.

- No supporting evidence for the suspected condition is found, and no treatment is currently required.

The fact that the patient may be scheduled for continuing observation in the office and/or clinic setting following discharge does not limit the use of this category.

Code V71.81, Observation for suspected child abuse or neglect, is used when child abuse is suspected but not found after the observation and evaluation is completed. This situation is most likely to occur during a visit to a physician's office, an emergency department, or a primary care clinic.

The observation codes are for use in very limited situations when a person is being observed for a suspected condition that is ruled out. The observation codes are not for use if an injury or illness or any signs or symptoms related to the suspected condition are present. In such cases, the diagnosis or symptom code should be assigned.

The category V71 observation code is to be used as the first-listed code or as principal diagnosis only. Additional codes may be used in addition to the observation code, but only if they are unrelated to the suspected condition being observed.

Codes in category V71 are indexed in the Alphabetic Index under "Admission (encounter), for, observation (without need for further medical care)" and "Observation (for)."

EXAMPLE: A patient is admitted to the hospital for observation following an automobile accident because serious head trauma is suspected; all diagnostic tests are negative for head injury: V71.4, Observation following other accident

Category V72, Special Investigations and Examinations

Category V72 includes codes to describe ancillary services provided to the patient, such as radiological examinations, laboratory examinations, and preoperative examinations. These codes are indexed in the Alphabetic Index under "Admission (encounter), for, examination" and "Examination."

Coding Guidelines

When only diagnostic services are provided during the outpatient encounter, sequence first the diagnosis, condition, problem, or other reason that is identified as chiefly responsible for the outpatient encounter. Codes for other appropriate diagnoses then should follow.

A code from category V72, Special investigations and examinations, is assigned as the reason for an encounter only when no problem, diagnosis, or condition is identified as the reason for the examination. Codes from the V72 category reflect "routine" services, or services that are ordered without medical necessity. Insurance companies that do not cover services without a patient's diagnosis or physical symptom or complaint frequently reject outpatient testing services that fall within this category. Codes from category V72 are rarely used for inpatient coding and are never assigned as an additional code.

A diagnosis code from category V72 reflects the reason for the service, which may be a procedure or a test. The procedure performed on the patient may also be coded with ICD-9-CM and/or Current Procedural Terminology (CPT). It is likely that the CPT procedure codes are stored in the facility's charge description master and printed directly on the patient's file or bill.

EXAMPLE: Patient visits the radiology department for chest x-ray. Because the patient has no other complaints and the x-ray is part of a routine physical examination, only the V code is appropriate: V72.5, Radiology examination, NEC

EXAMPLE: Patient visits the radiology department for chest x-ray to rule out pneumonia. Patient complains of cough and fever. Either of these symptoms should be listed first, rather than the V code. The pneumonia is not coded because it was not established during the encounter: 786.2, Cough; 780.6, Fever

EXAMPLE: Patient visits the laboratory department for routine blood work. Because the patient has no other complaints documented, only the V code is appropriate: V72.6, Laboratory examination

EXAMPLE: Patient visits the laboratory department with complaints of polydipsia. A blood glucose test is performed to rule out diabetes. The symptom code for polydipsia is listed first. Because the diabetes has not been established during this encounter, it is not coded: 783.5, Polydipsia

Several codes for women's health visits are included in category V72. For example, subcategory V72.3, Gynecological examination, offers two choices to describe a visit by a woman to her primary care or specialist physician. Code V72.31 is intended to describe a routine gynecological examination for a healthy woman that may include a Papanicolaou (Pap) cervical smear with pelvic examination. Code V72.32 is used to describe the continued monitoring of a woman who makes a visit to the physician's office for a Pap smear to confirm findings of a recent normal smear following an initial abnormal smear. Another common reason for a young woman's visit to a physician is to have a pregnancy test. Usually the test results are known at the conclusion of the visit. A positive test result is assigned a code from category V22, Normal pregnancy. If the pregnancy test is negative, code V72.41 is used to report the visit. If the results of the pregnancy test are not available and/or the pregnancy has not yet been confirmed, code V72.40 is used to report the visit.

During a pregnancy, it may be necessary to test a patient's Rh status. If a pregnant woman's blood group is Rh negative, knowing whether the father is Rh positive or Rh negative will help find the risk of Rh sensitization and whether or not the woman should receive Rh immunoglobulin to prevent sensitization for the rest of the pregnancy. The code V72.86, Encounter for blood typing, would be used for this type of encounter.

Frequently, patients are referred to physicians for consultations or to hospital outpatient departments for preoperative evaluations or clearances. For preoperative evaluations, the visits are coded and sequenced as follows:

1.   Code from category V72.8, Other specified examinations, to identify the preoperative consultation or visit. These include preoperative cardiovascular examinations, preoperative respiratory examinations, other specified preoperative examinations, and unspecified preoperative evaluations.

2.   Code to describe the condition for which the surgery is being performed.

3.   Code to describe any conditions found during the preoperative evaluation.

Categories V73–V82, Special Screening Examinations

The codes in categories V73 through V82 are used to identify screening examinations for specific conditions and disorders that are currently not active.

Screening is the testing for a disease or condition in reasonably healthy individuals so that early detection and treatment can be provided. The screening code may be the first-listed code if the reason for the visit is specifically the screening exam. It may be an additional code if the screening is done during an outpatient visit for other health problems.

If a patient has a physical sign or symptom and is referred for a test to rule out or to confirm a suspected condition, this is a diagnostic examination, not a screening. The screening codes should not be used for this situation. Rather, the patient's physical sign or symptom(s) could be coded as the reason for the test.

When the principal diagnosis is a code from category V72, an additional code from categories V73 through V82 may also be assigned to identify any special screening test performed. If a condition is established during the screening, the code for the condition should be reported rather than the screening code.

Codes in categories V73 through V82 are referenced in the Alphabetic Index under "Screening (for)."

> **EXAMPLE:** Patient visits the laboratory department for a diabetes blood test screening: V72.6, Laboratory examination; V77.1, Special screening for diabetes mellitus

Categories V83–V84, Genetic Carrier Status and Genetic Susceptibility to Disease

Codes in category V83, Genetic carrier status, are intended to describe a patient who is known to carry a particular gene that could cause a disease to be passed on to his or her children. The code does not mean the patient has this particular disease. It does not mean there is 100 percent certainty that the disease would be passed on genetically to the next generation. The code could be used to explain why a patient is receiving additional monitoring or testing.

Codes in category V84, Genetic susceptibility to disease, are intended to describe a patient who has a confirmed abnormal gene that makes the patient more susceptible to a particular disease. A patient who has a genetic susceptibility to a disease, particularly if it is a malignancy, may request prophylactic removal of an organ to prevent the disease from occurring. These codes can be used to identify encounters for prophylactic organ removal, including breast, ovary, prostate, endometrium, or other anatomical site.

Category V85, Body Mass Index

The body mass index (BMI) is the first determination of a patient's weight in proportion to height. BMI measures are calculated as kilograms per meters squared. The BMI adult codes are for use for individuals over 20 years of age. Codes in this category were created to be used in conjunction with a code from 278.0, Overweight and obesity, to provide specific information about a patient's weight. BMI codes can also be used for underweight patients. Examples of BMI codes are:

V85.0	Body Mass Index less than 19, adult	
V85.1	Body Mass Index between 19–24, adult	
V85.2	Body Mass Index between 25–29, adult	
	V85.21	Body Mass Index 25.0–25.9, adult
	V85.22	Body Mass Index 26.0–26.9, adult
	V85.23	Body Mass Index 27.0–27.9, adult
	V85.24	Body Mass Index 28.0–28.9, adult
	V85.25	Body Mass Index 29.0–29.9, adult

Sequencing of V Codes

V codes can be used in both inpatient and outpatient settings. Generally, V codes are used more frequently in outpatient settings. V codes may be used as either a first-listed code or secondary code, depending on the circumstances of the visit. Some V codes may only be listed first; others may only be listed as secondary codes.

V codes often describe the reason for the visit to be the performance of a particular procedure or service. V codes are diagnosis codes. The procedure or service must also be coded with a procedure code to fully describe the visit.

The list below describes the recommended sequencing of V codes (*Coding Clinic*, Fourth Quarter 1996; Fourth Quarter 1998; Fourth Quarter 2001; Fourth Quarter 2002; Fourth Quarter 2003; and ICD-9-CM Official Guidelines for Coding and Reporting, effective April 1, 2005).

First-Listed V Codes/Categories/Subcategories:

V20	Health supervision of infant or child
V22.0	Supervision of normal first pregnancy
V22.1	Supervision of other normal pregnancy
V24	Postpartum care and examination
V29	Observation and evaluation of newborns for suspected condition not found (Exception: A code from V30–V39 may be sequenced before the V29 if it is in the newborn record.)
V30–V39	Liveborn infants according to type of birth
V46.12	Encounter for respirator dependence during power failure
V56.0	Extracorporeal dialysis
V58.0	Radiotherapy
V58.1	Chemotherapy (**Note:** V58.0 and V58.1 can be used together on a record with either being sequenced first when a patient receives both radiation therapy and chemotherapy during the same visit.)
V59	Donors
V66	Convalescence and palliative care (except V66.7, Palliative care)
V68	Encounters for administrative purposes
V70	General medical examination (except V70.7, Examination of participant in clinical trial)
V71	Observation and evaluation for suspected conditions not found
V72	Special investigations and examinations (except V72.5, Radiological examination NEC, and V72.6, Laboratory examination)

First- or Additional-Listed V Codes/Categories/Subcategories:

V01	Contact with or exposure to communicable disease
V02	Carrier or suspected carrier of infectious diseases
V03–V06	Need for prophylactic vaccination and inoculations
V07	Need for isolation and other prophylactic measures
V08	Asymptomatic HIV infection status
V10	Personal history of malignant neoplasm
V12	Personal history of certain other diseases
V13	Personal history of other diseases (except V13.4, Personal history of arthritis and V13.69, Personal history of other congenital malformations)
V16–V19	Family history of disease
V23	Supervision of high-risk pregnancy

V25	Encounter for contraceptive management
V26	Procreative management (except V26.5, Sterilization status)
V28	Antenatal screening
V43.22	Fully implantable artificial heart status
V45.7	Acquired absence of organ
V49.81	Postmenopausal status (age-related) (natural)
V50	Elective surgery for purposes other than remedying health status
V52	Fitting and adjustment of prosthetic device and implant
V53	Fitting and adjustment of other device
V54	Other orthopedic aftercare
V55	Attention to artificial openings
V56	Encounter for dialysis or dialysis catheter care (except V56.0, Extracorporeal dialysis, can only be a first-listed code)
V57	Care involving use of rehabilitation procedures
V58.3	Attention to surgical dressings and sutures
V58.4	Other aftercare following surgery
V58.6	Long-term (current) drug use
V58.7	Aftercare following surgery to specified body systems, not elsewhere classified
V58.8	Other specified procedures and aftercare
V61	Other family circumstances
V63	Unavailability of other medical facilities for care
V65	Other persons seeking consultation without complaint or sickness
V67	Follow-up examination
V69	Problems related to lifestyle
V70.7	Examination of participant in clinical trial
V73–V82	Special screening examinations
V83	Genetic carrier status

V Codes/Categories/Subcategories as Additional Codes Only:

V09	Infection with drug-resistant microorganisms
V13.61	Personal history of hypospadias
V14	Personal history of allergy to medicinal agents
V15	Other personal history presenting hazards to health (except V15.7, Personal history of contraception)
V21	Constitutional states in development
V22.2	Pregnancy state, incidental
V26.5	Sterilization status
V27	Outcome of delivery
V42	Organ or tissue replaced by transplant
V43	Organ or tissue replaced by other means
V44	Artificial opening status
V45	Other postsurgical states (except V45.7, Acquired absence of organ)
V46	Other dependence on machines (Exception: V46.12, Encounter for respiratory dependence during power failure)
V49.6x	Upper limb amputation status
V49.7x	Lower limb amputation status
V49.82	Dental sealant status
V49.83	Awaiting heart transplant status
V60	Housing, household, and economic circumstances

V62	Other psychosocial circumstances
V64	Persons encountering health services for specified procedure, not carried out
V66.7	Palliative care
V84	Genetic susceptibility to disease

Nonspecific V Codes

Certain V codes are very nonspecific. It is unlikely these codes are appropriate for use in inpatient settings. Their use in the outpatient setting should be limited to situations when no further documentation is available for more precise coding. Otherwise, a code for a sign or symptom, or a code that describes any other reason for the visit, should be used.

V11	Personal history of mental disorder. A code from the mental disorders chapter with an in-remission fifth digit should be used instead.
V13.4	Personal history of arthritis
V13.69	Personal history of congenital malformations
V15.7	Personal history of contraception
V40	Mental and behavioral problems
V41	Problems with special senses and other special functions
V47	Other problems with internal organs
V48	Problems with head, neck, and trunk
V49	Problems with limbs and other problems

      Exceptions:

V49.6	Upper limb amputation status
V49.7	Lower limb amputation status
V49.81	Postmenopausal status (age-related) (natural)
V49.82	Dental sealant status
V49.83	Awaiting heart transplant status

V51	Aftercare involving the use of plastic surgery
V58.2	Blood transfusion, without reported diagnosis
V58.5	Orthodontics
V58.9	Unspecified aftercare
V72.5	Radiological examination, NEC
V72.6	Laboratory examination (Codes V72.5 and V72.6 are not to be used if any sign, symptoms, or reason for a test is documented.)

Review Exercise: Chapter 23

Assign ICD-9-CM diagnosis and procedure codes to the following:

1. Office visit for gynecological exam including Papanicolaou smear; gynecological exam with Pap smear of the cervix

   V72.31, 89.23, 91.46

2. Visit to emergency room after falling 10 feet at work; exam reveals no injuries

   V71.3   E884.9

3. Encounter for observation of suspected malignant neoplasm of the cervix; Pap smear performed and the findings are negative

   V71.1, 91.46

4. Visit to radiology department for barium swallow; abdominal pain; barium swallow performed and the findings are negative

   789.00,   87.61

5. Follow-up examination of colon adenocarcinoma with colon resection one year ago, no recurrence found; colonoscopy

   (V67.09, V10.05, 45.23)

6. Admission to inpatient hospice for palliative care for giant cell glioblastoma of brain; patient determined to be terminal

   191.9, V66.7

7. Routine general medical examination

   V70.0

8. Examination of eyes

   V72.0

9. Infant to clinic for developmental handicap screening

   V79.3

10. Encounter for laboratory test; patient complains of fatigue

    780.79

11. Screening for osteoporosis

    V82.81

12. Encounter for physical therapy; status post below-the-knee amputation six months ago; physical therapy

    V57.1, V49.75, 93.39

13. Status post artificial heart valve

    V43.3

14. Kidney donor; left nephrectomy

    V59.4, 55.51

15. Encounter for chemotherapy; breast carcinoma, upper inner quadrant; chemotherapy

    V58.1   174.2   99.25

References and Bibliography

American Health Information Management Association. 2000 (September). Where in the world is ICD-10. *Journal of the American Health Information Management Association* 71(8).

American Hospital Association. 1985–2005. *Coding Clinic for ICD-9-CM*. Chicago: American Hospital Association.

American Psychiatric Association. 2000. *Diagnostic and Statistical Manual of Mental Disorders-Text Revision*. 4th ed. Washington, D.C.: American Psychiatric Press.

Beers, Mark H., and Robert Berkow, eds. 2000. *The Merck Manual*. 17th ed. Rahway, N.J.: Merck & Co.

Braunwald, Eugene, Anthony Fauci, Dennis Kasper, Stephen Hauser, Dan Longo, and J. Jameson. 2001. *Harrison's Principles of Internal Medicine*. New York: McGraw-Hill.

Brown, Faye. 2005. *ICD-9-CM Coding Handbook, with Answers*. Chicago: American Hospital Association.

Canobbia, Mary M. 1990. *Cardiovascular Disorders*. Mosby's Clinical Nursing Series. Vol. 1. St. Louis: Mosby Year Book.

Dorland, W. A. Newman, ed. 2003. *Dorland's Illustrated Medical Dictionary*. 30th ed. Philadelphia: W. B. Saunders.

Ertl, Linda. 1992 (June). Clinical notes: Intestinal ostomies. *Journal of the American Health Information Management Association* 63(6): 18–22.

Graham, Launa L. 1999. *Understanding Clinical Disease Processes for ICD-9-CM Coding*. Chicago: American Health Information Management Association.

Grimes, Deanna, et al. 1990. *Infectious Diseases*. Mosby's Clinical Nursing Series. Vol. 3. St. Louis: Mosby Year Book.

ICD-9-CM Coordination and Maintenance Committee. 1999–2005. Excerpts (agendas, proposals, and background materials) from the "Diagnoses and Procedures" portion of meeting minutes. Available online at http://www.cdc.gov/nchs/about/otheract/icd9/maint/maint.htm.

Illinois Department of Public Health. 2003. *Birth Defects and Other Adverse Pregnancy Outcomes in Illinois, 1997–2001*. Epidemiologic Report Series 03:02. Springfield, Ill.: Illinois Department of Health, Division of Epidemiologic Studies.

Johnson, Paula, MD, et al. 1999. Cardiac Troponin T as a marker for myocardial ischemia in patients seen at the emergency department for acute chest pain. *American Heart Journal* 137(6): 1137–44.

Melloni, John. 2001. *Melloni's Illustrated Medical Dictionary*. 4th ed. Pearl River, N.Y.: The Parthenon Publishing Group.

Nicholas, Toula. 1992 (March). Clinical notes: Cardiac catheterization. *Journal of the American Health Information Management Association* 63(3): 25–26.

Prophet, Sue. 2002. ICD-10 on the horizon. *Journal of the American Health Information Management Association* 73(7): 36–41.

Puckett, Craig D. 1998. *The Educational Annotation of ICD-9-CM.* 5th ed. Reno: Channel Publishing.

Rice, Matthew, MD, and David MacDonald, MD. 1999. Appropriate roles of cardiac Troponins in evaluating patients with chest pain. *Journal of the American Board of Family Practice* 12 (3): 214–18.

Rogers, Vickie, and Ann Zeisset. 2004. *Applying Inpatient Coding Skills under Prospective Payment.* Chicago: American Health Information Management Association.

Stedman, Thomas. 2000. *Stedman's Medical Dictionary.* 27th ed. Baltimore: Williams & Wilkins.

U.S. Department of Health and Human Services. 2003 . *International Classification of Diseases, 9th Revision, Clinical Modification.* Washington, D.C.: U.S. Government Printing Office.

U. S. Department of Health and Human Services. 1994. *Living with Heart Disease: Is It Heart Failure?* Consumer Version, Clinical Practice Guideline, Number 11. Rockville, Md.: Agency for Health Care Policy and Research.

Way, Lawrence W., MD. 1996. *Current Surgical Diagnosis & Treatment.* 10th ed. New York City: McGraw-Hill Professional Publishing Group.

Coding Self-Test

Assign the appropriate ICD-9-CM codes (include procedure codes, M codes, E codes, and V codes, where applicable) to the following:

1. Complete elective abortion due to maternal rubella, fetus not damaged; aspiration curettage

    _____

2. Postpartum abscess of breast; patient discharged five days ago following spontaneous delivery of live triplets

    _____

3. Adenocarcinoma of descending colon with extension to mesenteric lymph nodes; permanent sigmoid colostomy

    _____

4. Paranoid schizophrenic patient in remission

    _____295.35_____

5. Obstructive hydrocephalus; ventriculoatrial shunt

    _____331.4, 02.32_____

6. Parkinsonism secondary to haloperidol drug therapy

    _____332.1, E939.2_____

7. Gangrene of lower leg due to uncontrolled type I diabetes

    _____250.73, 785.4_____

8. Twin delivered by cesarean delivery (in hospital) with hypoglycemia due to maternal diabetes; male stillborn

    _____

9. History of allergic reaction to sulfa

    _____V14.02_____

10. Renal dialysis session for patient with chronic kidney disease, stage V; hemodialysis

    _____V56.0, 585.5, 39.95_____

11. Chronic obstructive asthma with COPD

_493.20_

12. Unstable angina

_411.1_

13. Unexplained dizziness

_780.4_

14. Hypertensive heart and kidney disease with chronic kidney disease, stage III

_404.93, 585.3_

15. Iron deficiency anemia due to chronic blood loss

_280.0_

16. Cystic pancreatitis

_577.2_

17. Reye's syndrome

_331.81_

18. Deep third-degree burn of chest and right leg

_____

19. Chronic brain syndrome due to cerebral arteriosclerosis

_438.89 310.9_

20. Fracture of frontal bone with subarachnoid hemorrhage and concussion due to motor vehicle accident (patient driver of automobile)

_____

21. Infiltrative tuberculosis of both lungs, confirmed by bacterial culture; tuberculous spondylitis, bacterial and histological examinations not done at this time

_011.04, 015.01, 720.81_

22. Ovarian retention cyst; laparoscopic partial oophorectomy

_620.2, 65.25_

23. Lyme disease with associated arthritis

_____

24. Abnormal prothrombin time, cause to be determined

_790.92_

25. Newborn born in community hospital transferred to university medical center. Code for the infant at the university medical center treated for hypoplastic left heart syndrome.

_____

26. Ingestion of 30 amitriptyline (Elavil) tablets resulting in an overdose, determined to be a suicide attempt; tachycardia

_____

27. Fracture, right shoulder, as the result of a fall off a ladder, occurred at a private residence; closed reduction, humerus, upper end, with immobilization

_____

28. Inflamed seborrheic keratosis of right temple; cryotherapy of lesion on right temple

_____

29. Moderate mental retardation as the result of acute bacterial meningitis ten years ago

_____

30. Chlamydial vaginitis

_____099.53_____

31. Infiltrating duct carcinoma, upper outer quadrant, with metastases to bone

_____

32. Diabetic hypoglycemic shock in a patient with uncontrolled type I diabetes

_____250.83_____

33. Secondary thrombocytopenia due to hypersplenism; splenectomy

_____287.4____41.5_____

34. Pneumonia due to coagulase-positive staphylococcus aureus; fiber-optic bronchoscopy

_____482.41___33.22_____

35. Peptic ulcer of the lesser curvature of the stomach, acute, with hemorrhage; esophagogastro-duodenoscopy with closed biopsy of stomach

_____533.00___45.16_____

36. Rapidly progressive chronic glomerulonephritis; percutaneous renal biopsy

_____582.4 , 55.23_____

37. Coronary artery disease within previous vein bypass grafts; coronary artery bypass grafts with double internal mammary bypass and a single aortocoronary bypass with extracorporeal circulation

_____414.05 , 36.16 , 36.11_____

38. Patient with a history of bladder carcinoma seen for a follow-up examination related to his past partial cystectomy treatment; no recurrence found; cystoscopy with biopsy of bladder

_____V10.51, V67.09 , 57.33_____

39. Degenerative joint disease, localized in knees; total knee replacement, left knee

_____

40. Malignant lymphoma, undifferentiated Burkitt's type; bone marrow aspiration

_____200.2 , 41.39_____

41. Postcatheterization stricture of urethra with urinary incontinence; release of urethral stricture

_____598.2 , 788.30 , 58.5_____

42. Chronic hidradenitis suppurativa; wide excision of hidradenitis of right axilla; partial-thickness skin graft

_____

43. Heroin poisoning, accidental overdose; coma; multiple drug dependence including heroin and barbiturates

_____

44. Positive TB skin test

_____017.05_____

45. Gunshot wound of chest with massive intrathoracic injury to multiple organs; shot by another person with a handgun who was charged with attempted homicide; injury occurred on a public street; patient died during an exploratory thoracotomy

_____908.0 VE965.0, E967.1, E969, 34.02, E969_____

46. Patient admitted for her first round of chemotherapy after a total abdominal hysterectomy and salpingo-oophorectomy for ovarian carcinoma with known metastases to intra-pelvic lymph nodes; chemotherapy

_____99.25 V58.76 239.8_____

47. Congenital hypertrophic pyloric stenosis corrected by pyloromyotomy in a four-week-old infant

_____

48. Internal derangement of lateral meniscus, posterior horn, right knee due to past sports injury; arthroscopy, right knee

_____

49. Traumatic arthritis of left wrist secondary to old fracture-dislocation of wrist, which was the result of a fall

_____

50. Pregnancy, delivered at 35 weeks, single liveborn infant; postpartum fever of unknown origin; patient with known continuous marihuana drug dependence

_____

Appendix A

Microorganisms

Table of Microorganisms

Bacteria	Species	Common Diseases
Bacillus	B. anthracis	Cutaneous anthrax, eye infections, food poisoning, intestinal anthrax, pulmonary anthrax
Bacteriodes	B. fragilis B. melaninogenicus	Abscess of brain, liver, bacteremia, endocarditis, gangrene, peritonitis
Bordetella	B. parapertussis B. bronchiseptica	Whooping cough
Brucella	B. melitensis B. abortus B. suis	Undulant fever, brucellosis
Chlamydia	C. trachomatis C. psittaci	Conjunctivitis, lymphogranuloma venereum, trachoma, cervicitis, salpingitis, urethritis
Clostridium	C. botulinum C. perfringens C. tetani C. septicum	Botulism, gas gangrene, lockjaw
Enterobacter		Urinary tract infection, pneumonia
Escherichia coli (E. coli)		Appendicitis, cystitis, infantile diarrhea, peritonitis, pyelitis, pyelonephritis, postop wound infections
Hemophilus	H. aegyptius H. adrophilus H. ducreyi H. influenzae H. parainfluenzae	Chancres, conjunctivitis, endocarditis, chronic sinusitis, influenza, meningitis, mastoiditis, pneumonia, upper respiratory disease
Klebsiella	K. ozaenae K. rhinoscleromatis K. pneumoniae	Disorder of smelling faculties, nodules of nose, pneumonia, severe enteritis, upper respiratory disease
Mycobacterium	M. Leprae M. fortuitum	Cervical adenitis, leprosy, skin lesions, tuberculosis

(Continued on next page)

Table of Microorganisms (Continued)

Bacteria	Species	Common Diseases
Mycoplasma	M. hominis M. pneumoniae M. tuberculous	Cervicitis, pneumonia, prostatitis, urethritis
Neisseria	N. meningitidis N. pneumoniae	Gonorrhea, meningococcal meningitis, pulmonary infections, tooth abscesses, urinary tract infection
Proteus	P. vulgaris P. mirabilis P. morganii P. rettgeri P. inconstans	Kidney disease, urinary tract infection
Pseudomonas	P. aeruginosa P. maltophilia P. cepacia	Chronic otitis media, upper respiratory infections, urinary tract infection, wounds of burn sites, endocarditis
Rickettsiaceae	R. australis R. conorii R. prowazekii R. rickettsii R. typhi R. tsutsugamushi R. quintana	Spotted fever typhus, rickettsial pneumonitis
Salmonella	S. enteritis S. typhi S. arizonae S. cholerae—suis	Enteritis, endocarditis, liver infections, nephritis, meningitis, osteomyelitis, typhoid fever, typhoid ulcers
Shigella	S. dysenteriae S. flexneri S. boydii S. sonnei	Dysentery
Staphylococcus	S. aureus S. epidermis S. saprophyticus	Diarrhea, food poisoning, conjunctivitis, meningitis, skin infections, pneumonia, septicemia
Streptococcus—alpha	Group D (enterococcus)	Urinary tract infection, wound infection
Streptococcus—beta	Group A (S. pyogenes)	Pharyngitis, tonsillitis wound and skin infections, septicemia
	Group B (S. agalactiae)	Perinatal: pneumonia, meningitis, septicemia
	Group C	Pharyngitis, tonsillitis, sepsis, necrotizing fasciitis
Streptococcus pneumoniae		Pneumonia, septicemia, meningitis, otitis media
Streptococcus	S. viridans S. mitis S. bovis S. faecalis	Glomerulonephritis, puerperal fever, laryngitis, rheumatic fever, scarlet fever, sinusitis, tonsillitis
Treponema	T. pallidum T. pertenue T. carateum T. vincentii	Pinta (skin infection syphilis, trench mouth, yaw)

Classification of Bacteria

Gram-Negative Rods

Aerobic	*Facultative Anaerobic*	*Anaerobic*
Campylobacter	Enterobacteriaceae:	Bacteroides
Helicobacter	Escherichia	Fusobacterium
Legionella	Salmonella	
Brucella	Shigella	
Bordetella	Citrobacter	
Francisella	Klebsiella	
Pseudomonas	Enterobacter	
	Serratia	
	Proteus	
	Morganella	
	Yersinia	
	Vibrionaceae:	
	Vibrio	
	Aeromonas	
	Pasteurellaceae:	
	Haemophilus	
	Gardnerella	
	Pasteurella	

Gram-Negative Cocci

Aerobic	*Facultative Anaerobic*	*Anaerobic*
Neisseria		Veillonella
Branhamella (Moraxella)		

Gram-Positive Rods

Aerobic	*Facultative Anaerobic*	*Anaerobic*
Bacillus	Lactobacillus	Clostridium
Corynebacterium	Listeria	
Mycobacterium	Actinomyces	
Nocardia		

Gram-Positive Cocci

Aerobic	*Facultative Anaerobic*	*Anaerobic*
Peptostreptococcus	Staphylococcus	Peptococcus
	Streptococcus	

Miscellaneous

Arthropod Vector:	Rickettsia, Coxiella
No Arthropod Vector:	Chlamydia
Devoid of Cell Wall:	Mycoplasma, Ureaplasma
Microaerophilic:	Borrelia
Obligate Aerobic:	Leptospira
Living Cells Required:	Treponema

Appendix B

Commonly Used Drugs

Drug	Action	Use
Adriamycin	cytotoxic	used to produce regression antibiotic in disseminated neoplastic conditions
Albuterol (Ventolin, Proventil)	antiasthmatic/ bronchodilators	bronchospasms in reversible obstructive airway disease
Aldactazide	diuretic & antihypertensive	used for the rx of edematous conditions due to CHF, cirrhosis of the liver, and essential hypertension
Aldomet	antihypertensive	used in the management of hypertension
Aldoril	antihypertensive	used for rx of severe essential hypertension and in malignant hypertension
Alkeran	antineoplastic	used for palliation in multiple myeloma and nonresectable epithelial ovarian carcinoma
Allopurinol	unclassified agent	used in the treatment of gout
Alupent	bronchodilator	used in the rx of bronchial asthma and reversible bronchospasm in bronchitis and emphysema
Amikacin (Amikin)	antibiotic	used in the short-term rx of serious Gram-negative bacterial infections
Aminophylline	bronchodilator, pulmonary vasodilator, smooth muscle relaxant	used for relief and/or prevention of symptoms from asthma and reversible bronchospasms in bronchitis and emphysema
Amoxicillin (Trimox, Amoxil)	antibiotic	used in the rx of infections due to Gram-negative and Gram-positive organisms
Ampicillin	antibacterial	used in the rx of Gram-negative bacteria
Ancef	antibiotic	used in the rx of serious respiratory tract; urinary tract; biliary tract; skin, bone, and genital infections; septicemia; and endocarditis
Apresoline	antihypertensive	used for the management of essential hypertension
Ascriptin	analgesic, anti-inflammatory, antipyretic	used in the rx of rheumatoid arthritis, osteoarthritis, and other arthritic conditions

(Continued on next page)

Commonly Used Drugs (Continued)

Drug	Action	Use
Atarax	anxiolytic	used for the relief of anxiety and tension associated with psychoneurosis and as an adjunct in organic disease states in which anxiety is manifested
Ativan	anxiolytic	used for the management of anxiety disorders
Augmentin	antibiotic, anti-infective	UTI, lower respiratory tract infection, otitis media
Bactrim	antibacterial	used for the rx of urinary tract infections, acute otitis media, bronchitis in adults, and Pneumocystis carinii pneumonitis
Benadryl	antihistamine	used for the rx of perennial and seasonal allergies due to inhalant allergens and foods; motion sickness; and Parkinsonism
Bentyl	smooth muscle relaxant	used for the rx of functional bowel/ irritable bowel syndrome
Betadine	antiseptic	used for disinfection of topical wounds
Brethine	bronchodilator	used for the rx of bronchial asthmas and reversible bronchospasm in bronchitis and emphysema
Bronkosol	bronchodilator	used for the rx of bronchial asthma and reversible bronchospasm in bronchitis and emphysema
Cardizem	calcium channel blocker	angina, atrial fibrillation, atrial flutter
Chloromycetin	antibiotic	used for the rx of serious infections
Cimetidine (Tagamet)	histamine	used for the short-term rx of antagonist
Cipro	anti-infective, antibacterial	used for UTI, lower respiratory infection, bone and joint infection
Cisplatin	antineoplastic	used for testicular, ovarian, and bladder carcinomas
Clindamycin	antibiotic	used for the rx of bacterial and parasitic infections
Clinoril	anti-inflammatory	used for the rx of osteoarthritis and rheumatoid arthritis
Clonidine (Catapres)	antihypertensive	used for hypertension, reduces blood pressure rapidly
Colace	stool softener	used in constipation due to hard stools, in painful anorectal conditions, in cardiac and other conditions in which maximum ease of passage is desirable
Compazine	antiemetic, anxiolytic	used for control of severe nausea and vomiting, and for the short-term rx of generalized nonpsychotic anxiety

Commonly Used Drugs (Continued)

Drug	Action	Use
Coumadin	anticoagulant	used for prophylaxis and rx of venous thrombosis, atrial fibrillation with embolization, and pulmonary embolism
Cytoxan	antineoplastic	used to slow all growth in leukemia, myeloma, lymphoma, breast, ovarian, and lung cancers
Dalmane	hypnotic	used for the rx of insomnia
Darvocet-N	analgesic	used for relief of mild to moderate pain
Decadron	anti-inflammatory	used for rx of endocrine and allergic rheumatic disorders, ophthalmic, respiratory, and hematological disorders
Demerol	analgesic	used for relief of moderate to severe pain
Desyrel	antidepressant	used for rx of depression
Diabinese	antidiabetic	used to control mild to moderately severe adult-onset diabetes
Digitalis	cardiotonic	used to increase the force of myocardial contractions and as a conduction system depressant to decrease heart rate
Digoxin (Lanoxin)	cardiotonic	used in the rx of CHF
Dilantin	antiepileptic	used for control of tonic-clonic and psychomotor seizures
Dilaudid	narcotic, analgesic	used for the relief of pain
Diltiazem	calcium blocker	used to dilate coronary arteries in angina
Dolobid	analgesic, anti-inflammatory, antipyretic	used for management of acute or long-term osteoarthritis and mild to moderate pain
Dopamine	vasopressor	used to increase cardiac and urinary output in shock syndrome due to MIs, trauma, renal failure, and septicemia
Dyazide	diuretic/antihypertensive	used for rx of edema and hypertension
Ecotrin	analgesic	used for relief of minor aches and pains of arthritis and rheumatism
Elavil	antidepressant	used for relief of symptoms of depression
Epinephrine	bronchodilator, cardiotonic	most commonly used to relieve (Adrenaline) respiratory distress due to bronchospasm and to restore cardiac rhythm in cardiac arrest
Erythromycin	antibiotic	used for rx of upper and lower respiratory tract, skin, and soft tissue infections

(Continued on next page)

Commonly Used Drugs (Continued)

Drug	Action	Use
Euthroid	thyroid preparation	used for rx of hypothyroidism, simple goiter, and subacute or chronic thyroiditis
Feosol	hematinic	used for rx of iron deficiency anemia
Flexeril	skeletal muscle relaxant	used as adjunct to rest and physical therapy for relief of muscle spasm
5-Fluorouracil	antineoplastic	used for palliative management of carcinoma of colon, rectum, breast, stomach, and pancreas
Garamycin	aminoglycoside	used for rx of serious infections caused by susceptible strains of Pseudomonas, E. coli, Proteus, Klebsiella-Serratia, Citrobacter, and Staphylococcus
Glucophage	antidiabetic	used to treat NIDDM
Halcion	hypnotic	used for short-term management of insomnia characterized by difficulty in falling asleep
Haldol	tranquilizer	used for management of manifestations of psychiatric disorders
Heparin	anticoagulant	used for prophylaxis and rx of venous thrombosis, pulmonary embolism, prevention of cerebral thrombosis, and rx of consumptive coagulopathies
Hydralazine	antihypertensive	used in the management of hypertension
Hydrochlorothiazide	diuretic/ antihypertensive	used in the management of hypertension, also adjunctive therapy in edema associated with CHF, hepatic cirrhosis, and corticosteroid and estrogen therapy
Hydrocortisone	anti-inflammatory	used to relieve symptoms of rheumatic disorders; replacement therapy for endogenous hormones
Hydrodiuril	diuretic and hypertensive	used for adjunctive therapy in edema associated with CHF, hepatic cirrhosis, and corticosteroid and estrogen therapy; management of hypertension
Hygroton	diuretic and antihypertensive	used for management of hypertension, adjunctive therapy in edema associated with CHF, and renal dysfunction
Imuran	immunosuppressive	used in prevention of rejection in renal homotransplantation, and for management of severe, active rheumatoid arthritis
Inderal (Propranolol)	beta-adrenergic blocking agent	used for rx of hypertension, long-term management of angina pectoris due to coronary atherosclerosis and cardiac arrhythmias, myocardial infarction, and migraine

Commonly Used Drugs (Continued)

Drug	Action	Use
Insulin	antidiabetic	many varieties of injectable insulin including beef, pork, and human are available for treatment of diabetes
Isoptin (Verapamil)	calcium antagonist	used for conversion to sinus rhythm of paroxysmal supraventricular tachycardias
Isordil	smooth muscle relaxant	used for the rx of acute angina attacks
Kaon	potassium	used for rx of hypokalemia and digitalis intoxication
Keflex	antibiotic	used for rx of infections
Kefzol	antibiotic	used for rx of respiratory tract, genitourinary tract, biliary tract, skin and soft tissue, bone and joint infections, and endocarditis
Lanoxin	cardiotonic	used in treatment of arrhythmias and low-output cardiac failure
Lasix	diuretic	used in the rx of edema associated with CHF, cirrhosis of the liver, and renal disease including the nephrotic syndrome
Leukeran (Chlorambucil)	antineoplastic	used for rx of chronic lymphatic leukemia and malignant lymphomas
Librium	sedative	used for management of anxiety disorders and withdrawal symptoms of acute alcoholism
Lidocaine	antiarrhythmic	used for rx of ventricular arrhythmias
Lithium	psychotherapeutic	used in rx of manic episodes of manic-depressive illness
Lopressor	antihypertensive	used for management of hypertension
Lovastatin	cholesterol-lowering agent	used for reduction of elevated total LDL levels in patients with primary hypercholesterolemia
Mandol	antibiotic	used for rx of serious respiratory, urinary, skin, and bone infections, and peritonitis and septicemia
Meclomen	anti-inflammatory	used for rx of acute and chronic rheumatoid arthritis and osteoarthritis
Mellaril	tranquilizer	used for short-term rx of moderate to marked depression and for rx of symptoms such as agitation, anxiety, and tension; rx for behavioral problems in children
Metamucil	laxative	rx for chronic constipation

(Continued on next page)

Commonly Used Drugs (Continued)

Drug	Action	Use
Methotrexate	antineoplastic	
Minipress	antihypertensive	used for rx of gestational chorio-carcinoma, chorioadenoma destruens, and hydatidiform mole
Minoxidil	antihypertensive	used for rx of hypertension
Motrin	analgesic and antipyretic	used for relief of signs and symptoms of rheumatoid arthritis and osteoarthritis; rx for primary dysmenorrhea; and provides relief of mild to moderate pain
Mustargen	antineoplastic	used for rx of Hodgkin's disease, lymphosarcoma, chronic leukemias, and bronchogenic carcinoma
Mycostatin (Nystatin)	antibiotic	used for rx of candidiasis
Mylanta	antacid	used for relief of symptoms associated with gastric hyperacidity and trapped gas
Myleran	antineoplastic	used for rx of chronic myelogenous leukemia
Mylicon	antiflatulent	used for relief of the painful symptoms of excess gas in the digestive system
Nipride	hypotensive	used for immediate reduction of blood pressure
Nitroglycerin	muscle relaxant	used for prophylaxis and rx of angina pectoris
Norflex	analgesic and anticholinergic	used for relief of discomfort associated with acute painful musculoskeletal conditions
Norpace	antiarrhythmic	used for suppression and prevention of recurrence of some cardiac arrhythmias
Norpramin	antidepressant	used for relief of symptoms in various depressive syndromes, especially endogenous depression
Norvasc	calcium channel blocker	used for hypertension; angina
Oncovin (Vincristine)	antineoplastic	used in rx of acute leukemia and useful in combination with other drugs for some lymphomas and sarcomas
Orinase (Tolbutamide)	antidiabetic	used for management of diabetes mellitus of stable type without acute complications
Paxil	antidepressant	used for depression
Pentamidine	antiprotozoal	used against Pneumocystis carinii
Periactin	antihistamine	used for allergic reactions and urticaria
Persantine	coronary vasodilator	therapy for chronic angina pectoris

Commonly Used Drugs (Continued)

Drug	Action	Use
Phenergan	antihistamine	used for allergic rhinitis, control of nausea and vomiting, sedation, and motion sickness
Phenobarbital	anticonvulsant sedative and hypnotic	used for prophylactic management of all forms of epilepsy
Prednisone	glucocorticoid	used for its immunosuppressant effects and for relief of inflammations; used in arthritis, polymyositis, and other systemic diseases
Prilosec	anti-ulcer	used for gastric and duodenal ulcer; gastroesophageal reflux disease
Procan (Procainamide)	antiarrhythmic	used for rx of premature ventricular contractions, ventricular tachycardia, atrial fibrillation, and paroxysmal atrial tachycardia
Procardia (Nifedipine)	antianginal	used for rx of vasospastic angina and chronic stable angina
Prolixin	antipsychotic	used for management of chronic schizophrenia
Pronestyl	depresses excitability of cardiac muscle	used in rx of cardiac arrhythmias
Prozac	antidepressant	used for depression
Quinidine	antiarrhythmic	used in rx of cardiac arrhythmias
Ranitidine (Zantac)	antisecretory	used for short-term rx of active duodenal ulcer and rx of pathological hypersecretory states
Restoril	hypnotic	used for relief of insomnia
Riopan	antacid	used for relief of heartburn, sour stomach, acid indigestion, and upset stomach
Septra DS	antibacterial	used for rx of urinary tract infections and acute exacerbations of chronic bronchitis
Solu-Cortef	anti-inflammatory, adrenocortical steroid	used for acute exacerbations of allergies; rheumatic, respiratory, GI, and hematology disorders
Streptokinase	fibrinolytic	used for lysis of pulmonary embolism, deep vein thrombosis, arterial thrombosis and embolism, and coronary artery thrombosis
Surfak	stool softener	used for fecal softening without pro-pulsion action to accomplish defecation
Synthroid	hormone	used for replacement therapy for reduced or absent thyroid function of any etiology
Tenormin	antihypertensive	used for management of hypertension

(Continued on next page)

315

Commonly Used Drugs (Continued)

Drug	Action	Use
Theo-Dur	bronchodilator	used for relief of bronchial asthma symptoms and for reversible bronchospasm associated with chronic bronchitis and emphysema
Theophylline	bronchodilator, pulmonary vasodilator, smooth muscle relaxant	used for rx of bronchial obstruction in asthma and chronic obstructive pulmonary disease
Thiotepa	antineoplastic	used in rx of adenocarcinomas of breast and ovary and for controlling intracavitary effusions
Thorazine	psychotropic	used for the management of manifestations of psychotic disorders
Tobramycin	antibiotic	used for rx of serious bacterial infections
Tolectin	anti-inflammatory	used for relief of signs and symptoms of rheumatoid arthritis, osteoarthritis, and juvenile rheumatoid arthritis
Tonocard (Tocainide)	antiarrhythmic	used for rx of ventricular arrhythmias
Traxene	CNS-depressant	used for management of anxiety disorders indicated as adjunctive therapy in the management of partial seizures and for relief of acute alcohol withdrawal
Tylenol	analgesic/ antipyretic	used for relief of pain and/or fever
Valium	anxiolytic	used for management of anxiety disorders; relief of acute agitation, tremor, and hallucinosis in acute alcohol withdrawal
Vasotec	ace inhibitor	used for hypertension, heart failure
Veetids	anti-infective, antibiotic	used for mild to moderately severe infections
Velban	antineoplastic	used for palliative rx of a variety of malignant and neoplastic conditions
Vicodin	analgesic, antipyretic	used for relief of moderately severe pain
Wytensin	antihypertensive	used for rx of hypertension
Zantac	antisecretory	used for short-term rx of active duodenal ulcer
Zaroxolyn	diuretic/saluretic/ antihypertensive	used in management of hypertension and rx of edema
Zestril	ace inhibitor	used for hypertension, heart failure
Zithromax	antibiotic, anti-infective	used for skin infections, respiratory tract infections
Zocor	antilipemic agent	used for hypercholesterolemia
Zoloft	antidepressant	used for depression
Zovirax	antiviral	used in rx of herpes viruses

Appendix C

Morphology Terminology

Adenocarcinoma: Carcinoma derived from glandular tissue or in which the tumor cells form recognizable glandular structures. Adenocarcinomas may be classified according to the predominant pattern of cell arrangement, as papillary, alveolar, and so on, or according to a particular product of the cells, as mucinous adenocarcinoma.

Adenoma: A benign epithelial tumor in which the cells form recognizable glandular structures or in which the cells are clearly derived from glandular epithelium.

Adenoma, chromophobe: A tumor of the anterior lobe of the pituitary whose cells do not stain readily with either acid or basic dyes and whose presence may be associated with hypopituitarism.

Angioblastoma: Certain blood-vessel tumors of the brain; those arising in the cerebellum (cerebellar angioblastoma) may be cystic and associated with von Hippel-Lindau's disease; also, a blood-vessel tumor arising from the meninges of the brain or spinal cord (angioblastic meningioma).

Angioma: A tumor whose cells tend to form blood vessels (hemangioma) or lymph vessels (lymphangioma); a tumor made up of blood vessels or lymph vessels.

Angiosarcoma: A hemangiosarcoma.

Astrocytoma: A tumor composed of astrocytes; such tumors have been classified into Grades I–IV in order of increasing malignancy.

Carcinoma: A malignant new growth made up of epithelial cells tending to infiltrate the surrounding tissues and give rise to metastases.

Carcinoma, basal cell: An epithelial tumor that seldom metastasizes but has the potential for local invasion and destruction.

Carcinoma, cholangiocellular: Primary carcinoma of the liver originating in bile duct cells. Also called *cholangioma* and *cholangiocarcinoma*.

Carcinoma, embryonal: A highly malignant, primitive form of carcinoma, probably of germinal cell or teratomatous derivation, that usually arises in a gonad and rarely in other sites; a seminoma.

Carcinoma, epidermoid: Carcinoma in which the cells tend to differentiate in the same way that the cells of the epidermis do; that is, they tend to form prickle cells and undergo cornification.

Carcinoma, squamous cell: Carcinoma developed from squamous epithelium, and having cuboid cells.

Cholangiocarcinoma: Cholangiocellular carcinoma.

Cholangioma: Cholangiocellular carcinoma.

Chondroma: A tumor or tumor-like growth of cartilage cells that may remain within the substance of a cartilage or bone (true chondroma, or enchondroma) or may develop on the surface of a cartilage (ecchondroma, or ecchondrosis).

Chondrosarcoma: A malignant tumor derived from cartilage cells or their precursors. Also called *chondroma sarcomatosum.*

Choriocarcinoma: An epithelial malignancy of trophoblastic cells, formed by the abnormal proliferation of cuboidal and syncytial cells of the placental epithelium, without the production of chorionic villi. Almost all cases arise in the uterus, developing from hydatidiform mole (50 percent), following an abortion (25 percent), or during a normal pregnancy (22 percent). The remainder occur in ectopic pregnancies and in genital (ovarian and testicular) and extragenital teratomas. Also called *chorioblastoma, chorioepithelioma, chorionic carcinoma or epithelioma, deciduocellular sarcoma,* and *syncytioma malignum.*

Cystadenocarcinoma: Carcinoma and cystadenoma.

Cystadenoma: Adenoma associated with cystoma.

Cystadenoma, mucinous: A multilocular tumor produced by the epithelial cells of the ovary and having mucin-filled cavities; the great majority of these tumors are benign. Also called *mucinous cystadenoma.*

Cystadenoma, serous: A cystic tumor of the ovary that contains thin, clear, yellow serous fluid and varying amounts of solid tissue, with a malignant potential several times greater than that of mucinous cystadenoma.

Cystoma: A tumor containing cysts of neoplastic origin; a cystic tumor.

Disease, Hodgkin's: A form of malignant lymphoma characterized by painless, progressive enlargement of the lymph nodes, spleen, and general lymphoid tissue; other symptoms may include anorexia, lassitude, weight loss, fever, pruritus, night sweats, and anemia. The characteristic histologic feature is presence of Reed-Sternberg cells.

Disease, Von Recklinghausen's: A familial condition characterized by developmental changes in the nervous system, muscles, bones, and skin and marked superficially by the formation of multiple pedunculated soft tumors (neurofibromas) distributed over the entire body associated with areas of pigmentation. Also called *neurofibromatosis, multiple neuroma,* and *neuromatosis.*

Embryoma: A general term applied to neoplasms thought to derive from embryonic cells or tissues, including dermoid cysts, teratomas, embryonal carcinomas and sarcomas, nephroblastomas, hepatoblastomas, and so on.

Endothelioblastoma: A tumor derived from primitive vasoformative tissue with formation of usually small and slitlike vascular spaces lined by prominent endothelial cells, including hemangioendothelioma, angiosarcoma, lymphangioendothelioma, and lymphangiosarcoma.

Endothelioma: A tumor originating from the endothelial lining of blood vessels (hemangio-endothelioma), lymphatics (lymphangioendothelioma), or serous cavities (mesothelioma).

Ependymoma: A neoplasm composed of differentiated ependymal cells; most ependymomas grow slowly and are benign, but malignant varieties do occur.

Fibroblastoma: A tumor arising from a fibroblast; such tumors are now differentiated as fibromas or fibrosarcomas.

Fibroma: A tumor composed mainly of fibrous or fully developed connective tissue. Also called *fibroid.*

Fibrosarcoma: A sarcoma derived from fibroblasts that produce collagen.

Glioma: A tumor composed of tissue that represents neuroglia in any one of its stages of development; sometimes extended to include all the primary intrinsic neoplasms of the brain and spinal cord, including astrocytomas, ependymomas, neurocytomas, and so on.

Hemangioma: An extremely common benign tumor, occurring most often in infancy and childhood, made up of newly formed blood vessels, and resulting from malformation of angioblastic tissue of fetal life. Two main types exist—capillary and cavernous.

Hemangiosarcoma: A malignant tumor formed by the proliferation of endothelial and fibroblastic tissue.

Hepatoma: A tumor of the liver, especially hepatocellular carcinoma.

Hypernephroma: Renal cell carcinoma whose structure resembles the cortical tissue of the adrenal gland.

Keloid: A sharply elevated, irregularly shaped, progressively enlarging scar due to the formation of excessive amounts of collagen in the corium during connective tissue repair.

Leiomyoma: A benign tumor derived from smooth muscle, most commonly of the uterus. Also called *fibroid.*

Leiomyosarcoma: A sarcoma containing large spindle cells of smooth muscle, most commonly of the uterus or retroperitoneal region.

Leukemia: A progressive, malignant disease of the blood-forming organs, characterized by distorted proliferation and development of leukocytes and their precursors in the blood and bone marrow. Leukemia is classified clinically on the basis of (1) the duration and character of the disease—acute or chronic; (2) the type of cell involved—myeloid (myelogenous), lymphoid (lymphogenous), or monocytic; or (3) increase or no increase in the number of abnormal cells in the blood—leukemic or aleukemic (subleukemic).

Leukemia, acute nonlymphocytic (ANLL): Leukemia occurring most commonly after treatment with alkylating agents characterized by pancytopenia, megaloblastic bone marrow, nucleated red cells in treatment, with a short survival time.

Leukemia, adult T-cell: A form of leukemia with onset in adulthood, leukemic cells with T-cell properties, frequent dermal involvement, lymphadenopathy and hepatosplenomegaly, and a subacute or chronic course; it is associated with human T-cell leukemia-lymphoma virus.

Leukemia, aleukemic: Leukemia in which the total white blood cell count in the peripheral blood is either normal or below normal; it may be lymphocytic, monocytic, or myelogenous. Also called *subleukemic leukemia.*

Leukemia, basophilic: A disorder resembling acute or chronic leukemia in which the basophilic leukocytes predominate.

Leukemia, chronic granulocytic: A form of leukemia occurring mainly between the ages of twenty-five and sixty, usually associated with a unique chromosomal abnormality, in which the major clinical manifestations of malaise, hepatosplenomegaly, anemia, and leukocytosis are related to abnormal, excessive, unrestrained overgrowth of granulocytes in the bone marrow.

Leukemia, eosinophilic: A form of leukemia in which the eosinophil is the predominating cell. Although resembling chronic myelocytic leukemia in many ways, this form may follow an acute course despite the absence of predominantly blast forms in the peripheral blood.

Leukemia, hairy-cell: Leukemia marked by splenomegaly and by an abundance of large, mononuclear abnormal cells with numerous irregular cytoplasmic projections that give them a flagellated or hairy appearance in the bone marrow, spleen, liver, and peripheral blood. Also called *leukemic reticuloendotheliosis.*

Leukemia, leukopenic: *See* **leukemia, aleukemic.**

Leukemia, lymphatic: Leukemia associated with hyperplasia and overactivity of the lymphoid tissue, in which the leukocytes are lymphocytes or lymphoblasts. Also called *lymphoblastic leukemia, lymphocytic leukemia, lymphogenous leukemia, lymphoid leukemia.*

Leukemia, mast cell: A type of leukemia characterized by overwhelming numbers of tissue mast cells present in the peripheral blood.

Leukemia, monocytic: Leukemia in which the predominating leukocytes are identified as monocytes.

Leukemia, myelogenous: Leukemia arising from myeloid tissue in which the granular, polymorphonuclear leukocytes and their precursors are predominant. Also called *myelocytic leukemia, myeloid granulocytic leukemia.*

Leukemia, plasma cell: Leukemia in which the plasma cell is the predominating cell in the peripheral blood.

Lipoma: A benign tumor usually composed of mature fat cells.

Liposarcoma: A malignant tumor derived from primitive or embryonal lipoblastic cells that exhibit varying degrees of lipoblastic and/or lipomatous differentiation.

Lymphangioma: A benign tumor representing a congenital malformation of the lymphatic system, made up of newly formed lymph-containing vascular spaces and channels. Also called *angiomalymphaticum.*

Lymphangiosarcoma: A malignant tumor of lymphatic vessels, usually arising in a limb that is the site of chronic lymphedema.

Lymphoblastoma: Lymphoblastic lymphoma.

Lymphoma: Any neoplastic disorder of the lymphoid tissue; the term *lymphoma* often is used alone to denote malignant lymphoma.

Lymphoma, Burkitt's: A form of undifferentiated malignant lymphoma, usually found in central Africa—but also reported from other areas—and manifested most often as a large osteolytic lesion in the jaw or as an abdominal mass. The Epstein-Barr virus, a herpes virus, has been isolated from Burkitt's lymphoma and has been implicated as a causative agent.

Lymphoma, diffuse: Malignant lymphoma in which the neoplastic cells diffusely infiltrate the entire lymph node, without any definite organized pattern. Also called *lymphatic sarcoma* and *lymphosarcoma.*

Lymphoma, granulomatous: Hodgkin's disease.

Lymphoma, histiocytic: Malignant lymphoma characterized by the presence of large-sized tumor cells, resembling histiocytes morphologically but considered to be of lymphoid origin, that are irregular in shape with relatively abundant, frequently acidophilic cytoplasm. Also called *reticulum cell sarcoma.*

Lymphoma, lymphoblastic: A malignant lymphoma composed of a diffuse, relatively uniform proliferation of cells with round or convoluted nuclei and scanty cytoplasm that are cytologically similar to the lymphoblasts seen in acute lymphocytic leukemia.

Lymphoma, malignant: A group of malignant neoplasms characterized by the proliferation of cells native to the lymphoid tissues (lymphocytes, histiocytes, and their precursors and derivatives). The group is divided into two major clinicopathologic categories—Hodgkin's disease and non-Hodgkin's lymphoma.

Lymphoma, nodular: Malignant lymphoma in which the lymphomatous cells are clustered into identifiable nodules within the lymph nodes that somewhat resemble the germinal centers of lymph node follicles. Nodular lymphomas usually occur in older persons, commonly involving many (or all) nodes as well as possibly extranodal sites. Also called *Brill-Symmers' or Symmers' disease, follicular lymphoma,* and *giant follicle lymphoma.*

Lymphomas, non-Hodgkin's: A heterogeneous group of malignant lymphomas, the only common feature being an absence of the giant Reed-Sternberg cells characteristic of Hodgkin's disease. They arise from the lymphoid components of the immune system and present a clinical picture broadly similar to that of Hodgkin's disease, except the disease is initially more widespread, with the most common manifestation being painless enlargement of one or more peripheral lymph nodes.

Lymphosarcoma: A diffuse lymphoma.

Medulloblastoma: A cerebellar tumor composed of undifferentiated neuroepithelial cells that is highly radiosensitive.

Melanoblastoma: Malignant melanoma.

Melanoma: A tumor arising from the melanocytic system of the skin and other organs. When used alone, the term refers to malignant melanoma.

Melanoma, malignant: A malignant neoplasm of melanocytes, arising de novo or from a preexisting benign nevus, that occurs most often in the skin but also may involve the oral cavity, esophagus, anal canal, vagina, leptomeninges, and the conjunctiva or eye. Also called *melanotic carcinoma, melanoblastoma,* and *melanocarcinoma.*

Meningioma: A hard, slow-growing, usually vascular tumor occurring mainly along the meningeal vessels and superior longitudinal sinus, invading the dura and skull, and leading to erosion and thinning of the skull.

Mycosis fungoides: A chronic or rapidly progressive form of cutaneous T-cell lymphoma (formerly thought to be of fungal origin) that in some cases evolves into generalized lymphoma with a tendency for nodal, hematogenous, and visceral involvement.

Myeloma: A tumor composed of cells of the type normally found in the bone marrow. *See* **myeloma, multiple.**

Myeloma, multiple: A disseminated malignant neoplasm of plasma cells characterized by multiple bone marrow tumor foci and secretion of an M component, associated with widespread osteolytic lesions appearing radiographically as punched-out defects and resulting in bone pain, pathologic fractures, hypercalcemia, and normochromic, normocytic anemia. Spread to extraosseous sites occurs frequently in advanced disease. Depression of immunoglobulin levels results in increased susceptibility to infection. Bence Jones proteinuria is present in many cases and occasionally results in systemic amyloidosis. Renal failure resulting from calcium nephropathy or extensive cast formation occurs in about 20 percent of cases.

Myoma: A tumor made up of muscular elements.

Myxoblastoma: *See* **myxoma.**

Myxoma: A tumor composed of primitive connective tissue cells and stroma resembling mesenchyme.

Myxosarcoma: A sarcoma containing myxomatous tissue.

Neuroblastoma: A sarcoma of nervous system origin, composed chiefly of neuroblasts and affecting mostly infants and children up to ten years of age. Most of such tumors arise in the autonomic nervous system (sympathicoblastoma) or in the adrenal medulla.

Neurofibroma: A tumor of peripheral nerves caused by abnormal proliferation of Schwann cells.

Neuroma: A tumor or new growth largely made up of nerve cells and nerve fibers; a tumor growing from a nerve.

Nevus: Any congenital lesion of the skin; for example, a birthmark.

Osteoblastoma: A benign, painful, rather vascular tumor of bone characterized by the formation of osteoid tissue and primitive bone. Also called *giant osteoid osteoma.*

Osteochondroma: Osteoma blended with chondroma, a benign tumor consisting of projecting adult bone capped by cartilage.

Osteoclastoma: Giant cell tumor of bone.

Osteoma: A tumor composed of bone tissue; a hard tumor of bonelike structure developing on a bone (homoplastic osteoma) and sometimes on other structures (heteroplastic osteoma).

Osteoma, osteoid: A small, benign, but painful, circumscribed tumor of spongy bone occurring especially in the bones of the extremities and vertebrae, most often in young persons.

Osteosarcoma: Osteogenic sarcoma.

Papilloma: A benign epithelial neoplasm producing finger-like or verrucous projections from the epithelial surface.

Pheochromocytoma: A usually benign, well-encapsulated, lobular, vascular tumor of chromaffin tissue of the adrenal medulla or sympathetic paraganglia. The cardinal symptom, reflecting the increased secretion of epinephrine and norepinephrine, is hypertension, which may be persistent or intermittent. During severe attacks, there may be headache, sweating, palpitation, apprehension, tremor, pallor or flushing of the face, nausea and vomiting, pain in the chest and abdomen, and paresthesias of the extremities.

Rhabdomyoma: A benign tumor derived from striated muscle.

Rhabdomyosarcoma: A highly malignant tumor of striated muscle derived from primitive mesenchymal cells and exhibiting differentiation along rhabdomyoblastic lines, including, but not limited to, the presence of cells with recognizable cross-striations.

Sarcoma: A tumor made up of a substance like the embryonic connective tissue; tissue composed of closely packed cells embedded in a fibrillar or homogenous substance. Sarcomas are often highly malignant.

Sarcoma, Ewing's: *See* **tumor, Ewing's.**

Sarcoma, Kaposi's: A multicentric, malignant neoplastic vascular proliferation characterized by the development of bluish-red cutaneous nodules, usually on the lower extremities, most often on the toes or feet, and slowly increasing in size and number and spreading to more proximal sites.

Sarcoma, osteogenic: A malignant primary tumor of bone composed of a malignant connective tissue stroma with evidence of malignant osteoid, bone, and/or cartilage formation. Also called *osteolytic sarcoma* and *osteoid sarcoma.*

Seminoma: A radiosensitive, malignant neoplasm of the testis, thought to be derived from primordial germ cells of the sexually undifferentiated embryonic gonad, occurring as a gray to yellow-white nodule or mass.

Teratoma: A true neoplasm made up of a number of different types of tissue, none of which is native to the area where it occurs; most often found in the ovary or testis.

Teratoma, malignant: A solid, malignant ovarian tumor resembling a dermoid cyst but composed of immature embryonal and/or extraembryonal elements derived from all three germ layers. Also called *immature teratoma* and *solid teratoma.*

Teratoma, mature: A benign teratoma of the ovary, usually found in young women. Also called *benign cystic teratoma, cystic teratoma,* and *dermoid cyst.*

Tumor, Ewing's: A malignant tumor of the bone that always arises in medullary tissue, occurring more often in cylindrical bones, with pain, fever, and leukocytosis as prominent symptoms. Also called *Ewing's sarcoma.*

Tumor, giant cell, of bone: A bone tumor composed of cellular spindle cell stroma containing scattered multinucleated giant cells resembling osteoclasts; symptoms may include local pain and tenderness, functional disability, and, occasionally, pathologic fractures.

Tumor, Krukenberg's: A special type of carcinoma of the ovary, usually metastatic, from cancer of the gastrointestinal tract, especially of the stomach.

Tumor, mixed: A tumor composed of more than one type of neoplastic tissue, especially "a complex embryonal tumor of local origin, which reproduces the normal development of the tissues and organs of the affected part" (Ewing).

Tumor, Wilms': A rapidly developing malignant mixed tumor of the kidneys, made up of embryonal elements. It usually affects children before the fifth year but may occur in the fetus and, rarely, in later life.

Appendix D

Sample UB-92 and CMS-1500 Billing Forms

Sample UB-92 billing form

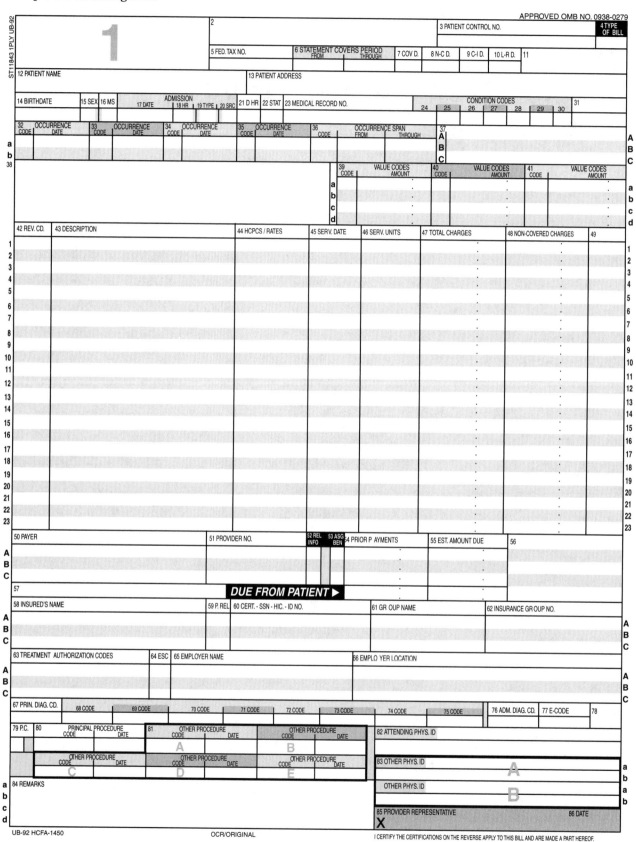

Sample CMS-1500 form

PLEASE
DO NOT
STAPLE
IN THIS
AREA

CARRIER →

| | PICA | | | | | **HEALTH INSURANCE CLAIM FORM** | | PICA | | |

| MEDICARE | MEDICAID | CHAMPUS | CHAMPVA | GROUP HEALTH PLAN | FECA BLK LUNG | OTHER | 1a. INSURED'S I.D. NUMBER (FOR PROGRAM IN ITEM 1) |

1. MEDICARE   MEDICAID   CHAMPUS   CHAMPVA   GROUP HEALTH PLAN   FECA BLK LUNG   OTHER   1a. INSURED'S I.D. NUMBER   (FOR PROGRAM IN ITEM 1)
   (Medicare #) (Medicaid #) (Sponsor's SSN) (VA File #) (SSN or ID) (SSN) (ID)

2. PATIENT'S NAME (Last Name, First Name, Middle Initial)

3. PATIENT'S BIRTH DATE   MM DD YY   SEX   M   F

4. INSURED'S NAME (Last Name, First Name, Middle Initial)

5. PATIENT'S ADDRESS (No., Street)

6. PATIENT RELATIONSHIP TO INSURED   Self   Spouse   Child   Other

7. INSURED'S ADDRESS (No., Street)

CITY   STATE

8. PATIENT STATUS   Single   Married   Other   Employed   Full-Time Student   Part-Time Student

CITY   STATE

ZIP CODE   TELEPHONE (Include Area Code) (   )

ZIP CODE   TELEPHONE (INCLUDE AREA CODE) (   )

9. OTHER INSURED'S NAME (Last Name, First Name, Middle Initial)

10. IS PATIENT'S CONDITION RELATED TO:

11. INSURED'S POLICY GROUP OR FECA NUMBER

a. OTHER INSURED'S POLICY OR GROUP NUMBER

a. EMPLOYMENT? (CURRENT OR PREVIOUS)   YES   NO

a. INSURED'S DATE OF BIRTH   MM DD YY   SEX   M   F

b. OTHER INSURED'S DATE OF BIRTH   MM DD YY   SEX   M   F

b. AUTO ACCIDENT?   PLACE (State)   YES   NO

b. EMPLOYER'S NAME OR SCHOOL NAME

c. EMPLOYER'S NAME OR SCHOOL NAME

c. OTHER ACCIDENT?   YES   NO

c. INSURANCE PLAN NAME OR PROGRAM NAME

d. INSURANCE PLAN NAME OR PROGRAM NAME

10d. RESERVED FOR LOCAL USE

d. IS THERE ANOTHER HEALTH BENEFIT PLAN?   YES   NO   **If yes**, return to and complete item 9 a-d.

READ BACK OF FORM BEFORE COMPLETING & SIGNING THIS FORM.
12. PATIENT'S OR AUTHORIZED PERSON'S SIGNATURE I authorize the release of any medical or other information necessary to process this claim. I also request payment of government benefits either to myself or to the party who accepts assignment below.

SIGNED _____   DATE _____

13. INSURED'S OR AUTHORIZED PERSON'S SIGNATURE I authorize payment of medical benefits to the undersigned physician or supplier for services described below.

SIGNED _____

PATIENT AND INSURED INFORMATION →

14. DATE OF CURRENT: MM DD YY   ◄ ILLNESS (First symptom) OR INJURY (Accident) OR PREGNANCY(LMP)

15. IF PATIENT HAS HAD SAME OR SIMILAR ILLNESS. GIVE FIRST DATE   MM DD YY

16. DATES PATIENT UNABLE TO WORK IN CURRENT OCCUPATION   MM DD YY   FROM   TO   MM DD YY

17. NAME OF REFERRING PHYSICIAN OR OTHER SOURCE

17a. I.D. NUMBER OF REFERRING PHYSICIAN

18. HOSPITALIZATION DATES RELATED TO CURRENT SERVICES   MM DD YY   FROM   TO   MM DD YY

19. RESERVED FOR LOCAL USE

20. OUTSIDE LAB?   YES   NO $ CHARGES

21. DIAGNOSIS OR NATURE OF ILLNESS OR INJURY. (RELATE ITEMS 1,2,3 OR 4 TO ITEM 24E BY LINE)

1. |___.___   3. |___.___

2. |___.___   4. |___.___

22. MEDICAID RESUBMISSION CODE   ORIGINAL REF. NO.

23. PRIOR AUTHORIZATION NUMBER

24. A DATE(S) OF SERVICE			B Place of Service	C Type of Service	D PROCEDURES, SERVICES, OR SUPPLIES (Explain Unusual Circumstances)		E DIAGNOSIS CODE	F $ CHARGES	G DAYS OR UNITS	H EPSDT Family Plan	I EMG	J COB	K RESERVED FOR LOCAL USE
From MM DD YY	To MM DD YY				CPT/HCPCS	MODIFIER							
1													
2													
3													
4													
5													
6													

25. FEDERAL TAX I.D. NUMBER   SSN   EIN

26. PATIENT'S ACCOUNT NO.

27. ACCEPT ASSIGNMENT? (For govt. claims, see back)   YES   NO

28. TOTAL CHARGE $

29. AMOUNT PAID $

30. BALANCE DUE $

31. SIGNATURE OF PHYSICIAN OR SUPPLIER INCLUDING DEGREES OR CREDENTIALS (I certify that the statements on the reverse apply to this bill and are made a part thereof.)

SIGNED _____   DATE _____

32. NAME AND ADDRESS OF FACILITY WHERE SERVICES WERE RENDERED (If other than home or office)

33. PHYSICIAN'S, SUPPLIER'S BILLING NAME, ADDRESS, ZIP CODE & PHONE #

PIN#   GRP#

PHYSICIAN OR SUPPLIER INFORMATION →

(APPROVED BY AMA COUNCIL ON MEDICAL SERVICE 8/88)   **PLEASE PRINT OR TYPE**   APPROVED OMB-0938-0008 FORM CMS-1500 (12/90),   FORM RRB-1500, APPROVED OMB-1215-0055 FORM OWCP-1500,   APPROVED OMB-0720-0001 (CHAMPUS)

Appendix E

Ethics in Coding

Preamble to the American Health Information Management Association Code of Ethics

The ethical obligations of the health information management (HIM) professional include the protection of patient privacy and confidential information; disclosure of information; development, use, and maintenance of health information systems and health records; and the quality of information. Both handwritten and computerized medical records contain many sacred stories—stories that must be protected on behalf of the individual and the aggregate community of persons served in the healthcare system. Healthcare consumers are increasingly concerned about the loss of privacy and the inability to control the dissemination of their protected information. Core health information issues include what information should be collected, how the information should be handled, who should have access to the information, and under what conditions the information should be disclosed.

Ethical obligations are central to the professional's responsibility, regardless of the employment site or the method of collection, storage, and security of health information. Sensitive information (genetic, adoption, drug, alcohol, sexual, and behavioral information) requires special attention to prevent misuse. Entrepreneurial roles require expertise in the protection of the information in the world of business and interactions with consumers.

Professional Values

The mission of the HIM profession is based on core professional values developed since the inception of the Association in 1928. These values and the inherent ethical responsibilities for AHIMA members and credentialed HIM professionals include providing service; protecting medical, social, and financial information; promoting confidentiality; and preserving and securing health information. Values to the healthcare team include promoting the quality and advancement of healthcare, demonstrating HIM expertise and skills, and promoting interdisciplinary cooperation and collaboration. Professional values in relationship to the employer include protecting committee deliberations and complying with laws, regulations, and policies. Professional values related to the public include advocating change, refusing to participate or conceal unethical practices, and reporting violations of practice standards to the proper authorities. Professional values to individual and professional associations include obligations to be honest, bringing honor to self, peers and profession, committing to continuing education and lifelong learning, performing Association duties honorably, strengthening professional membership, representing the profession to the public, and promoting and participating in research.

These professional values will require a complex process of balancing the many conflicts that can result from competing interests and obligations of those who seek access to health information and require an understanding of ethical decision-making.

Purpose of the American Health Information Management Association Code of Ethics

The HIM professional has an obligation to demonstrate actions that reflect values, ethical principles, and ethical guidelines. The American Health Information Management Association (AHIMA) Code of Ethics sets forth these values and principles to guide conduct. The code is relevant to all AHIMA members and credentialed HIM professionals and students, regardless of their professional functions, the settings in which they work, or the populations they serve.

The AHIMA Code of Ethics serves six purposes:

- Identifies core values on which the HIM mission is based.

- Summarizes broad ethical principles that reflect the profession's core values and establishes a set of ethical principles to be used to guide decision-making and actions.

- Helps HIM professionals identify relevant considerations when professional obligations conflict or ethical uncertainties arise.

- Provides ethical principles by which the general public can hold the HIM professional accountable.

- Socializes practitioners new to the field to HIM's mission, values, and ethical principles.

- Articulates a set of guidelines that the HIM professional can use to assess whether they have engaged in unethical conduct.

The code includes principles and guidelines that are both enforceable and aspirational. The extent to which each principle is enforceable is a matter of professional judgment to be exercised by those responsible for reviewing alleged violations of ethical principles.

The Use of the Code

Violation of principles in this code does not automatically imply legal liability or violation of the law. Such determination can only be made in the context of legal and judicial proceedings. Alleged violations of the code would be subject to a peer review process. Such processes are generally separate from legal or administrative procedures and insulated from legal review or proceedings to allow the profession to counsel and discipline its own members although in some situations, violations of the code would constitute unlawful conduct subject to legal process.

Guidelines for ethical and unethical behavior are provided in this code. The terms "shall and shall not" are used as a basis for setting high standards for behavior. This does not imply that everyone "shall or shall not" do everything that is listed. For example, not everyone participates in the recruitment or mentoring of students. A HIM professional is not being unethical if this is not part of his or her professional activities; however, if students are part of one's professional responsibilities, there is an ethical obligation to follow the guidelines stated in the code. This concept is true for the entire code. If someone does the stated activities, ethical behavior is the standard. The guidelines are not a comprehensive list. For example, the statement "protect all confidential information to include personal, health, financial, genetic, and outcome information" can also be interpreted as "shall not fail to protect all confidential information to include personal, health, financial, genetic, and outcome information."

A code of ethics cannot guarantee ethical behavior. Moreover, a code of ethics cannot resolve all ethical issues or disputes or capture the richness and complexity involved in striving to make responsible choices within a moral community. Rather, a code of ethics sets forth values and ethical principles, and offers ethical guidelines to which professionals aspire and by which their actions can be judged. Ethical behaviors result from a personal commitment to engage in ethical practice.

Professional responsibilities often require an individual to move beyond personal values. For example, an individual might demonstrate behaviors that are based on the values of honesty, providing service to others, or demonstrating loyalty. In addition to these, professional values might require promoting confidentiality, facilitating interdisciplinary collaboration, and refusing to participate or conceal unethical practices. Professional values could require a more comprehensive set of values than what an individual needs to be an ethical agent in their personal lives.

The AHIMA Code of Ethics is to be used by AHIMA and individuals, agencies, organizations, and bodies (such as licensing and regulatory boards, insurance providers, courts of law, agency boards of directors, government agencies, and other professional groups) that choose to adopt it or use it as a frame of reference. The AHIMA Code of Ethics reflects the commitment of all to uphold the profession's values and to act ethically. Individuals of good character who discern moral questions and, in good faith, seek to make reliable ethical judgments, must apply ethical principles.

The code does not provide a set of rules that prescribe how to act in all situations. Specific applications of the code must take into account the context in which it is being considered and the possibility of conflicts among the code's values, principles, and guidelines. Ethical responsibilities flow from all human relationships, from the personal and familial to the social and professional. Further, the AHIMA Code of Ethics does not specify which values, principles, and guidelines are the most important and ought to outweigh others in instances when they conflict.

Code of Ethics 2004

Ethical Principles: The following ethical principles are based on the core values of the American Health Information Management Association and apply to all health information management professionals.

Health information management professionals:

> *I. Advocate, uphold, and defend the individual's right to privacy and the doctrine of confidentiality in the use and disclosure of information.*

> *II. Put service and the health and welfare of persons before self-interest and conduct themselves in the practice of the profession so as to bring honor to themselves, their peers, and to the health information management profession.*

   III. *Preserve, protect, and secure personal health information in any form or medium and hold in the highest regard the contents of the records and other information of a confidential nature, taking into account the applicable statutes and regulations.*

   IV. *Refuse to participate in or conceal unethical practices or procedures.*

   V. *Advance health information management knowledge and practice through continuing education, research, publications, and presentations.*

   VI. *Recruit and mentor students, peers and colleagues to develop and strengthen professional workforce.*

   VII. *Represent the profession accurately to the public.*

   VIII. *Perform honorably health information management association responsibilities, either appointed or elected, and preserve the confidentiality of any privileged information made known in any official capacity.*

   IX. *State truthfully and accurately their credentials, professional education, and experiences.*

   X. *Facilitate interdisciplinary collaboration in situations supporting health information practice.*

   XI. *Respect the inherent dignity and worth of every person.*

How to Interpret the Code of Ethics

The following ethical principles are based on the core values of the American Health Information Management Association and apply to all health information management professionals. Guidelines included for each ethical principle are a non-inclusive list of behaviors and situations that can help to clarify the principle. They are not to be meant as a comprehensive list of all situations that can occur.

I. Advocate, uphold, and defend the individual's right to privacy and the doctrine of confidentiality in the use and disclosure of information.

Health information management professionals **shall:**

1.1. Protect all confidential information to include personal, health, financial, genetic, and outcome information.

1.2. Engage in social and political action that supports the protection of privacy and confidentiality, and be aware of the impact of the political arena on the health information system. Advocate for changes in policy and legislation to ensure protection of privacy and confidentiality, coding compliance, and other issues that surface as advocacy issues as well as facilitating informed participation by the public on these issues.

1.3. Protect the confidentiality of all information obtained in the course of professional service. Disclose only information that is directly relevant or necessary to achieve the purpose of disclosure. Release information only with valid consent from a patient or a person legally authorized to consent on behalf of a patient or as authorized by federal or state regulations. The need-to-know criterion is essential when releasing health information for initial disclosure and all redisclosure activities.

1.4. Promote the obligation to respect privacy by respecting confidential information shared among colleagues, while responding to requests from the legal profession, the media, or other non-healthcare related individuals, during presentations or teaching and in situations that could cause harm to persons.

II. Put service and the health and welfare of persons before self-interest and conduct themselves in the practice of the profession so as to bring honor to themselves, their peers, and to the health information management profession.

Health information management professionals **shall:**

2.1. Act with integrity, behave in a trustworthy manner, elevate service to others above self-interest, and promote high standards of practice in every setting.

2.2. Be aware of the profession's mission, values, and ethical principles, and practice in a manner consistent with them by acting honestly and responsibly.

2.3. Anticipate, clarify, and avoid any conflict of interest, to all parties concerned, when dealing with consumers, consulting with competitors, or in providing services requiring potentially conflicting roles (for example, finding out information about one facility that would help a competitor). The conflicting roles or responsibilities must be clarified and appropriate action must be taken to minimize any conflict of interest.

2.4. Ensure that the working environment is consistent and encourages compliance with the AHIMA Code of Ethics, taking reasonable steps to eliminate any conditions in their organizations that violate, interfere with, or discourage compliance with the code.

2.5. Take responsibility and credit, including authorship credit, only for work they actually perform or to which they contribute. Honestly acknowledge the work of and the contributions made by others verbally or written, such as in publication.

Health information management professionals **shall not:**

2.6. Permit their private conduct to interfere with their ability to fulfill their professional responsibilities.

2.7. Take unfair advantage of any professional relationship or exploit others to further their personal, religious, political, or business interests.

III. Preserve, protect, and secure personal health information in any form or medium and hold in the highest regard the contents of the records and other information of a confidential nature obtained in the official capacity, taking into account the applicable statutes and regulations.

Health information management professionals **shall:**

3.1. Protect the confidentiality of patients' written and electronic records and other sensitive information. Take reasonable steps to ensure that patients' records are stored in a secure location and that patients' records are not available to others who are not authorized to have access.

3.2. Take precautions to ensure and maintain the confidentiality of information transmitted, transferred, or disposed of in the event of a termination, incapacitation, or death of a healthcare provider to other parties through the use of any media. Disclosure of identifying information should be avoided whenever possible.

3.3. Inform recipients of the limitations and risks associated with providing services via electronic media (such as computer, telephone, fax, radio, and television).

IV. *Refuse to participate in or conceal unethical practices or procedures.*

Health information management professionals **shall:**

4.1. Act in a professional and ethical manner at all times.

4.2. Take adequate measures to discourage, prevent, expose, and correct the unethical conduct of colleagues.

4.3. Be knowledgeable about established policies and procedures for handling concerns about colleagues' unethical behavior. These include policies and procedures created by AHIMA, licensing and regulatory bodies, employers, supervisors, agencies, and other professional organizations.

4.4. Seek resolution if there is a belief that a colleague has acted unethically or if there is a belief of incompetence or impairment by discussing their concerns with the colleague when feasible and when such discussion is likely to be productive. Take action through appropriate formal channels, such as contacting an accreditation or regulatory body and/or the AHIMA Professional Ethics Committee.

4.5. Consult with a colleague when feasible and assist the colleague in taking remedial action when there is direct knowledge of a health information management colleague's incompetence or impairment.

Health information management professionals **shall not:**

4.6. Participate in, condone, or be associated with dishonesty, fraud and abuse, or deception. A non-inclusive list of examples includes:

- Allowing patterns of retrospective documentation to avoid suspension or increase reimbursement

- Assigning codes without physician documentation

- Coding when documentation does not justify the procedures that have been billed

- Coding an inappropriate level of service

- Miscoding to avoid conflict with others

- Engaging in negligent coding practices

- Hiding or ignoring review outcomes, such as performance data

- Failing to report licensure status for a physician through the appropriate channels

- Recording inaccurate data for accreditation purposes

- Hiding incomplete medical records

- Allowing inappropriate access to genetic, adoption, or behavioral health information
- Misusing sensitive information about a competitor
- Violating the privacy of individuals

V. Advance health information management knowledge and practice through continuing education, research, publications, and presentations.

Health information management professionals **shall:**

5.1. Develop and enhance continually their professional expertise, knowledge, and skills (including appropriate education, research, training, consultation, and supervision). Contribute to the knowledge base of health information management and share with colleagues their knowledge related to practice, research, and ethics.

5.2. Base practice decisions on recognized knowledge, including empirically based knowledge relevant to health information management and health information management ethics.

5.3. Contribute time and professional expertise to activities that promote respect for the value, integrity, and competence of the health information management profession. These activities may include teaching, research, consultation, service, legislative testimony, presentations in the community, and participation in their professional organizations.

5.4. Engage in evaluation or research that ensures the anonymity or confidentiality of participants and of the data obtained from them by following guidelines developed for the participants in consultation with appropriate institutional review boards. Report evaluation and research findings accurately and take steps to correct any errors later found in published data using standard publication methods.

5.5. Take reasonable steps to provide or arrange for continuing education and staff development, addressing current knowledge and emerging developments related to health information management practice and ethics.

Health information management professionals **shall not:**

5.6. Design or conduct evaluation or research that is in conflict with applicable federal or state laws.

5.7. Participate in, condone, or be associated with fraud or abuse.

VI. Recruit and mentor students, peers and colleagues to develop and strengthen professional workforce.

Health information management professionals **shall:**

6.1. Evaluate students' performance in a manner that is fair and respectful when functioning as educators or clinical internship supervisors.

6.2. Be responsible for setting clear, appropriate, and culturally sensitive boundaries for students.

6.3. Be a mentor for students, peers and new health information management professionals to develop and strengthen skills.

6.4. Provide directed practice opportunities for students.

Health information management professionals **shall not:**

6.5. Engage in any relationship with students in which there is a risk of exploitation or potential harm to the student.

VII. *Accurately represent the profession to the public.*

Health information management professionals **shall:**

7.1 Be an advocate for the profession in all settings and participate in activities that promote and explain the mission, values, and principles of the profession to the public.

VIII. *Perform honorably health information management association responsibilities, either appointed or elected, and preserve the confidentiality of any privileged information made known in any official capacity.*

Health information management professionals **shall:**

8.1. Perform responsibly all duties as assigned by the professional association.

8.2. Resign from an Association position if unable to perform the assigned responsibilities with competence.

8.3. Speak on behalf of professional health information management organizations, accurately representing the official and authorized positions of the organizations.

IX. *State truthfully and accurately their credentials, professional education, and experiences.*

Health information management professionals **shall:**

9.1. Make clear distinctions between statements made and actions engaged in as a private individual and as a representative of the health information management profession, a professional health information organization, or the health information management professional's employer.

9.2. Claim and ensure that their representations to patients, agencies, and the public of professional qualifications, credentials, education, competence, affiliations, services provided, training, certification, consultation received, supervised experience, other relevant professional experience are accurate.

9.3. Claim only those relevant professional credentials actually possessed and correct any inaccuracies occurring regarding credentials.

X. *Facilitate interdisciplinary collaboration in situations supporting health information practice.*

Health information management professionals **shall:**

10.1. Participate in and contribute to decisions that affect the well-being of patients by drawing on the perspectives, values, and experiences of those involved in decisions related to patients. Professional and ethical obligations of the interdisciplinary team as a whole and of its individual members should be clearly established.

XI. *Respect the inherent dignity and worth of every person.*

Health information management professionals **shall:**

11.1. Treat each person in a respectful fashion, being mindful of individual differences and cultural and ethnic diversity.

11.2. Promote the value of self-determination for each individual.

Adapted with permission from the Code of Ethics of the National Association of Social Workers.

Resources

National Association of Social Workers. "Code of Ethics." 1999. Available at http://www.naswdc.org.

Harman, L.B. (Ed.). *Ethical challenges in the management of health information.* Gaithersburg, MD: Aspen, 2001.

AHIMA Code of Ethics, 1957, 1977, 1988, and 1998.

Appendix F

AHIMA Practice Brief on Data Quality

Managing and Improving Data Quality (Updated)

Complete and accurate diagnostic and procedural coded data is necessary for research, epidemiology, outcomes and statistical analyses, financial and strategic planning, reimbursement, evaluation of quality of care, and communication to support the patient's treatment.

Consistency of coding has been a major AHIMA initiative in the quest to improve data quality management in healthcare service reporting. The Association has also taken a stand on the quality of healthcare data and information.[1]

Data Quality Mandates

Adherence to industry standards and approved coding principles that generate coded data of the highest quality and consistency remains critical to the healthcare industry and the maintenance of information integrity throughout healthcare systems. HIM professionals must continue to meet the challenges of maintaining an accurate and meaningful database reflective of patient mix and resource use. As long as diagnostic and procedural codes serve as the basis for payment methodologies, the ethics of clinical coders and healthcare organization billing processes will be challenged.

Ensuring accuracy of coded data is a shared responsibility between HIM professionals, clinicians, business services staff, and information systems integrity professionals. The HIM professional has the unique responsibility of administration, oversight, analysis, and/or coding clinical data in all healthcare organizations. Care must be taken in organizational structures to ensure that oversight of the coding and data management process falls within the HIM department's responsibility area so data quality mandates are upheld and appropriate HIM principles are applied to business practices.

Clinical Collaboration

The Joint Commission and the Medicare Conditions of Participation as well as other accreditation agencies require final diagnoses and procedures to be recorded in the medical record and authenticated by the responsible practitioner. State laws also provide guidelines concerning the content of the health record as a legal document.

Clinical documentation primarily created by physicians is the cornerstone of accurate coding, supplemented by appropriate policies and procedures developed by facilities to meet patient care requirements. Coded data originates from the collaboration between clinicians and HIM professionals with clinical terminology, classification system, nomenclature, data analysis, and compliance policy expertise.

Thus, the need for collaboration, cooperation, and communication between clinicians and support personnel continues to grow as information gathering and storage embrace new technology. Movement of the coding process into the business processing side of a healthcare organization must not preclude access to and regular communication with clinicians.

Clinical Database Evaluation

Regulatory agencies are beginning to apply data analysis tools to monitor data quality and reliability for reimbursement appropriateness and to identify unusual claims data patterns that may indicate payment errors or health insurance fraud. Examples include the Hospital Payment Monitoring Program tool First Look Analysis Tool for Hospital Outlier Monitoring (FATHOM), used by Quality Improvement Organizations, and the comprehensive error rate testing (CERT) process to be used by Centers for Medicare & Medicaid Services carriers to produce national, contractor, provider type, and benefit category-specific paid claims error rates.

Ongoing evaluation of the clinical database by health information managers facilitates ethical reporting of clinical information and early identification of data accuracy problems for timely and appropriate resolution. Pattern analysis of codes is a useful tool for prevention of compliance problems by identifying and correcting clinical coding errors.

Coding errors have multiple causes, some within the control of HIM processes and others that occur outside the scope of HIM due to inadequacy of the source document or the lack of information integrity resulting from inappropriate computer programming routines or software logic.

Data Quality Management and Improvement Initiatives

The following actions are required in any successful program:

- Evaluation and trending of diagnosis and procedure code selections, the appropriateness of reimbursement group assignment, and other coded data elements such as discharge status are required. This action ensures that clinical concept validity, appropriate code sequencing, specific code use requirements, and clinical pertinence are reflected in the codes reported

- Reporting data quality review results to organizational leadership, compliance staff, and the medical staff. This stresses accountability for data quality to everyone involved and allows the root causes of inconsistency or lack of reliability of data validity to be addressed. If the source for code assignment is inadequate or invalid, the results may reflect correct coding by the coding professional, but still represent a data quality problem because the code assigned does not reflect the actual concept or event as it occurred

- Following up on and monitoring identified problems. HIM professionals must resist the temptation to overlook inadequate documentation and report codes without appropriate clinical foundation within the record just to speed up claims processing, meet a business requirement, or obtain additional reimbursement. There is an ethical duty as members of the healthcare team to educate physicians on appropriate documentation practices and maintain high standards for health information practice. Organizational structures must support these efforts by the enforcement of medical staff rules and regulations and continuous monitoring of clinical pertinence of documentation to meet both business and patient care requirements

HIM clinical data specialists who understand data quality management concepts and the relationship of clinical code assignments to reimbursement and decision support for healthcare will have important roles to play in the healthcare organizations of the future. Continuing education and career boosting specialty advancement programs are expected to be the key to job security and professional growth as automation continues to change healthcare delivery, claims processing, and compliance activities.[2]

Data Quality Recommendations

HIM coding professionals and the organizations that employ them are accountable for data quality that requires the following behaviors.

HIM professionals should:

- Adopt best practices made known in professional resources and follow the code of ethics for the profession or their specific compliance programs.[3] This guidance applies to all settings and all health plans

- Use the entire health record as part of the coding process in order to assign and report the appropriate clinical codes for the standard transactions and codes sets required for external reporting and meeting internal abstracting requirements

- Adhere to all official coding guidelines published in the HIPAA standard transactions and code sets regulation. ICD-9-CM guidelines are available for downloading at www.cdc.gov/nchs/data/icd9/icdguide.pdf. Additional official coding advice is published in the quarterly publication AHA *Coding Clinic for ICD-9-CM*. CPT guidelines are located within the CPT code books and additional information and coding advice is provided in the AMA monthly publication *CPT Assistant*. Modifications to the initial HIPAA standards for electronic transactions or adoption of additional standards are submitted first to the designated standard maintenance organization. For more information, go to http://aspe.os. dhhs.gov/admnsimp/final/dsmo.htm.

- Develop appropriate facility or practice-specific guidelines when available coding guidelines do not address interpretation of the source document or guide code selection in specific circumstances. Facility practice guidelines should not conflict with official coding guidelines

- Maintain a working relationship with clinicians through ongoing communication and documentation improvement programs

- Report root causes of data quality concerns when identified. Problematic issues that arise from individual physicians or groups of clinicians should be referred to medical staff leadership or the compliance office for investigation and resolution

- Query when necessary. Best practices and coding guidelines suggest that when coding professionals encounter conflicting or ambiguous documentation in a source document, the physician must be queried to confirm the appropriate code selection[4]

- Consistently seek out innovative methods to capture pertinent information required for clinical code assignment to minimize unnecessary clinician inquiries. Alternative methods of accessing information necessary for code assignment may prevent the need to wait for completion of the health record, such as electronic access to clinical reports

- Ensure that clinical code sets reported to outside agencies are fully supported by documentation within the health record and clearly reflected in diagnostic statements and procedure reports provided by a physician

- Provide the physician the opportunity to review reported diagnoses and procedures on pre- or post-claim or post-bill submission, via mechanisms such as:

  —providing a copy (via mail, fax, or electronic transmission) of the sequenced codes and their narrative descriptions, taking appropriate care to protect patient privacy and security of the information

  —placing the diagnostic and procedural listing within the record and bringing it to the physician's attention within the appropriate time frame for correction when warranted

- Create a documentation improvement program or offer educational programs concerning the relationship of health record entries and health record management to data quality, information integrity, patient outcomes, and business success of the organization

- Conduct a periodic or ongoing review of any automated billing software (chargemasters, service description masters, practice management systems, claims scrubbers, medical necessity software) used to ensure code appropriateness and validity of clinical codes

- Require a periodic or ongoing review of encounter forms or other resource tools that involve clinical code assignment to ensure validity and appropriateness

- Complete appropriate continuing education and training to keep abreast of clinical advancements in diagnosis and treatment, billing and compliance issues, regulatory requirements, and coding guideline changes, and to maintain professional credentials

HIM coding professionals and the organizations that employ them have the responsibility to not engage in, promote, or tolerate the following behaviors that adversely affect data quality. HIM professionals should not:

- Make assumptions requiring clinical judgment concerning the etiology or context of the condition under consideration for code reporting

- Misrepresent the patient's clinical picture through code assignment for diagnoses/procedures unsupported by the documentation in order to maximize reimbursement, affect insurance policy coverage, or because of other third-party payer requirements. This includes falsification of conditions to meet medical necessity requirements when the patient's condition does not support health plan coverage for the service in question or using a specific code requested by a payer when, according to official coding guidelines, a different code is mandatory

- Omit the reporting of clinical codes that represent actual clinical conditions or services but negatively affect a facility's data profile, negate health plan coverage, or lower the reimbursement potential

- Allow changing of clinical code assignments under any circumstances without consultation with the coding professional involved and the clinician whose services are being reported. Changes are allowed only with subsequent validation of the documentation supporting the need for code revision

- Fail to use the physician query process outlined by professional practice standards or required by quality improvement organizations under contract for federal and state agencies that reimburse for healthcare services

- Assign codes to an incomplete record without organizational policies in place to ensure the codes are reviewed after the records are complete. Failure to confirm the accuracy and completeness of the codes submitted for a reimbursement claim upon completion of the medical record can increase both data quality and compliance risks[5]

- Promote or tolerate the falsification of clinical documentation or misrepresentation of clinical conditions or service provided

Prepared by AHIMA's Coding Products and Services team:

Kathy Brouch, RHIA, CCS
Susan Hull, MPH, RHIA, CCS
Karen Kostick, RHIT, CCS, CCS-P
Rita Scichilone, MHSA, RHIA, CCS, CCS-P
Mary Stanfill, RHIA, CCS, CCS-P
Ann Zeisset, RHIT, CCS, CCS-P

Notes

1. For details, see AHIMA's Position Statements on Consistency of Healthcare Diagnostic and Procedural Coding and on the Quality of Healthcare Data and Information at www.ahima.org/dc/positions.

2. For more information on AHIMA's specialty advancement programs, go to http://campus.ahima.org. Institutes for Healthcare Data Analytics and Clinical Data Management are planned for the 2003 AHIMA National Convention. Visit www.ahima.org/convention for more information.

3. AHIMA's Standards of Ethical Coding are available at www.ahima.org/infocenter/guidelines.

4. Prophet, Sue. "Practice Brief: Developing a Physician Query Process." *Journal of AHIMA* 72, no. 9 (2001): 88I–M.

5. More guidelines for HIM policy and procedure development are available in *Health Information Management Compliance: A Model Program for Healthcare Organizations* by Sue Prophet, AHIMA, 2002. Coding from incomplete records is also discussed in the AHIMA Practice Brief "Developing a Coding Compliance Document" in the July/August 2001 *Journal of AHIMA* (vol. 72, no. 7, prepared by AHIMA's Coding Practice Team).

Reference

AHIMA Coding Products and Services Team. "Managing and Improving Data Quality (Updated) (AHIMA Practice Brief)." *Journal of AHIMA* 74, no.7 (July/August 2003): 64A–C.

Appendix G

ICD-10-CM and ICD-10-PCS

Destination 10: Healthcare Organization Preparation for ICD-10-CM and ICD-10-PCS (AHIMA Practice Brief)

Editor's note: This update supplants the September 1998 practice brief "Preparing Your Organization for a New Coding System."

In November 2003 the National Committee on Vital and Health Statistics (NCVHS) submitted a letter to Health and Human Services Secretary Tommy Thompson recommending that the regulatory process be initiated for the adoption of ICD-10-CM and ICD-10-PCS as replacements for the current uses of ICD-9-CM. In this letter, NCVHS stated that the updated ICD systems can better accommodate advances in medicine, reduce the number of rejected claims, and improve reimbursement, care quality, safety, and disease management.

Exactly how will ICD-10-CM and ICD-10-PCS be adopted? Here's what will happen:

1. The secretary accepts the NCVHS recommendation.

2. The federal government publishes a notice of proposed rule making (NPRM) calling for public comment on their policy plus the published ICD-10-CM and ICD-10-PCS materials incorporated by reference.

3. The public at large has at least 30, but more likely 60, days to submit comments on the NPRM and its incorporated materials.

4. The federal government analyzes the public comments. Based on this analysis, any necessary changes are made.

5. The federal government publishes a final rule containing its updated policy, explanations thereof, plus the implementation date.

6. The standard HIPAA compliance clock for new transactions begins—two years for all but small health plans, who get three years.

While the HIPAA-mandated process will take time, experience with the transactions and code sets final rule has shown that careful planning and preparation are required for effective implementation. In addition, transitioning to ICD-10-CM and ICD-10-PCS is more complex than implementation of new code sets in the past because the uses of coded data today are more complex than those for which ICD-9-CM was designed. (See Figure G.1, Uses of Coded Data.)

Figure G.1. **Uses of coded data**

Today, coded data are used for:

- Measuring the quality, safety (or medical errors), and efficacy of care
- Making clinical decisions based on output from multiple systems
- Designing payment systems and processing claims for reimbursement
- Conducting research, epidemiological studies, and clinical trials
- Setting health policy
- Designing healthcare delivery systems
- Monitoring resource utilization
- Improving clinical, financial, and administrative performance
- Identifying fraudulent or abusive practices
- Managing care and disease processes
- Tracking public health and risks
- Providing data to consumers regarding costs and outcomes of treatment options

Source: "Testimony of the American Health Information Management Association to the National Committee on Vital and Health Statistics on ICD-10-CM." May 29, 2002. Available at www.ahima.org.

AHIMA believes an implementation plan established well in advance of the scheduled implementation date within the requirements of HIPAA is necessary to ensure a successful transition to ICD-10-CM and ICD-10-PCS. While this practice brief is not a comprehensive document of everything that needs to be done to prepare, the three major stages for the process outlined below illustrate the journey ahead for specific travelers working in healthcare organizations. Additional details for each phase will be available through the FORE Library: HIM Body of Knowledge.

So what should your healthcare organization do to set priorities for the various stages of the transition? And what should HIM professionals be doing to prepare?

Three Years Out

The first stage involves two major tasks: creating an implementation planning team and starting the initial education process. Together, these actions demonstrate a clear direction on the healthcare organization's road map.

Team Design

As in any other major undertaking, putting together a team to oversee the implementation is key to success. Members of the planning team should at least include senior management, medical staff, financial management, HIM, and information systems (IS) management. This group would develop the organization's plan and identify the actions, persons responsible, and deadlines for the various tasks required to complete the process. In addition, this plan should include estimated budget needs for each year leading up to implementation for early financial planning.

Team members should keep current on the status for adoption and maintain a broad understanding of ICD-10-CM and ICD-10-PCS. (See Figure G.2, Web Sites to Watch.)

Preliminary Educational Needs

Another major task in the first stage is education. HIM professionals should educate personnel in their organizations about the impending changes.

Individuals throughout the organization need to be aware of the upcoming changes. (See Figure G.3, Who Needs to Know?)

Figure G.2.   Web sites to watch

Use these Web sites to stay current on the status of the coding systems, as well as the anticipated release dates:

- **NCVHS**   http://aspe.os.dhhs.gov/ncvhs
- **CMS**   www.cms.hhs.gov/providers/pufdownload/icd10.asp
- **National Center for Health Statistics**   www.cdc.gov/nchswww/about/otheract/icd9/abticd10.htm
- **HHS Administrative Simplification**   http://aspe.os.dhhs.gov/admnsimp
  At this site, you can subscribe to the HIPAA-REGS listserv. It will notify you when documents related to the administrative simplification law are published.

Figure G.3.   Who needs to know?

Colleagues throughout the organization need to be aware of the ICD-10 transition team. Remember to provide information on how HIM can help their departments in the transition. Individuals needing to know about the upcoming changes include:

- Senior management
- Clinicians
- IS personnel
- Quality management personnel
- Utilization management personnel
- Release of information personnel
- Ancillary department personnel
- Data quality management personnel

- Data security personnel
- Data analysts
- Researchers
- Billing personnel
- Accounting personnel
- Compliance personnel
- Auditors

It is advisable to briefly review the regulations on electronic transactions and code sets with senior management, paying specific attention to the section on code sets, particularly the process for adoption of new code sets. Senior management should also be briefed on the proposed and final rules regarding adoption of ICD-10-CM and ICD-10-PCS. A short overview of the differences between the code sets might be helpful to justify the time, effort, and resources that will be required to implement the changes.

Because these systems code to a greater degree of specificity, clinical documentation must be examined to ensure that it is comprehensive enough to actually assign a code. HIM professionals should assess the adequacy of medical record documentation to support the assignment of codes from ICD-10-CM and ICD-10-PCS in their healthcare organizations. The need to assess and improve documentation prior to implementation is absolutely critical. This requires HIM professionals to become familiar enough with ICD-10-CM and ICD-10-PCS to be able to review medical record documentation and identify areas where improvement is needed (for example, certain specialties or types of records that are more problematic than others).

The results of this gap analysis would then be used to focus the documentation improvement efforts in the clinician education programs. While the results of a study performed by AHIMA in the summer of 2003 indicate that ICD-10-CM codes could be applied to today's medical records without changing documentation practices, improved documentation would result in higher coding specificity, and therefore higher data quality, in some cases.[1] Therefore, identification of areas in need of documentation improvement and the subsequent clinician education must begin early in order to effect real change in documentation practices. AHIMA plans to publish a clinical documentation assessment tool in 2004 to assist with this evaluation.

The education of IS staff will be vital. IS personnel will need to understand the logic and hierarchical structure of ICD-10-CM and ICD-10-PCS. IS department members will be particularly interested in the specifications of the coding system and may want to address the following questions:

1. How many digits? ICD-10-CM has seven characters, with a decimal point after the third character. ICD-10-PCS has seven characters and no decimal point.

2. Is it alphabetic, numeric, or a combination? Both of the new systems mix alphabetic and numeric characters.

3. Can it be obtained in a machine-readable form? To date, the only distribution has been via the Internet (see the aforementioned Web sites).

4. What coding systems will it replace, and when will it replace them? ICD-10-CM and ICD-10-PCS are slated as replacements for the current uses of ICD-9-CM no sooner than October 2006.

5. Is a crosswalk available? Official sources say these will be developed.

It is essential that IS staff be made aware of these changes, as they will have to implement them into a software application or an interface between two systems. A recommended step is for HIM and IS to work together to identify all systems and software in which ICD-9-CM codes are currently used.

Both IS staff and analysts will need to understand the data comparability issues as data between the two systems are compared over time. Data users will specifically need to understand the definition and composition of categories in the classification. Caution should be used when conducting longitudinal data analysis, as diagnoses and procedures may be classified differently in the two systems or code definitions may have changed, making it easy to misinterpret data.

Others need to know the differences between the code sets, the effect on their work, and the time frames involved in the coming changes. ICD-10-CM maintains many similarities to ICD-9-CM; it has the same hierarchical structure and many of the same conventions. Primarily, changes in ICD-10-CM are in its organization and structure, code composition, and level of detail. The process for selecting a diagnosis code using ICD-10-CM is not expected to change drastically.

ICD-10, as developed by the World Health Organization, does not include a classification for procedures. The US government, specifically the Centers for Medicare and Medicaid Services (CMS), contracted with 3M Health Information Systems to create a procedure coding system, ICD-10-PCS.

Overall, the current drafts of ICD-10-CM and ICD-10-PCS contain a significant increase in codes over ICD-9-CM. The level of specificity in ICD-10-CM and ICD-10-PCS will provide increased clinical detail, addition of information relevant to ambulatory and managed care encounters, enhanced system flexibility, and better reflection of current medical knowledge. Payers, policy makers, and providers will have more detailed information for establishing appropriate reimbursement rates, evaluating and improving the quality of patient care, improving efficiencies in healthcare delivery, reducing costs, and effectively monitoring resource and service utilization.

Two Years Out

The second stage also involves two major tasks: identifying and budgeting required IS changes and assessing, budgeting, and implementing clinician and coder education in the areas identified.

IS Changes

Building on the work in stage one, a more detailed analysis needs to occur in the second year of preparation. A budget for the required changes must also be established. The examination should include the following questions:

- What software changes are needed?

- What changes are required to accommodate multiple systems and applications that use coded data?

- What needs to be done to increase system storage capacity to support both coding systems for an adequate period?

If the facility uses commercial software, HIM professionals should ensure that their software provider is keeping up with the announced changes. This is one area (like the transactions and code sets final rule) in which assuming that someone else is fixing the problem has the potential to do real damage to the facility. Imagine the consequences if your vendor was not prepared and your facility could not submit claims or get reimbursed. Areas to discuss with your vendor include:

- Who will pay for systems upgrades?

- Are the upgrades included in an annual maintenance contract?

- If costs will be incurred by the organization, what are those projected costs and when will they be incurred?

Clinician and Coder Education

Implementation of any new coding system requires educational programs for clinicians responsible for documentation, coders, and a growing number of data users throughout the healthcare industry. The range of users and settings for which programs have to be designed and provided is much wider for ICD-10-CM than ICD-10-PCS.

Using the documentation gap analysis recommended in stage one, focused clinician education continues in those areas in need of improvement. In addition, reanalysis should be done to ascertain success of earlier efforts and assist in refocusing educational programs.

Because ICD-10-CM and ICD-10-PCS allow greater specificity, clinicians must change behaviors in documentation so the appropriate code can be selected (a goal consistent with the industry's goals to eliminate medical error). Clinicians will need to be actively involved in the educational process. This will allow them to understand the importance of complete and accurate documentation to support the level of specificity in ICD-10-CM and ICD-10-PCS.

Initial reports indicate the transition will require an expanded coder knowledge base, specifically in the following areas: detailed knowledge of anatomy and medical terminology; comprehension of operative reports; comprehension, interpretation, and application of standardized ICD-10-PCS definitions; and increased interaction and collaboration with medical staff.[2] It will be necessary to assess the clinical knowledge of the coding staff so that areas of weakness are identified and focused education can occur prior to implementation.

Coder education is a critical step during the third stage, but budgeting will be done in the first stages. Questions to consider when budgeting are:

1. Will you outsource the education or conduct it internally?

2. What are the costs and benefits of these two options?

3. When will the education need to be done?

4. Who will need what level of education?

5. What options (for example, Web-based training) are available for education?

6. How will workload be managed while coders are receiving education?

Although it would be technically possible for coding professionals to use a paper-based version of the ICD-10 systems, given the size and structure of the systems, most coding professionals and healthcare organizations will find them easiest to use in electronic format. Alternatives to manual use of these classification systems should be seriously considered, and the necessary vendors should be contacted.

One Year Out

The third stage involves three major tasks: implementation of required IS changes, follow-up assessment of documentation practices, and intensive education of the organization's coders.

Implement system changes following the detailed analysis of required IS changes that was compiled in stage two. A full reassessment after education should be done one year out to verify that goals are being achieved. A follow-up assessment of documentation practices after the clinician education is complete must be done to determine where improvements have occurred and where enhancements are necessary. Changing clinician documentation patterns will involve continuing education and reinforcement of the ICD-10-CM and ICD-10-PCS requirements for code specificity.

HIM professionals will want to familiarize themselves with the coding systems and any new and revised coding and reporting guidelines. Since ICD-10-CM has the same hierarchical structure and many of the same conventions as ICD-9-CM, experienced coding professionals will not require the same level of extensive education as they would for an entirely new coding system. They will primarily need to be educated in changes in structure, disease classification, definitions, and guidelines. However, ICD-10-PCS does vary from the "look and feel" of ICD-9-CM and will require coders to be educated in its intricacies and guidelines.

Remember that conducting education too far in advance of implementation can adversely affect its effectiveness. Coder education should be provided three months prior to ICD-10-CM implementation, according to 59 percent of respondents to the study conducted by AHIMA on ICD-10-CM.[3]

It is virtually impossible to make changes of this magnitude without encountering some obstacles. The key to managing the process is a good map that establishes "mile markers" to identify steps and priorities early. This method enables everyone to plan and prepare, thus minimizing problems. Watch the *Journal* for further details of AHIMA's strategy for training and provision of tools to facilitate implementation, such as a clinical knowledge assessment (individual practitioner), clinical documentation assessment evaluation (facility or enterprise), and organizational readiness report card (facility). Recommended steps to be undertaken by AHIMA members and other segments of the healthcare industry during each of the years leading up to implementation will also be detailed.

Notes

1. American Hospital Association (AHA) and American Health Information Management Association (AHIMA). "ICD-10-CM Field Testing Project. Report on Findings: Perceptions, Ideas and Recommendations from Coding Professionals across the Nation." Chicago: 2003. Available in the FORE Library: HIM Body of Knowledge at www.ahima.org.

2. Powell, Sharon, Barbara Steinbeck, and Thelma M. Grant. "Will You Be Ready? Preparing Now for ICD-10-PCS Implementation." Paper from the proceedings of the annual conference of the American Health Information Management Association, Chicago, 2002.

3. AHA and AHIMA. "ICD-10-CM Field Testing Project."

Prepared by

AHIMA's Coding Products and Services Team:

Kathy Giannangelo, RHIA, CCS
Susan Hull, MPH, RHIA, CCS
Karen Kostick, RHIT, CCS, CCS-P
Rita Scichilone, MHSA, RHIA, CCS, CCS-P
Mary Stanfill, RHIA, CCS, CCS-P
Sarah D. Wills-Dubose, MA, MEd, RHIA
Ann Zeisset, RHIT, CCS, CCS-P

Acknowledgment

Sue Bowman, RHIA, CCS

Source: AHIMA's Coding Products and Services Team. "Destination 10: Healthcare Organization Preparation for ICD-10-CM and ICD-10-PCS" (AHIMA Practice Brief). *Journal of AHIMA* 75, no. 3 (March 2004): 56A–D.

Preparing for the ICD-10 Journey

by Sue Bowman, RHIA, CCS

After years of doubt as to whether ICD-10 was ever going to be implemented in the United States, the journey toward replacement of ICD-9-CM has finally gotten under way. The historic decision of the National Committee on Vital and Health Statistics (NCVHS) to send a letter to the Secretary of Health and Human Services (HHS) recommending the initiation of the regulatory process for the concurrent adoption of ICD-10-CM and ICD-10-PCS begins the process.

Time to Dust off Your ICD-10 Knowledge

The practice brief "Destination 10: Healthcare Organization Preparation for ICD-10-CM and ICD-10-PCS," in this issue, describes the regulatory process required for ICD-10 to be adopted and the ways in which ICD-10 and ICD-10-PCS represent an improvement over ICD-9-CM.

Given the years of uncertainty surrounding ICD-10 implementation, many HIM professionals' interest in and knowledge of ICD-10 have dwindled with time. Now it is time to recall those forgotten memories and refresh our knowledge of the ICD-10-CM and ICD-10-PCS coding systems.

As HIM professionals across the country prepare to lead ICD-10 implementation teams in their organizations, they need to take steps to become "experts" on how ICD-10-CM and ICD-10-PCS differ from ICD-9-CM. The basic understanding HIM managers need to lead implementation efforts is not the same type of knowledge as the in-depth skills in code application that those involved directly in the day-to-day coding function will need.

This article reviews the structure and unique characteristics of ICD-10-CM and ICD-10-PCS. It is not intended to be comprehensive. Use the resources listed in "To Learn More," below, to continue to increase your familiarity with ICD-10-CM and ICD-10-PCS.

How Is ICD-10-CM Different?

ICD-10-CM has many similarities to ICD-9-CM. For example, it has the same hierarchical structure and many of the same conventions, instructional notes, and guidelines. ICD-10-CM will have much the same "look and feel" as ICD-9-CM; however, it includes a number of notable differences:

- ICD-10-CM is entirely alphanumeric (all letters except U are used).
- ICD-10-CM codes may be up to seven characters in length.
- Some chapters have been restructured in ICD-10-CM.
- Some diseases have been reclassified in ICD-10-CM.
- New features have been added to ICD-10-CM.

Conditions with a recently discovered etiology or new treatment protocol have been reassigned to a more appropriate chapter. For example, gout is in the endocrine chapter in ICD-9-CM but in the musculoskeletal chapter in ICD-10-CM. And some conditions have been grouped in a more logical fashion than in ICD-9-CM.

"Excludes" notes were expanded to provide guidance on the hierarchy of chapters and clarify priority of code assignments. Also, two types of Excludes notes are clearly distinguished to eliminate confusion as to the meaning of the exclusion. An early draft of ICD-10-CM referred to three types of Excludes notes, but subsequent system revisions resulted in the use of only two types. An "excludes1" note designates codes that can never be used together. An "excludes2" note is used to clarify that the excluded condition is not a part of or included in the code.

In addition to the alphanumeric structure, ICD-10-CM embodies other differences in code structure. An "x" is used as a placeholder to save space for future expansion. So, for example, there may be a six-character code for which there is no fifth character subclassification at the present time. In this case, an "x" is used in the fifth character position. An example is code S63.8x1a, Sprain of other part of right wrist and hand, initial encounter.

Another change in ICD-10-CM is the use of extensions, which provide additional information in certain circumstances. Extensions are used in the obstetrics, injury, and external cause chapters and always occupy the final (seventh) character position in a code. The example above, code S63.8x1a, includes the extension "a" for "initial encounter." The other applicable extensions for category S63 are "d" (subsequent encounter) and "q" (sequela).

Other notable changes in ICD-10-CM include:

- Injuries are grouped by body part rather than category of injury.

- Factors influencing health status and contact with health services (known as V codes in ICD-9-CM) and external causes of morbidity and mortality (known as E codes in ICD-9-CM) are considered part of the main classification in ICD-10-CM, not "supplementary" classifications.

- Codes for postoperative complications have been expanded and moved to the appropriate procedure-specific body system chapter, and a new concept of "postprocedural disorders" has been added.

- Combination codes have been created for commonly occurring symptoms/diagnoses and etiologies/manifestations.

What about ICD-10-PCS?

ICD-10-PCS was developed specifically as a replacement for ICD-9-CM Volume 3. Four major objectives guided the development of ICD-10-PCS:

- Completeness: a unique code should exist for all substantially different procedures.

- Expandability: as new procedures are developed, the system structure should allow them to be easily incorporated as unique codes.

- Multiaxial: each code character should have the same meaning within the specific procedure section and across procedure sections, to the extent possible.

- Standardized terminology: each term should be assigned a specific meaning, and the coding system should not include multiple meanings for the same term.

ICD-10-PCS has a seven-character alphanumeric code structure. Unlike ICD-9-CM, ICD-10-PCS codes do not exist as "finished" codes in the tabular listing. Rather, they exist as groups of interchangeable coding components called "characters," which must be assembled into a code for each distinct procedure performed. So, in essence, the correct code is "built" for each procedure being coded.

Procedures are divided into 17 sections that relate to the type of procedure. (See Figure G.4, Sections of ICD-10-PCS.) The first character of the procedure code identifies the section.

The medical and surgical section contains 30 root operations (See Figure G.5, Medical and Surgical Root Operations.) Definitions of these operations can be found in the ICD-10-PCS training manual. (See Figure G.6, To Learn More.) No diagnostic information is contained in ICD-10-PCS codes.

The ICD-10-PCS system contains an index and a tabular listing. The index allows codes to be located by looking up terms alphabetically. The main terms are root operations. However, common operative names, such as hysterectomy, can also be looked up, where a cross-reference directs the coder to the appropriate root operation term. The index provides only the first three or four characters of the procedure code. One must always refer to the tabular listing to obtain the complete code.

The tabular listing is arranged by sections, and most sections are subdivided by body system. There are separate tables for each root operation in a body system. The name of the section, body system, and root operation and its definition are listed at the top of each table. This list is followed by a grid, with the columns representing the last four characters of the code and the rows specifying the allowable combinations of these four characters. As demonstrated

Figure G.4.   Sections of ICD-10-PCS

0	Medical and Surgical	B	Extracorporeal Assistance and Performance
1	Obstetrics	C	Extracorporeal Therapies
2	Placement	D	Laboratory
3	Administration	F	Mental Health
4	Measurement and Monitoring	G	Chiropractic
5	Imaging	H	Miscellaneous
6	Nuclear Medicine	J	Substance Abuse Treatment
7	Radiation Oncology		
8	Osteopathic		
9	Physical Rehabilitation and Diagnostic Audiology		

Characters 2 through 7 have a standard meaning within each section but may have different meanings across sections. The characters for the medical and surgical section are:

1 = section	5 = approach
2 = body system	6 = device
3 = root operation	7 = qualifier
4 = body part	

Figure G.5.   Medical and surgical root operations

0	Alteration	B	Excision	N	Release
1	Bypass	C	Extirpation	P	Removal
2	Change	D	Extraction	Q	Repair
3	Control	F	Fragmentation	R	Replacement
4	Creation	G	Fusion	S	Reposition
5	Destruction	H	Insertion	T	Resection
6	Detachment	J	Inspection	V	Restriction
7	Dilation	K	Map	W	Revision
8	Division	L	Occlusion	X	Transfer
9	Drainage	M	Reattachment	Y	Transplantation

Figure G.6. **To learn more**

- The ICD-10-CM draft and ICD-10-CM official guidelines for coding and reporting are available at www.cdc.gov/nchs/about/otheract/icd9/icd10cm.htm.

- "ICD-10-CM Overview: Deciphering the Code" is an Internet-based continuing education course (approved for eight AHIMA continuing education credits) and is available from AHIMA at the following link: campus.ahima.org/campus/course_info/ICD10OVER/ICD10O_info.html.

- The ICD-10-PCS final draft and training manual is available at www.cms.hhs.gov/paymentsystems/icd9/icd10.asp.

- *ICD-10-CM Preview*, by Anita Hazelwood and Carol Venable, can be ordered from the AHIMA Web site: www.ahima.org.

- Six 2004 regional coding community seminars will include a two-hour segment on ICD-10-CM and ICD-10-PCS. More information is available at www.ahima.org/coding/coding_meetings.cfm.

- AHIMA's "Statement in Support of Prompt Adoption of ICD-10-CM and ICD-10-PCS Medical Code Set Standards in the United States" is available at www.ahima.org/dc/positions.

- AHIMA's testimony on ICD-10-CM and ICD-10-PCS before NCVHS is available at www.ahima.org/dc.

- "CodeWrite," the online coding newsletter available to members of the Coding Community of Practice (CoP) and frequently distributed to coding roundtable participants in print form, will feature a regular column on practical application of ICD-10-CM and ICD-10-PCS codes. Members can log in at www.ahima.org.

- The ICD-10 Implementation CoP offers an opportunity to network with colleagues on CD-10 implementation strategies and ensures ready access to a wealth of CD-10 resources. Members can log in at www.ahima.org.

during the testing of ICD-10-PCS by the Clinical Data Abstraction Centers, the format of the tabular listing facilitates bypassing the index entirely and going directly to the tabular listing to assign a code.

Future articles in this column will address implementation strategies organizations should undertake during the next few years to ensure a successful and smooth transition to the new code sets.

Sue Bowman (sue.bowman@ahima.org) is director of coding policy and compliance at AHIMA.

Source: Bowman, Sue. "Preparing for the ICD-10 Journey." (ICD-10: Mapping Our Course column) *Journal of AHIMA* 75, no. 3 (March 2004): 60–62.

Taking the Next Step Forward for ICD-10

by Dan Rode, MBA, FHFMA

In November 2003 the National Committee on Vital and Health Statistics (NCVHS) agreed to recommend that the secretary of Health and Human Services (HHS) adopt the ICD-10-CM and the ICD-10-PCS classification standards as replacement for the ICD-9-CM classification currently used in the US.

The work of many AHIMA volunteers, staff, and other members of the healthcare industry made this professional milestone happen. But the NCVHS agreement is just the beginning. The next step is yours.

Conversion Process Has Roots in HIPAA

Congress passed HIPAA in 1996 to ensure that the healthcare industry would have standards to promote administrative simplification. HIPAA requires that any standard transactions be approved by the secretary of HHS. The secretary must also approve any code sets used in HIPAA transactions—including the eight transaction sets currently in use, such as ICD-9-CM.

HIPAA also established a process for the secretary to approve such code sets. The first step is the advisory process, which NCVHS has just completed. The next step is the regulatory process.

Most HIM professionals who have come into contact with the various elements of Medicare or Medicaid are familiar with the regulatory process. First, the secretary will issue a "notice of proposed rule making" (NPRM) to upgrade the coding systems from ICD-9-CM.

This NPRM will give a history of the issue and explain why these particular rules or regulations are being considered. It will also cite the regulations being proposed and the department's rationale behind them. In addition, it will cite specific sections of HIPAA for reference, name the bodies overseeing the maintenance of the classification systems, and describe potential economic impact. Finally, it will provide a comment period for the public to review the proposed rule and make any recommendations for changes, deletions, or additions. The period for comment will be 30 to 60 days.

Once the comment period is closed, all two-way dialogue between HHS and the public ceases. If the department has a question, it can "fact find" for an answer, but no additional comments can be made or considered, unsolicited, until a final notice is published. The waiting period for a final rule can vary tremendously, as we have seen with other HIPAA regulations. It could be as short as 30 days or it could be years.

The final rule is the last step. It may appear in several iterations, and there may be a version that allows additional comments, should HHS decide to add to the regulation significant changes not considered in the NPRM. The final rule states the final regulations: what they are, how they were reached, and when compliance is required.

Why ICD-10 Can't Wait

AHIMA members know that conversion to the ICD-10-CM and ICD-10-CPS systems is key in the nation's move toward a national health information infrastructure (NHII) and a standard electronic health record. For this conversion to take place, however, every HIM professional must respond to an NPRM. If the industry fails to champion the replacement of ICD-9-CM, the secretary could decide not to move forward in a timely fashion with adoption and implementation of the ICD-10 systems. Any delay in such adoption could mean significantly higher costs for eventual implementation—and we'll be no closer to an NHII or an EHR.

AHIMA has offered testimony in the past, and it continues to work with the coding authorities and others to accelerate an appropriate final rule as soon as possible—ideally, in 2004.

Such a NPRM is likely to include a description of the two classification code set standards (or at least an indicator where the standards can be found); description of the data elements and the impact on known HIPAA transaction standards; how uniform and standardized guidance will be handled, per HIPAA; the maintenance process for both (most likely similar to the coordination and maintenance process we know today); the anticipated implementation process, and the implementation dates.

There will be some differences in implementation between these two classification code set standards and the transaction sets. Namely:

- Conversion or final implementation would be the same date for all covered entities. We expect this to be an October 1 date to coincide with the existing maintenance update.

- The recommended implementation period will probably be two years from the final rule date—coordinated with the October 1 change. Most testimony for conversion indicated a two-year period would be necessary.

- The rule would allow for maintenance to the codes to occur in the classification system during implementation. This has to occur because code sets cannot be frozen during the implementation period and be kept up to date.

What HIM Professionals Can Do to Help

How can HIM professionals help? No matter what your job, your role in this process is important. Here are some things HIM professionals can do to support the process:

- **Get up to speed on ICD-10.** You don't have to know how to code with these classification systems, but you do have to know what the systems achieve, what components of healthcare they affect, why a 30-year-old classification system does not represent 21st-century medicine, and so on. You can find resources describing the issue in the Communities of Practice, the FORE Library: HIM Body of Knowledge, and elsewhere on AHIMA's Web site (www.ahima.org). You can also find articles in past and upcoming issues of the *Journal of AHIMA*. AHIMA will continue to prepare materials to educate its members, but you have to be the authority. Others in the industry will be seeking you out to question this change. Be prepared to discuss the NPRM. Read the rule when it is published, understand how you and your organization will be affected, and lend your voice in support.

- **Know what these classification systems do** and how they will affect your organization or institution. Conversion to ICD-10 will, to some extent, affect everyone. Administrators, information systems managers, financial and billing managers, and doctors will want to know how it will affect computer systems, data collection, documentation, billing, data reporting, and so forth. HIM professionals will need to help their organizations understand how this change will affect the organization and what the benefits are.

- **Comment on the NPRM.** Your expertise and your voice are very necessary for this process. While an association like AHIMA can promote adoption, it can only write one letter. In the face of opposition from groups such as the Blue Cross and Blue Shield Association and the American Association of Health Plans/Health Insurance Association of America, the voice of AHIMA members is particularly needed. These groups have opposed upgrading ICD-9-CM based on cost, but they fail to acknowledge the value of detailed standardized classification of diseases and inpatient procedures. The secretary must see that upgrading ICD-9-CM has the full support of the industry. Your voice must be heard.

Moving Forward: You Won't Go It Alone

You will not be alone in the professional effort to adopt and implement ICD-10-CM and ICD-10-PCS. AHIMA has been very involved in the creation and testing of these two classification systems, and the association intends to be 46,000 members strong in making this change a credit to our profession. Several AHIMA tools are at your disposal regarding the history and arguments for upgrading ICD-9-CM, as well as information and education resources regarding the replacement classification systems.

For instance, a Community of Practice for those interested in ICD-10-CM and PCS implementation has been established. The Coding Roundtables will also offer a means for two-way communication. This is a time for the HIM profession to shine, take the lead, and help bring in these changes in a professional, timely, and efficient manner. Together we can take the next steps.

Dan Rode (dan.rode@ahima.org) is AHIMA's vice president of policy and government relations.

Source: Rode, Dan. "Taking the Next Step Forward for ICD-10." *Journal of AHIMA* 75, no. 1 (January 2004): 14–15.

From V Codes to Z Codes: Transitioning to ICD-10

by Karen M. Kostick, RHIT, CCS, CCS-P

V codes, described in the ICD-9-CM chapter "Supplementary Classification of Factors Influencing Health Status and Contact with Health Services," are often misunderstood in reporting healthcare services. These codes are designed for occasions when circumstances other than a disease or injury result in an encounter or are recorded by providers as problems or factors that influence care.

ICD-9-CM codes such as V01.82, Exposure to SARS-associated coronavirus, and V01.81, Contact with or exposure to anthrax, are examples of how V codes capture significant US healthcare statistics. Although health plans have sometimes been reluctant to accept V codes as justification for reimbursement, these codes play a key role in classifying selected services and capturing important information.

Under ICD-10-CM, these services will be reported under a new set of codes—Z codes—with some significant changes.

V Codes in ICD-9-CM

The official coding guidelines that became effective on October 1, 2002, include coding guidelines for V codes throughout Sections I–IV. Section I C, "Chapter or Disease Specific Coding Guidelines," includes a clarification note for coders and states that unless otherwise indicated, the coding guidelines for this section apply to all healthcare settings. Complete copies of the guidelines are available from the National Center for Health Statistics (NCHS) Web site at www.cdc.gov/nchs.

Section I includes a new section titled "Classification of Factors Influencing Health Status and Contact with Health Service (C-18)." This section provides coding guidelines for frequently used V code categories. V codes reviewed in Section II, "Selection of Principal Diagnosis(es)," and Section III, "Reporting Additional Diagnoses," apply to the inpatient, short-term acute care setting. Section IV, "Diagnostic Coding and Reporting Guidelines for Outpatient Services," provides V code instructions for the outpatient and physician office setting. The outpatient setting includes reporting by home health agencies.

Changes in ICD-10-CM

The selected ICD-9-CM V code coding guidelines included in this article preview coding practices in ICD-10-CM for factors influencing health status and contact with health services. The coding guidelines between the two coding classification systems are the same unless otherwise specified.

A significant change between the two coding classifications is that ICD-9-CM's supplementary codes are incorporated into the main classification in ICD-10-CM. The ICD-10-CM Tabular List categorizes codes to represent reasons for encounters as "Z" codes instead of "V" codes. ICD-10-CM codes in general may have up to seven characters, but Z codes under categories Z00–Z99 consist of three to six character codes. Additional ICD-10-CM information is available for downloading from the NCHS Web site.

Screening, Routine Examination

Screening visits provide healthy patients early detection tests such as a mammogram or a colonoscopy. Screening codes can be used as either a first listed or additional code depending on the reason for the encounter. If the reason for the encounter is specifically the screening exam, the screening code is the first listed code and any condition discovered during the screening may be listed as an additional diagnosis.

A procedure code is required to validate the screening exam. Screening visit codes do not apply when a diagnostic test is ordered for a patient to evaluate a complaint or an abnormality detected by a physician. For these visits, the sign or symptom is used to report the reason for the test. (See "Outpatient Facility-Screening Scenario".)

Routine and administrative examinations are performed without relationship to treatment or diagnosis of an illness or symptom, or performed at the request of third parties such as employers or schools. Routine examination codes should be used as first listed codes only. This category should not be used if the examination is for diagnosing a possible condition or for providing treatment. Instead a sign or symptom code is used to report the reason for the visit.

Codes within ICD-10-CM categories Z00 and Z01, Persons encountering health services for examinations, are available when the encounter is for an examination "with abnormal findings" and "without abnormal findings." A note instructs the coder to use an additional code to identify any abnormal findings based on the results of the examination.

Aftercare Versus Follow-up Visits

Aftercare codes identify specific types of continuing care after the initial treatment of an injury or disease. In 2002, two V code subcategories for orthopedic aftercare (V54.1 and V54.2) were added to specify encounters following initial treatment of fractures. Coding guidelines state that a fracture code from the main classification can only be used for an initial encounter. Subsequent encounters that usually occur in an outpatient, home health, or long-term care facility now have the ability to report the type and site of fractures within the new subcategory sections.

Orthopedic aftercare visit coding guidelines differ in ICD-10-CM in that Z codes should not be used if treatment is directed at the current injury. If treatment is directed at the current injury, the injury code should be reported with an extension as the seventh character to signify the subsequent encounter. The purpose of assigning the extension is to be able to track the continuity of care while identifying the type of injury.

While aftercare codes are used for a resolving or long-term condition, follow-up codes are used for conditions that have completed treatment or for cancer patients to monitor the recurrence of cancer after treatment has been completed. ICD-9-CM coding guidelines state that follow-up codes are listed first unless a condition has recurred on the follow-up visit, then the diagnosis code should be listed first in place of the follow-up code. ICD-10-CM coding guidelines differ in that if a condition is found to have recurred on a follow-up visit, the follow-up code is still used and the diagnosis code is listed second. Personal history codes should be assigned as an additional code with follow-up examinations.

History, Status Codes

Personal and family history codes are important pieces of information that support the need for screening exams and follow-up exams. The Centers for Medicare and Medicaid Services (CMS) requires history V codes when appropriate in conjunction with mammograms, Pap tests, pelvic exams, and colon cancer screenings. You can read the CMS coding policies at: www.cms.hhs.gov/medlearn/womens_health.pdf.

Some status codes support increased healthcare costs, as the status can affect the treatment plans and its outcome as noted in the official coding guidelines. Status codes can also be used to track public health issues. For example, the status codes for infection with drug-resistance microorganism are assigned as an additional code for infectious conditions to indicate the presence of drug-resistance of the infectious organism. It is evident ICD-10-CM offers additional codes and a greater level of specificity to report health status and contact with health services in the revised classification. However, in a couple areas, ICD-9-CM is more specific than ICD-10-CM, as noted in "Inpatient, Acute Care-Status Scenario," with regard to the ICD-10-CM category for infection with drug-resistance microorganisms.

Outpatient Prenatal Visits

An area to pay close attention to when reporting prenatal visits in ICD-9-CM is category V23, Supervision of high-risk pregnancy. Coding guidelines for high-risk prenatal visits instruct that a code from category V23 be assigned as the first-listed or principal diagnosis unless a pertinent excludes note applies. If a V23 category excludes note applies codes from Chapter 11, Complications of Pregnancy, Childbirth, and the Puerperium Chapter (630–677) may be listed as a first-listed or principal diagnosis code.

If appropriate, Chapter 11 codes may be assigned as additional codes with category 23. ICD-10-CM does not include codes for supervision of high-risk pregnancy in the chapter to report factors influencing health status and contact with health services (Z00–Z99). Rather, these codes are incorporated in the chapter for conditions related to pregnancy and childbirth. ICD-10-CM high-risk pregnancy codes are available for patients who have had complications in the past and are categorized by first, second, and third trimester.

Advocating Coding Consistency

The HIPAA standard transactions and code sets regulation includes a requirement that the official coding guidelines are used along with ICD-9-CM for reporting. This represents an important step in the adoption of uniform code reporting requirements across all payers. Coding for reimbursement is addressed in the American Hospital Association's (AHA) 2000 3rd Quarter *Coding Clinic,* including problems that arise between providers and payers in relation to coding guidelines and payer coding policies.

AHA provides helpful tips on how to effectively settle coding conflicts with payers. When payers deny a particular claim, it is recommended that you first identify whether it is really a coding conflict and not a coverage matter. A payer may be using the correct coding guidelines but may not be covering certain services such as a routine or follow-up examination.

If you determine that a health plan reporting policy conflicts with the official coding guidelines, AHA advises you to obtain the payer policy in writing and advocate adherence to official coding guidelines. Coding professionals may influence the fiscal intermediary or carrier to apply official coding guidelines to ensure reliable claims data. These coding practices are also referenced in the AHIMA Standards of Ethical Coding.

Outpatient Facility—Screening Scenario

Asymptomatic 67-year-old female patient presents to the outpatient radiology department for a bilateral mammogram. The physician's order documented breast cancer screening. The radiology report notes clusters of microcalcification in the left breast.

First-Listed Diagnosis	ICD-9-CM:	V76.12 Other screening mammogram
	ICD-10-CM:	Z12.31 Encounter for screening mammogram for malignancy of breast
Additional Diagnosis	ICD-9-CM:	793.81 Mammographic microcalcification
	ICD-10-CM:	R92.0 Mammographic microcalcification found on diagnostic imaging of breast
Procedure	CPT:	76092 Screening mammography, bilateral

Physician Office—Routine Exam Scenario

45-year-old established patient presented to her physician's office for a routine physical exam. During the examination the physician identified an enlarged thyroid. The physician ordered a laboratory test and requested to see the patient in two weeks.

First-Listed Diagnosis	ICD-9-CM:	V70.0 Routine general medical examination at a health-care facility
	ICD-10-CM:	Z00.011 Encounter for general medical examination with abnormal findings
Additional Diagnosis	ICD-9-CM:	240.9 Goiter, unspecified
	ICD-10-CM:	E04.9 Nontoxic goiter, unspecified

Home Health—Aftercare Visit Scenario

74-year-old patient fell at home and sustained a subtrochanteric fracture of the left femur and was discharged home. Physician ordered physical therapy for difficulty in walking and exercise three times a week for one month

First-Listed Diagnosis	ICD-9-CM:	V57.1 Other physical therapy
	ICD-10-CM:	S72.22xd Displaced subtrochanteric fracture of left femur, subsequent encounter for closed fracture with routine healing
Additional Diagnosis	ICD-9-CM:	719.7 Difficulty in walking V54.13 Aftercare for healing traumatic fracture of hip
	ICD-10-CM:	R26.2 Difficulty in walking, not elsewhere classified

Inpatient, Acute Care—Status Scenario

A 54-year-old male is admitted into the hospital with a principal diagnosis of surgical site infection secondary to a recent right side below the knee amputation. Patient is a type I diabetic with diabetic peripheral vascular disease and congestive heart failure. The patient sought treatment when the wound began to exude purulent drainage. On the second day of his hospitalization he had developed nausea, uncontrolled diabetes, and ketoacidosis.

Moist saline dressings were applied twice daily to the wound. Wound culture tested positive for Staphylococcus aureus and was resistant to flucloxacillin. Ciprofloxacin effectively treated the infection. Diabetic ketoacidosis managed well and blood glucose was brought under control. Patient was discharged to a rehabilitation facility for continued wound management.

Principal Dx	ICD-9-CM:	997.62 Amputation stump infection
	ICD-10-CM:	T87.43 Infection of amputation stump, right lower extremity
Additional Dx	ICD-9-CM:	041.11 Staphylococcus aureus V09.0 Infection with microorganisms resistant to penicillins 250.13 Diabetes with ketoacidosis 250.73 Diabetes uncontrolled with peripheral circulatory disorders 443.81 Peripheral angiopathy in diseases classified elsewhere 428.0 Congestive heart failure, unspecified
	ICD-10-CM:	B95.6 Staphylococcus aureus as the cause of diseases classified elsewhere Z16 Infection with drug-resistant microorganisms E10.10 Type 1 diabetes mellitus with ketoacidosis without coma E10.51 Type 1 diabetes mellitus with diabetic peripheral angiopathy without gangrene I50.9 Congestive heart failure, NOS

References

AHA. *Coding Clinic,* 1996, 4th Quarter.

AHA. *Coding Clinic,* 2002, 4th Quarter.

AHIMA's Standards of Ethical Coding are available at www.ahima.org/infocenter/guidelines/standards.cfm.

CMS. Medicare Preventive Services Education Program. "Women's Health." Available at www.cms.hhs.gov/medlearn/womens_health.pdf.

Hazelwood, Anita, and Carol Venable. *ICD-10-CM Preview.* Chicago: AHIMA, 2003.

ICD-9-CM Official Guidelines For Coding and Reporting (Effective October 1, 2002). Available at www.cdc.gov/nchs/datawh/ftpserv/ftpicd9/ftpicd9.htm#guidelines.

ICD-10-CM Official Guidelines. Available at www.cdc.gov/nchs/about/otheract/icd9/abticd10.htm.

Karen Kostick (karen.kostick@ahima.org) is a coding practice manager at AHIMA.

Source: Kostick, Karen M. "From V Codes to Z Codes: Transitioning to ICD-10." *Journal of AHIMA* 75, no. 2 (February 2004): 65–68.

Appendix H

Developing a Physician Query Process

by Sue Bowman, RHIA, CCS

Principles of Medical Record Documentation

Medical record documentation is used for a multitude of purposes, including:

- Serving as a means of communication between the physician and the other members of the healthcare team providing care to the patient

- Serving as a basis for evaluating the adequacy and appropriateness of patient care

- Providing data to support insurance claims

- Assisting in protecting the legal interests of patients, healthcare professionals, and healthcare facilities

- Providing clinical data for research and education

To support these various uses, it is imperative that medical record documentation be complete, accurate, and timely. Facilities are expected to comply with a number of standards regarding medical record completion and content promulgated by multiple regulatory agencies.

Joint Commission on Accreditation of Healthcare Organizations

The Joint Commission's 2000 Hospital Accreditation Standards state, "the medical record contains sufficient information to identify the patient, support the diagnosis, justify the treatment, document the course and results, and promote continuity among health care providers" (IM.7.2).[1] The Joint Commission Standards also state, "medical record data and information are managed in a timely manner" (IM.7.6).

Timely entries are essential if a medical record is to be useful in a patient's care. A complete medical record is also important when a patient is discharged, because information in the record may be needed for clinical, legal, or performance improvement purposes. The Joint Commission requires hospitals to have policy and procedures on the timely entry of all significant clinical information into the patient's medical record, and they do not consider a medical record complete until all final diagnoses and complications are recorded without the use of symbols or abbreviations.

Joint Commission standards also require medical records to be reviewed on an ongoing basis for completeness of timeliness of information, and action is taken to improve the quality and timeliness of documentation that affects patient care (IM.7.10). This review must address the presence, timeliness, legibility, and authentication of the final diagnoses and conclusions at termination of hospitalization.

Medicare

The Medicare Conditions of Participation require medical records to be accurately written, promptly completed, properly filed and retained, and accessible.[2] Records must document, as appropriate, complications, hospital-acquired infections, and unfavorable reactions to drugs and anesthesia. The conditions also stipulate that all records must document the final diagnosis with completion of medical records within 30 days following discharge.

Relationship between Coding and Documentation

Complete and accurate diagnostic and procedural coded data must be available, in a timely manner, in order to:

- Improve the quality and effectiveness of patient care

- Ensure equitable healthcare reimbursement

- Expand the body of medical knowledge

- Make appropriate decisions regarding healthcare policies, delivery systems, funding, expansion, and education

- Monitor resource utilization

- Permit identification and resolution of medical errors

- Improve clinical decision making

- Facilitate tracking of fraud and abuse

- Permit valid clinical research, epidemiological studies, outcomes and statistical analyses, and provider profiling

- Provide comparative data to consumers regarding costs and outcomes, average charges, and outcomes by procedure

Physician documentation is the cornerstone of accurate coding. Therefore, assuring the accuracy of coded data is a shared responsibility between coding professionals and physicians. Accurate diagnostic and procedural coded data originate from collaboration between physicians, who have a clinical background, and coding professionals, who have an understanding of classification systems.

Expectations of Physicians

Physicians are expected to provide complete, accurate, timely, and legible documentation of pertinent facts and observations about an individual's health history, including past and present illnesses, tests, treatments, and outcomes. Medical record entries should be documented at the time service is provided. Medical record entries should be authenticated.

If subsequent additions to documentation are needed, they should be identified as such and dated. (Often these expectations are included in the medical staff or house staff rules and regulations.) Medical record documentation should:

- Address the clinical significance of abnormal test results

- Support the intensity of patient evaluation and treatment and describe the thought processes and complexity of decision making

- Include all diagnostic and therapeutic procedures, treatments, and tests performed, in addition to their results

- Include any changes in the patient's condition, including psychosocial and physical symptoms

- Include all conditions that coexist at the time of admission, that subsequently develop, or that affect the treatment received and the length of stay. This encompasses all conditions that affect patient care in terms of requiring clinical evaluation, therapeutic treatment, diagnostic procedures, extended length of hospital stay, or increased nursing care and monitoring[3]

- Be updated as necessary to reflect all diagnoses relevant to the care or services provided

- Be consistent and discuss and reconcile any discrepancies (this reconciliation should be documented in the medical record)

- Be legible and written in ink, typewritten, or electronically signed, stored, and printed

Expectations of Coding Professionals

The AHIMA Code of Ethics sets forth ethical principles for the HIM profession. HIM professionals are responsible for maintaining and promoting ethical practices. This Code of Ethics states, in part: "Health information management professionals promote high standards for health information management practice, education, and research."

Another standard in this code states, "Health information management professionals strive to provide accurate and timely information." Data accuracy and integrity are fundamental values of HIM that are advanced by:

- Employing practices that produce complete, accurate, and timely information to meet the health and related needs of individuals

- Following the guidelines set forth in the organization's compliance plan for reporting improper preparation, alteration, or suppression of information or data by others

- Not participating in any improper preparation, alteration, or suppression of health record information or other organization data

A conscientious goal for coding and maintaining a quality database is accurate clinical and statistical data. AHIMA's Standards of Ethical Coding were developed to guide coding professionals in this process. As stated in the standards, coding professionals are expected to support the importance of accurate, complete, and consistent coding practices for the production of quality healthcare data. These standards also indicate that coding professionals should only assign and report codes that are clearly and consistently supported by physician documentation in the medical record. It is the responsibility of coding professionals to assess physician documentation to assure that it supports the diagnosis and procedure codes reported on claims.

Dialogue between coding professionals and clinicians is encouraged, because it improves coding professionals' clinical knowledge and educates the physicians on documentation practice issues. AHIMA's Standards of Ethical Coding state that coding professionals are expected to consult physicians for clarification and additional documentation prior to code assignment when there is conflicting or ambiguous data in the health record. Coding professionals should also assist and educate physicians by advocating proper documentation practices, further specificity, and resequencing or inclusion of diagnoses or procedures when needed to more accurately reflect the acuity, severity, and the occurrence of events. It is recommended that coding be performed by credentialed HIM professionals.[4]

It is inappropriate for coding professionals to misrepresent the patient's clinical picture through incorrect coding or add diagnoses or procedures unsupported by the documentation to maximize reimbursement or meet insurance policy coverage requirements. Coding professionals should not change codes or the narratives of codes on the billing abstract so that meanings are misrepresented. Diagnoses or procedures should not be inappropriately included or excluded, because payment or insurance policy coverage requirements will be affected. When individual payer policies conflict with official coding rules and guidelines, these policies should be obtained in writing whenever possible.

Reasonable efforts should be made to educate the payer on proper coding practices in order to influence a change in the payer's policy.

Proper Use of Physician Queries

The process of querying physicians is an effective and, in today's healthcare environment, necessary mechanism for improving the quality of coding and medical record documentation and capturing complete clinical data. Query forms have become an accepted tool for communicating with physicians on documentation issues influencing proper code assignment. Query forms should be used in a judicious and appropriate manner. They must be used as a communication tool to improve the accuracy of code assignment and the quality of physician documentation, not to inappropriately maximize reimbursement. The query process should be guided by AHIMA's Standards of Ethical Coding and the official coding guidelines. An inappropriate query—such as a form that is poorly constructed or asks leading questions—or overuse of the query process can result in quality-of-care, legal, and ethical concerns.

The Query Process

The goal of the query process should be to improve physician documentation and coding professionals' understanding of the unique clinical situation, not to improve reimbursement. Each facility should establish a policy and procedure for obtaining physician clarification of documentation that affects code assignment. The process of querying physicians must be a patient-specific process, not a general process. Asking "blanket" questions is not appropriate. Policies regarding the circumstances when physicians will be queried should be designed to promote timely, complete, and accurate coding and documentation.

Physicians should not be asked to provide clarification of their medical record documentation without the opportunity to access the patient's medical record.

Each facility also needs to determine if physicians will be queried concurrently (during the patient's hospitalization) or after discharge. Both methods are acceptable. Querying physicians concurrently allows the documentation deficiency to be corrected while the patient is still in-house and can positively influence patient care.

The policy and procedure should stipulate who is authorized to contact the physician for clarifications regarding a coding issue. Coding professionals should be allowed to contact physicians directly for clarification, rather than limiting this responsibility to supervisory personnel or a designated individual.

The facility may wish to use a designated physician liaison to resolve conflicts between physicians and coding professionals. The appropriate use of the physician liaison should be described in the facility's policy and procedures.

Query Format

Each facility should develop a standard format for the query form. No "sticky notes" or scratch paper should be allowed. Each facility should develop a standard design and format for physician queries to ensure clear, consistent, appropriate queries.

The query form should:

- Be clearly and concisely written

- Contain precise language

- Present the facts from the medical record and identify why clarification is needed

- Present the scenario and state a question that asks the physician to make a clinical interpretation of a given diagnosis or condition based on treatment, evaluation, monitoring, and/or services provided. "Open-ended" questions that allow the physician to document the specific diagnosis are preferable to multiple-choice questions or questions requiring only a "yes" or "no" response. Queries that appear to lead the physician to provide a particular response could lead to allegations of inappropriate upcoding.

- Be phrased such that the physician is allowed to specify the correct diagnosis. It should not indicate the financial impact of the response to the query. The form should not be designed so that all that is required is a physician signature.

- Include:

  —Patient name

  —Admission date

  —Medical record number

  —Name and contact information (phone number and e-mail address) of the coding professional

  —Specific question and rationale (that is, relevant documentation or clinical findings)

  —Place for physician to document his or her response

  —Place for the physician to sign and date his or her response

The query forms should not:

- "Lead" the physician

- Sound presumptive, directing, prodding, probing, or as though the physician is being led to make an assumption

- Ask questions that can be responded to in a "yes" or "no" fashion

- Indicate the financial impact of the response to the query

- Be designed so that all that is required is a physician signature

When Is a Query Appropriate?

Physicians should be queried whenever there is conflicting, ambiguous, or incomplete information in the medical record regarding any significant reportable condition or procedure. Querying the physician only when reimbursement is affected will skew national healthcare data and might lead to allegations of upcoding.

Every discrepancy or issue not addressed in the physician documentation should not necessarily result in the physician being queried. Each facility needs to develop policies and procedures regarding the clinical conditions and documentation situations warranting a request for physician clarification. For example, insignificant or irrelevant findings may not warrant querying the physician regarding the assignment of an additional diagnosis code.

Also, if the maximum number of codes that can be entered in the hospital information system has already been assigned, the facility may decide that it is not necessary to query the physician regarding an additional code. Facilities need to balance the value of marginal data being collected against the administrative burden of obtaining the additional documentation.

Members of the medical staff in consultation with coding professionals should develop the specific clinical criteria for a valid query. The specific clinical documentation that must be present in the patient's record to generate a query should be described. For example, anemia, septicemia, and respiratory failure are conditions that often require physician clarification. The medical staff can assist the coding staff in determining when it would be appropriate to query a physician regarding the reporting of these conditions by describing the specific clinical indications in the medical record documentation that raise the possibility that the condition in question may be present.

When Is a Query Not Necessary?

Queries are not necessary if a physician involved in the care and treatment of the patient, including consulting physicians, has documented a diagnosis and there is no conflicting documentation from another physician. Medical record documentation from any physician involved in the care and treatment of the patient, including documentation by consulting physicians, is appropriate for the basis of code assignment. If documentation from different physicians conflicts, seek clarification from the attending physician, as he or she is ultimately responsible for the final diagnosis.

Queries are also not necessary when a physician has documented a final diagnosis and clinical indicators—such as test results—do not appear to support this diagnosis. While coding professionals are expected to advocate complete and accurate physician documentation and to collaborate with physicians to realize this goal, they are not expected to challenge the physician's medical judgment in establishing the patient's diagnosis. However, because a discrepancy between clinical findings and a final diagnosis is a clinical issue, a facility may choose to establish a policy that the physician will be queried in these instances.

Documentation of Query Response

The physician's response to the query must be documented in the patient's medical record. Each facility must develop a policy regarding the specific process for incorporating this additional documentation in the medical record. For example, this policy might stipulate that the physician is required to add the additional information to the body of the medical record. As an alternative, a form, such as a medical record "progress note" form, might be attached to the query form and the attachment is then filed in the medical record. However, another alternative is to file the query form itself in the permanent medical record. Any documentation obtained post-discharge must be included in the discharge summary or identified as a late entry or addendum.

Any decision to file this form in the medical record should involve the advice of the facility's corporate compliance officer and legal counsel, due to potential compliance and legal risks related to incorporating the actual query form into the permanent medical record (such as its potential use as evidence of poor documentation in an audit, investigation, or malpractice suit, risks related to naming a nonclinician in the medical record, or quality of care concerns if the physician response on a query form is not clearly supported by the rest of the medical record documentation).

If the query form will serve as the only documentation of the physician's clarification, the use of "open-ended" questions (that require the physician to specifically document the additional information) are preferable to multiple choice questions or the use of questions requiring only a "yes" or "no" answer. The query form would need to be approved by the medical staff/medical records committee before implementation of a policy allowing this form to be maintained in the medical record. Also keep in mind that the Joint Commission hospital accreditation standards stipulate that only authorized individuals may make entries in medical records (IM.7.1.1). Therefore, the facility needs to consider modifying the medical staff bylaws to specify coding professionals as individuals authorized to make medical record entries prior to allowing query forms to become a permanent part of the medical record.

Auditing, Monitoring, and Corrective Action

Ideally, complete and accurate physician documentation should occur at the time care is rendered. The need for a query form results from incomplete, conflicting, or ambiguous documentation, which is an indication of poor documentation. Therefore, query form usage should be the exception rather than the norm. If physicians are being queried frequently, facility management or an appropriate medical staff committee should investigate the reasons why.

A periodic review of the query practice should include a determination of what percentage of the query forms are eliciting negative and positive responses from the physicians. A high negative response rate may be an indication that the coding staff are not using the query process judiciously and are being overzealous.

A high positive response rate may indicate that there are widespread poor documentation habits that need to be addressed. It may also indicate that the absence of certain reports (for example, discharge summary, operative report) at the time of coding is forcing the coding staff to query the physicians to obtain the information they need for proper coding. If this is the case, the facility may wish to reconsider its policy regarding the availability of certain reports prior to coding. Waiting for these reports may make more sense in terms of turnaround time and productivity rather than finding it necessary to frequently query the physicians. The question of why final diagnoses are not available at the time of discharge may arise at the time of an audit, review by the peer review organization, or investigation.

The use of query forms should also be monitored for patterns, and any identified patterns should be used to educate physicians on improving their documentation at the point of care. If a pattern is identified, such as a particular physician or diagnosis, appropriate steps should be taken to correct the problem so the necessary documentation is present prior to coding in the future and the need to query this physician, or to query physicians regarding a particular diagnosis, is reduced. Corrective action might include targeted education for one physician or education for the entire medical staff on the proper documentation necessary for accurate code assignment.

Patterns of poor documentation that have not been addressed through education or other corrective action are signs of an ineffective compliance program. The Department of Health and Human Services Office of Inspector General has noted in its Compliance Program Guidance for Hospitals that "accurate coding depends upon the quality of completeness of the physician's documentation" and "active staff physician participation in educational programs focusing on coding and documentation should be emphasized by the hospital."[5]

The format of the queries should also be monitored on a regular basis to ensure that they are not inappropriately leading the physician to provide a particular response. Inappropriately written queries should be used to educate the coding staff on a properly written query. Patterns of inappropriately written queries should be referred to the corporate compliance officer.

Prepared by

Sue Prophet, RHIA, CCS

Acknowledgments

AHIMA Advocacy and Policy Task Force
AHIMA's Coding Practice Team
AHIMA Coding Policy and Strategy Committee
AHIMA Society for Clinical Coding
Dan Rode, MBA, FHFMA

Notes

1. Joint Commission on Accreditation of Healthcare Organizations. *Comprehensive Accreditation Manual for Hospitals: The Official Handbook.* Oakbrook Terrace, IL: Joint Commission, 2000.

2. Health Care Financing Administration, Department of Health and Human Services. "Conditions of Participation for Hospitals." *Code of Federal Regulations,* 2000. 42 CFR, Chapter IV, Part 482.

3. ICD-9-CM Official Guidelines for Coding and Reporting developed and approved by the American Hospital Association, American Health Information Management Association, Health Care Financing Administration, and the National Center for Health Statistics.

4. AHIMA is the professional organization responsible for issuing several credentials in health information management: Registered Health Information Administrator (RHIA), Registered Health Information Technician (RHIT), Certified Coding Specialist (CCS), and Certified Coding Specialist—Physician-based (CCS-P).

5. Office of Inspector General, Department of Health and Human Services. *Compliance Program Guidance for Hospitals.* Washington, DC: Office of Inspector General, 1998.

References

AHIMA Code of Ethics, 1998.

AHIMA Standards of Ethical Coding, 1999.

AHIMA Coding Policy and Strategy Committee. "Practice Brief: Data Quality." *Journal of AHIMA* 67, no. 2 (1996).

Article Citation

Prophet, Sue. "Developing a Physician Query Process (AHIMA Practice Brief)." *Journal of AHIMA* 72, no. 9 (2001): 88I–M.

Appendix I

ICD-9-CM Official Guidelines for Coding and Reporting

ICD-9-CM Official Guidelines for Coding and Reporting appear as published on the CMS Web site: www.cms.gov.

ICD-9-CM Official Guidelines for Coding and Reporting

Effective April 1, 2005
Narrative changes appear in bold text
The guidelines have been updated to include the V Code Table

The Centers for Medicare and Medicaid Services (CMS) and the National Center for Health Statistics (NCHS), two departments within the U. S. Federal Government's Department of Health and Human Services (DHHS) provide the following guidelines for coding and reporting using the International Classification of Diseases, 9th Revision, Clinical Modification (ICD-9-CM). These guidelines should be used as a companion document to the official version of the ICD-9-CM as published on CD-ROM by the U.S. Government Printing Office (GPO).

These guidelines have been approved by the four organizations that make up the Cooperating Parties for the ICD-9-CM: the American Hospital Association (AHA), the American Health Information Management Association (AHIMA), CMS, and NCHS. These guidelines are included on the official government version of the ICD-9-CM, and also appear in *"Coding Clinic for ICD-9-CM"* published by the AHA.

These guidelines are a set of rules that have been developed to accompany and complement the official conventions and instructions provided within the ICD-9-CM itself. These guidelines are based on the coding and sequencing instructions in Volumes I, II and III of ICD-9-CM, but provide additional instruction. **Adherence to these guidelines when assigning ICD-9-CM diagnosis and procedure codes is required under the Health Insurance Portability and Accountability Act (HIPAA). The diagnosis codes (Volumes 1-2) have been adopted under HIPAA for all healthcare settings. Volume 3 procedure codes have been adopted for inpatient procedures reported by hospitals**. A joint effort between the healthcare provider and the coder is essential to achieve complete and accurate documentation, code assignment, and reporting of diagnoses and procedures. These guidelines have been developed to assist both the healthcare provider and the coder in identifying those diagnoses and procedures that are to be reported. The importance of consistent, complete documentation in the medical record cannot be overemphasized. Without such documentation accurate coding cannot be achieved. **The entire record should be reviewed to determine the specific reason for the encounter and the conditions treated.**

The term encounter is used for all settings, including hospital admissions. In the context of these guidelines, the term provider is used throughout the guidelines to mean physician or any qualified health care practitioner who is legally accountable for establishing the patient's diagnosis. Only this set of guidelines, approved by the Cooperating Parties, is official.

The guidelines are organized into sections. Section I includes the structure and conventions of the classification and general guidelines that apply to the entire classification, and chapter-specific guidelines that correspond to the chapters as they are arranged in the classification. Section II includes guidelines for selection of principal diagnosis for non-outpatient settings. Section III includes guidelines for reporting additional diagnoses in non-outpatient settings. Section IV is for outpatient coding and reporting.

Section I. Conventions, general coding guidelines and chapter specific guidelines

The conventions, general guidelines and chapter-specific guidelines are applicable to all health care settings unless otherwise indicated.

A. Conventions for the ICD-9-CM

The conventions for the ICD-9-CM are the general rules for use of the classification independent of the guidelines. These conventions are incorporated within the index and tabular of the ICD-9-CM as instructional notes. The conventions are as follows:

1. Format:

The ICD-9-CM uses an indented format for ease in reference

2. Abbreviations

a. Index abbreviations

NEC "Not elsewhere classifiable"
This abbreviation in the index represents "other specified" when a specific code is not available for a condition the index directs the coder to the "other specified" code in the tabular.

b. Tabular abbreviations

NEC "Not elsewhere classifiable"
This abbreviation in the tabular represents "other specified". When a specific code is not available for a condition the tabular includes an NEC entry under a code to identify the code as the "other specified" code (See Section I.A.5.a."Other" codes).

NOS "Not otherwise specified"
This abbreviation is the equivalent of unspecified. (See Section I.A.5.b., "Unspecified" codes)

3. Punctuation

[ ] Brackets are used in the tabular list to enclose synonyms, alternative wording or explanatory phrases. Brackets are used in the index to identify manifestation codes. (See Section I.A.6. "Etiology/manifestations")

( ) Parentheses are used in both the index and tabular to enclose supplementary words that may be present or absent in the statement of a disease or procedure without affecting the code number to which it is assigned. The terms within the parentheses are referred to as nonessential modifiers.

: Colons are used in the Tabular list after an incomplete term which needs one or more of the modifiers following the colon to make it assignable to a given category.

4. Includes and Excludes Notes and Inclusion terms

Includes: This note appears immediately under a three-digit code title to further define, or give examples of, the content of the category.

Excludes: An excludes note under a code indicates that the terms excluded from the code are to be coded elsewhere. In some cases the codes for the excluded terms should not be used in conjunction with the code from which it is excluded. An example of this is a congenital condition excluded from an acquired form of the same condition. The congenital and acquired codes should not be used together. In other cases, the excluded terms may be used together with an excluded code. An example of this is when fractures of different bones are coded to different codes. Both codes may be used together if both types of fractures are present.

Inclusion terms: List of terms are included under certain four and five digit codes. These terms are the conditions for which that code number is to be used. The terms may be synonyms of the code title, or, in the case of "other specified" codes, the terms are a list of the various conditions assigned to that code. The inclusion terms are not necessarily exhaustive. Additional terms found only in the index may also be assigned to a code.

5. Other and Unspecified codes

a. "Other" codes

Codes titled "other" or "other specified" (usually a code with a 4th digit 8 or fifth-digit 9 for diagnosis codes) are for use when the information in the medical record provides detail for which a specific code does not exist. Index entries with NEC in the line designate "other" codes in the tabular. These index entries represent specific disease entities for which no specific code exists so the term is included within an "other" code.

b. "Unspecified" codes

Codes (usually a code with a 4th digit 9 or 5th digit 0 for diagnosis codes) titled "unspecified" are for use when the information in the medical record is insufficient to assign a more specific code.

6. Etiology/manifestation convention ("code first", "use additional code" and "in diseases classified elsewhere" notes)

Certain conditions have both an underlying etiology and multiple body system manifestations due to the underlying etiology. For such conditions, the ICD-9-CM has a coding convention that requires the underlying condition be sequenced first followed by the manifestation. Wherever such a combination exists, there is a "use additional code" note at the etiology code, and a "code first" note at the manifestation code. These instructional notes indicate the proper sequencing order of the codes, etiology followed by manifestation.

In most cases the manifestation codes will have in the code title, "in diseases classified elsewhere." Codes with this title are a component of the etiology/ manifestation convention. The code title indicates that it is a manifestation code. "In diseases classified elsewhere" codes are never permitted to be used as first listed or principal diagnosis codes. They must be used in conjunction with an underlying condition code and they must be listed following the underlying condition.

There are manifestation codes that do not have "in diseases classified elsewhere" in the title. For such codes a "use additional code" note will still be present and the rules for sequencing apply.

In addition to the notes in the tabular, these conditions also have a specific index entry structure. In the index both conditions are listed together with the etiology code first followed by the manifestation codes in brackets. The code in brackets is always to be sequenced second.

The most commonly used etiology/manifestation combinations are the codes for Diabetes mellitus, category 250. For each code under category 250 there is a use additional code note for the manifestation that is specific for that particular diabetic manifestation. Should a patient have more than one manifestation of diabetes, more than one code from category 250 may be used with as many manifestation codes as are needed to fully describe the patient's complete diabetic condition. The **category** 250 diabetes codes should be sequenced first, followed by the manifestation codes.

"Code first" and "Use additional code" notes are also used as sequencing rules in the classification for certain codes that are not part of an etiology/ manifestation combination. See - Section I.B.9. "Multiple coding for a single condition".

7. "And"

The word "and" should be interpreted to mean either "and" or "or" when it appears in a title.

8. **"With"**

   The word "with" in the alphabetic index is sequenced immediately following the main term, not in alphabetical order.

9. **"See" and "See Also"**

   The "see" instruction following a main term in the index indicates that another term should be referenced. It is necessary to go to the main term referenced with the "see" note to locate the correct code.

   A "see also" instruction following a main term in the index instructs that there is another main term that may also be referenced that may provide additional index entries that may be useful. It is not necessary to follow the "see also" note when the original main term provides the necessary code.

B. General Coding Guidelines

1. **Use of Both Alphabetic Index and Tabular List**

   Use both the Alphabetic Index and the Tabular List when locating and assigning a code. Reliance on only the Alphabetic Index or the Tabular List leads to errors in code assignments and less specificity in code selection.

2. **Locate each term in the Alphabetic Index**

   Locate each term in the Alphabetic Index and verify the code selected in the Tabular List. Read and be guided by instructional notations that appear in both the Alphabetic Index and the Tabular List.

3. **Level of Detail in Coding**

   Diagnosis and procedure codes are to be used at their highest number of digits available.

   ICD-9-CM diagnosis codes are composed of codes with either 3, 4, or 5 digits. Codes with three digits are included in ICD-9-CM as the heading of a category of codes that may be further subdivided by the use of fourth and/or fifth digits, which provide greater detail.

   A three-digit code is to be used only if it is not further subdivided. Where fourth-digit subcategories and/or fifth-digit subclassifications are provided, they must be assigned. A code is invalid if it has not been coded to the full number of digits required for that code. For example, Acute myocardial infarction, code 410, has fourth digits that describe the location of the infarction (e.g., 410.2, Of inferolateral wall), and fifth digits that identify the episode of care. It would be incorrect to report a code in category 410 without a fourth and fifth digit.

ICD-9-CM Volume 3 procedure codes are composed of codes with either 3 or 4 digits. Codes with two digits are included in ICD-9-CM as the heading of a category of codes that may be further subdivided by the use of third and/or fourth digits, which provide greater detail.

4. Code or codes from 001.0 through V84.8

The appropriate code or codes from 001.0 through V84.8 must be used to identify diagnoses, symptoms, conditions, problems, complaints or other reason(s) for the encounter/visit.

5. Selection of codes 001.0 through 999.9

The selection of codes 001.0 through 999.9 will frequently be used to describe the reason for the admission/encounter. These codes are from the section of ICD-9-CM for the classification of diseases and injuries (e.g., infectious and parasitic diseases; neoplasms; symptoms, signs, and ill-defined conditions, etc.).

6. Signs and symptoms

Codes that describe symptoms and signs, as opposed to diagnoses, are acceptable for reporting purposes when a related definitive diagnosis has not been established (confirmed) by the provider. Chapter 16 of ICD-9-CM, Symptoms, Signs, and Ill-defined conditions (codes 780.0 - 799.9) contain many, but not all codes for symptoms.

7. Conditions that are an integral part of a disease process

Signs and symptoms that are integral to the disease process should not be assigned as additional codes.

8. Conditions that are not an integral part of a disease process

Additional signs and symptoms that may not be associated routinely with a disease process should be coded when present.

9. Multiple coding for a single condition

In addition to the etiology/manifestation convention that requires two codes to fully describe a single condition that affects multiple body systems, there are other single conditions that also require more than one code. "Use additional code" notes are found in the tabular at codes that are not part of an etiology/manifestation pair where a secondary code is useful to fully describe a condition. The sequencing rule is the same as the etiology/manifestation pair - , "use additional code" indicates that a secondary code should be added.

For example, for infections that are not included in chapter 1, a secondary code from category 041, Bacterial infection in conditions classified elsewhere and of unspecified site, may be required to identify the bacterial organism causing the infection. A "use additional code" note will normally be found at the infectious disease code, indicating a need for the organism code to be added as a secondary code.

"Code first" notes are also under certain codes that are not specifically manifestation codes but may be due to an underlying cause. When a "code first" note is present and an underlying condition is present the underlying condition should be sequenced first.

"Code, if applicable, any causal condition first", notes indicate that this code may be assigned as a principal diagnosis when the causal condition is unknown or not applicable. If a causal condition is known, then the code for that condition should be sequenced as the principal or first-listed diagnosis.

Multiple codes may be needed for late effects, complication codes and obstetric codes to more fully describe a condition. See the specific guidelines for these conditions for further instruction.

10.   Acute and Chronic Conditions

If the same condition is described as both acute (subacute) and chronic, and separate subentries exist in the Alphabetic Index at the same indentation level, code both and sequence the acute (subacute) code first.

11.   Combination Code

A combination code is a single code used to classify:
Two diagnoses, or
A diagnosis with an associated secondary process (manifestation)
A diagnosis with an associated complication

Combination codes are identified by referring to subterm entries in the Alphabetic Index and by reading the inclusion and exclusion notes in the Tabular List.

Assign only the combination code when that code fully identifies the diagnostic conditions involved or when the Alphabetic Index so directs. Multiple coding should not be used when the classification provides a combination code that clearly identifies all of the elements documented in the diagnosis. When the combination code lacks necessary specificity in describing the manifestation or complication, an additional code should be used as a secondary code.

12.   Late Effects

A late effect is the residual effect (condition produced) after the acute phase of an illness or injury has terminated. There is no time limit on when a late effect code can be used. The residual may be apparent early, such as in cerebrovascular accident cases, or it may occur months or years later, such as that due to a previous injury. Coding of late effects generally requires two codes sequenced in the following order: The condition or nature of the late effect is sequenced first. The late effect code is sequenced second.

An exception to the above guidelines are those instances where the code for late effect is followed by a manifestation code identified in the Tabular List and title, or the late effect code has been expanded (at the fourth and fifth-digit levels) to include the manifestation(s). The code for the acute phase of an illness or injury that led to the late effect is never used with a code for the late effect.

13.   Impending or Threatened Condition

Code any condition described at the time of discharge as "impending" or "threatened" as follows:

    If it did occur, code as confirmed diagnosis.

    If it did not occur, reference the Alphabetic Index to determine if the condition has a subentry term for "impending" or "threatened" and also reference main term entries for "Impending" and for "Threatened."

    If the subterms are listed, assign the given code.

    If the subterms are not listed, code the existing underlying condition(s) and not the condition described as impending or threatened.

C. Chapter-Specific Coding Guidelines

In addition to general coding guidelines, there are guidelines for specific diagnoses and/or conditions in the classification. Unless otherwise indicated, these guidelines apply to all health care settings. Please refer to Section II for guidelines on the selection of principal diagnosis.

1.   Chapter 1: Infectious and Parasitic Diseases (001-139)

a.   Human Immunodeficiency Virus (HIV) Infections

1)   Code only confirmed cases

Code only confirmed cases of HIV infection/illness. This is an exception to the hospital inpatient guideline Section II, H.

In this context, "confirmation" does not require documentation of positive serology or culture for HIV; the provider's diagnostic statement that the patient is HIV positive, or has an HIV-related illness is sufficient.

2)   Selection and sequencing of HIV codes

(a)   Patient admitted for HIV-related condition

If a patient is admitted for an HIV-related condition, the principal diagnosis should be 042, followed by additional diagnosis codes for all reported HIV-related conditions.

(b)   **Patient with HIV disease admitted for unrelated condition**

If a patient with HIV disease is admitted for an unrelated condition (such as a traumatic injury), the code for the unrelated condition (e.g., the nature of injury code) should be the principal diagnosis. Other diagnoses would be 042 followed by additional diagnosis codes for all reported HIV-related conditions.

(c)   **Whether the patient is newly diagnosed**

Whether the patient is newly diagnosed or has had previous admissions/encounters for HIV conditions is irrelevant to the sequencing decision.

(d)   **Asymptomatic human immunodeficiency virus**

V08 Asymptomatic human immunodeficiency virus [HIV] infection, is to be applied when the patient without any documentation of symptoms is listed as being "HIV positive," "known HIV," "HIV test positive," or similar terminology. Do not use this code if the term "AIDS" is used or if the patient is treated for any HIV-related illness or is described as having any condition(s) resulting from his/her HIV positive status; use 042 in these cases.

(e)   **Patients with inconclusive HIV serology**

Patients with inconclusive HIV serology, but no definitive diagnosis or manifestations of the illness, may be assigned code 795.71, Inconclusive serologic test for Human Immunodeficiency Virus [HIV].

(f)   **Previously diagnosed HIV-related illness**

Patients with any known prior diagnosis of an HIV-related illness should be coded to 042. Once a patient has developed an HIV-related illness, the patient should always be assigned code 042 on every subsequent admission/encounter. Patients previously diagnosed with any HIV illness (042) should never be assigned to 795.71 or V08.

(g) HIV Infection in Pregnancy, Childbirth and the Puerperium

During pregnancy, childbirth or the puerperium, a patient admitted (or presenting for a health care encounter) because of an HIV-related illness should receive a principal diagnosis code of 647.6X, Other specified infectious and parasitic diseases in the mother classifiable elsewhere, but complicating the pregnancy, childbirth or the puerperium, followed by 042 and the code(s) for the HIV-related illness(es). Codes from Chapter 15 always take sequencing priority.

Patients with asymptomatic HIV infection status admitted (or presenting for a health care encounter) during pregnancy, childbirth, or the puerperium should receive codes of 647.6X and V08.

(h) Encounters for testing for HIV

If a patient is being seen to determine his/her HIV status, use code V73.89, Screening for other specified viral disease. Use code V69.8, Other problems related to lifestyle, as a secondary code if an asymptomatic patient is in a known high risk group for HIV. Should a patient with signs or symptoms or illness, or a confirmed HIV related diagnosis be tested for HIV, code the signs and symptoms or the diagnosis. An additional counseling code V65.44 may be used if counseling is provided during the encounter for the test.

When a patient returns to be informed of his/her HIV test results use code V65.44, HIV counseling, if the results of the test are negative.

If the results are positive but the patient is asymptomatic use code V08, Asymptomatic HIV infection. If the results are positive and the patient is symptomatic use code 042, HIV infection, with codes for the HIV related symptoms or diagnosis. The HIV counseling code may also be used if counseling is provided for patients with positive test results.

b. Septicemia, Systemic Inflammatory Response Syndrome (SIRS), Sepsis, Severe Sepsis, and Septic Shock

1) Sepsis as principal diagnosis or secondary diagnosis

(a) Sepsis as principal diagnosis

If sepsis is present on admission, and meets the definition of principal diagnosis, the underlying systemic infection code (e.g., 038.xx, 112.5, etc) should be assigned as the principal diagnosis, followed by code 995.91, Systemic inflammatory response syndrome due to infectious process without organ dysfunction, as required by the sequencing rules in the Tabular List. Codes from subcategory 995.9 can never be assigned as a principal diagnosis.

(b) Sepsis as secondary diagnoses

When sepsis develops during the encounter (it was not present on admission), the sepsis codes may be assigned as secondary diagnoses, following the sequencing rules provided in the Tabular List.

(c) Documentation unclear as to whether sepsis present on admission

If the documentation is not clear whether the sepsis was present on admission, the provider should be queried. After provider query, if sepsis is determined at that point to have met the definition of principal diagnosis, the underlying systemic infection (038.xx, 112.5, etc) may be used as principal diagnosis along with code 995.91, Systemic inflammatory response syndrome due to infectious process without organ dysfunction.

2) **Septicemia/Sepsis**

In most cases, it will be a code from category 038, Septicemia, that will be used in conjunction with a code from subcategory 995.9 such as the following:

(a) **Streptococcal sepsis**

If the documentation in the record states streptococcal sepsis, codes 038.0 and code 995.91 should be used, in that sequence.

(b) **Streptococcal septicemia**

If the documentation states streptococcal septicemia, only code 038.0 should be assigned, however, the provider should be queried whether the patient has sepsis, an infection with SIRS.

(c)   **Sepsis or SIRS must be documented**

Either the term sepsis or SIRS must be documented, to assign a code from subcategory 995.9.

3)   **Terms sepsis, severe sepsis, or SIRS**

If the terms sepsis, severe sepsis, or SIRS are used with an underlying infection other than septicemia, such as pneumonia, cellulitis or a nonspecified urinary tract infection, a code from category 038 should be assigned first, then code 995.91, followed by the code for the initial infection. The use of the terms sepsis or SIRS indicates that the patient's infection has advanced to the point of a systemic infection so the systemic infection should be sequenced before the localized infection. The instructional note under subcategory 995.9 instructs to assign the underlying systemic infection first.

Note: The term urosepsis is a nonspecific term. If that is the only term documented then only code 599.0 should be assigned based on the default for the term in the ICD-9-CM index, in addition to the code for the causal organism if known.

4)   **Severe sepsis**

For patients with severe sepsis, the code for the systemic infection (e.g., 038.xx, 112.5, etc) or trauma should be sequenced first, followed by either code 995.92, Systemic inflammatory response syndrome due to infectious process with organ dysfunction, or code 995.94, Systemic inflammatory response syndrome due to noninfectious process with organ dysfunction. Codes for the specific organ dysfunctions should also be assigned.

5)   **Septic shock**

(a)   **Sequencing of septic shock**

Septic shock is a form of organ dysfunction associated with severe sepsis. A code for the initiating underlying systemic infection followed by a code for SIRS (code 995.92) must be assigned before the code for septic shock. As noted in the sequencing instructions in the Tabular List, the code for septic shock cannot be assigned as a principal diagnosis.

(b)   **Septic Shock without documentation of severe sepsis**

Septic shock cannot occur in the absence of severe sepsis. A code from subcategory 995.9 must be sequenced before the code for septic shock. The use additional code notes and the code first note provide sequencing instructions.

6) **Sepsis and septic shock associated with abortion**

Sepsis and septic shock associated with abortion, ectopic pregnancy, and molar pregnancy are classified to category codes in Chapter 11 (630-639).

7) **Negative or inconclusive blood cultures**

Negative or inconclusive blood cultures do not preclude a diagnosis of septicemia or sepsis in patients with clinical evidence of the condition, however, the provider should be queried.

8) **Newborn sepsis**

See Section I.C.15.j for information on the coding of newborn sepsis.

9) **Sepsis due to a Postprocedural Infection**

Sepsis resulting from a postprocedural infection is a complication of care. For such cases code 998.59, Other postoperative infections, should be coded first followed by the appropriate codes for the sepsis. The other guidelines for coding sepsis should then be followed for the assignment of additional codes.

10) **External cause of injury codes with SIRS**

An external cause code is not needed with codes 995.91, Systemic inflammatory response syndrome due to infectious process without organ dysfunction, or code 995.92, Systemic inflammatory response syndrome due to infectious process with organ dysfunction.

Refer to Section I.C.19.a.7 for instruction on the use of external cause of injury codes with codes for SIRS resulting from trauma.

2. Chapter 2: Neoplasms (140-239)

General guidelines

Chapter 2 of the ICD-9-CM contains the codes for most benign and all malignant neoplasms. Certain benign neoplasms, such as prostatic adenomas, may be found in the specific body system chapters. To properly code a neoplasm it is necessary to determine from the record if the neoplasm is benign, in-situ, malignant, or of uncertain histologic behavior. If malignant, any secondary (metastatic) sites should also be determined.

The neoplasm table in the Alphabetic Index should be referenced first. However, if the histological term is documented, that term should be referenced first, rather than going immediately to the Neoplasm Table, in order to determine which column in the Neoplasm Table is appropriate. For example, if the documentation indicates "adenoma," refer to the term in the Alphabetic Index to review the entries under this term and the instructional note to "see also neoplasm, by site, benign." The table provides the proper code based on the type of neoplasm and the site. It is important to select the proper column in the table that corresponds to the type of neoplasm. The tabular should then be referenced to verify that the correct code has been selected from the table and that a more specific site code does not exist.

See Section I. C. 18.d.4. for information regarding V codes for genetic susceptibility to cancer.

a. **Treatment directed at the malignancy**

If the treatment is directed at the malignancy, designate the malignancy as the principal diagnosis.

b. **Treatment of secondary site**

When a patient is admitted because of a primary neoplasm with metastasis and treatment is directed toward the secondary site only, the secondary neoplasm is designated as the principal diagnosis even though the primary malignancy is still present.

c. **Coding and sequencing of complications**

Coding and sequencing of complications associated with the malignancies or with the therapy thereof are subject to the following guidelines:

1) **Anemia associated with malignancy**

When admission/encounter is for management of an anemia associated with the malignancy, and the treatment is only for anemia, the anemia is designated at the principal diagnosis and is followed by the appropriate code(s) for the malignancy.

2) **Anemia associated with chemotherapy**

When the admission/encounter is for management of an anemia associated with chemotherapy or radiotherapy and the only treatment is for the anemia, the anemia is sequenced first followed by the appropriate code(s) for the malignancy.

3) **Management of dehydration due to the malignancy**

When the admission/encounter is for management of dehydration due to the malignancy or the therapy, or a combination of both, and only the dehydration is being treated (intravenous rehydration), the dehydration is sequenced first, followed by the code(s) for the malignancy.

4) **Treatment of a complication resulting from a surgical procedure**

When the admission/encounter is for treatment of a complication resulting from a surgical procedure, designate the complication as the principal or first-listed diagnosis if treatment is directed at resolving the complication.

d. **Primary malignancy previously excised**

When a primary malignancy has been previously excised or eradicated from its site and there is no further treatment directed to that site and there is no evidence of any existing primary malignancy, a code from category V10, Personal history of malignant neoplasm, should be used to indicate the former site of the malignancy. Any mention of extension, invasion, or metastasis to another site is coded as a secondary malignant neoplasm to that site. The secondary site may be the principal or first-listed with the V10 code used as a secondary code.

e. **Admissions/Encounters involving chemotherapy and radiation therapy**

1) **Episode of care involves surgical removal of neoplasm**

When an episode of care involves the surgical removal of a neoplasm, primary or secondary site, followed by adjunct chemotherapy or radiation treatment, the neoplasm code should be assigned as principal or first-listed diagnosis, using codes in the 140-198 series or where appropriate in the 200-203 series.

2) **Patient admission/encounter solely for administration of chemotherapy**

If a patient admission/encounter is solely for the administration of chemotherapy or radiation therapy code V58.0, Encounter for radiation therapy, or V58.1, Encounter for chemotherapy, should be the first-listed or principal diagnosis. If a patient receives both chemotherapy and radiation therapy both codes should be listed, in either order of sequence.

3) Patient admitted for radiotherapy/chemotherapy and develops complications

When a patient is admitted for the purpose of radiotherapy or chemotherapy and develops complications such as uncontrolled nausea and vomiting or dehydration, the principal or first-listed diagnosis is V58.0, Encounter for radiotherapy, or V58.1, Encounter for chemotherapy, followed by any codes for the complications.

See Section I.C.18.d.8. for additional information regarding aftercare V codes.

f. Admission/encounter to determine extent of malignancy

When the reason for admission/encounter is to determine the extent of the malignancy, or for a procedure such as paracentesis or thoracentesis, the primary malignancy or appropriate metastatic site is designated as the principal or first-listed diagnosis, even though chemotherapy or radiotherapy is administered.

g. Symptoms, signs, and ill-defined conditions listed in Chapter 16

Symptoms, signs, and ill-defined conditions listed in Chapter 16 characteristic of, or associated with, an existing primary or secondary site malignancy cannot be used to replace the malignancy as principal or first-listed diagnosis, regardless of the number of admissions or encounters for treatment and care of the neoplasm.

h. Encounter for prophylactic organ removal

For encounters specifically for prophylactic removal of breasts, ovaries, or another organ due to a genetic susceptibility to cancer or a family history of cancer, the principal or first listed code should be a code from subcategory V50.4, Prophylactic organ removal, followed by the appropriate genetic susceptibility code and the appropriate family history code.

If the patient has a malignancy of one site and is having prophylactic removal of another site to prevent either a new primary malignancy or metastatic disease, a code for the malignancy should also be assigned in addition to a code from subcategory V50.4. A V50.4 code should not be assigned if the patient is having organ removal for treatment of a malignancy, such as the removal of the testes for the treatment of prostate cancer.

3. Chapter 3: Endocrine, Nutritional, and Metabolic Diseases and Immunity Disorders (240-279)

a. Diabetes mellitus

Codes under category 250, Diabetes mellitus, identify complications/manifestations associated with diabetes mellitus. A fifth-digit is required for all category 250 codes to identify the type of diabetes mellitus and whether the diabetes is controlled or uncontrolled.

1) Fifth-digits for category 250:

The following are the fifth-digits for the codes under category 250:

0   type II or unspecified type, not stated as uncontrolled
1   type I, [juvenile type], not stated as uncontrolled
2   type II or unspecified type, uncontrolled
3   type I, [juvenile type], uncontrolled

The age of a patient is not the sole determining factor, though most type I diabetics develop the condition before reaching puberty. For this reason type I diabetes mellitus is also referred to as juvenile diabetes.

2) Type of diabetes mellitus not documented

If the type of diabetes mellitus is not documented in the medical record the default is type II.

3) Diabetes mellitus and the use of insulin

All type I diabetics must use insulin to replace what their bodies do not produce. However, the use of insulin does not mean that a patient is a type I diabetic. Some patients with type II diabetes mellitus are unable to control their blood sugar through diet and oral medication alone and do require insulin. If the documentation in a medical record does not indicate the type of diabetes but does indicate that the patient uses insulin, the appropriate fifth-digit for type II must be used. For type II patients who routinely use insulin, code V58.67, Long-term (current) use of insulin, should also be assigned to indicate that the patient uses insulin. Code V58.67 should not be assigned if insulin is given temporarily to bring a type II patient's blood sugar under control during an encounter.

4) **Assigning and sequencing diabetes codes and associated conditions**

When assigning codes for diabetes and its associated conditions, the code(s) from category 250 must be sequenced before the codes for the associated conditions. The diabetes codes and the secondary codes that correspond to them are paired codes that follow the etiology/manifestation convention of the classification (See Section I.A.6., Etiology/manifestation convention). Assign as many codes from category 250 as needed to identify all of the associated conditions that the patient has. The corresponding secondary codes are listed under each of the diabetes codes.

5) **Diabetes mellitus in pregnancy and gestational diabetes**

(a) For diabetes mellitus complicating pregnancy, see Section I.C.11.f., Diabetes mellitus in pregnancy.

(b) For gestational diabetes, see Section I.C.11, g., Gestational diabetes.

6) **Insulin pump malfunction**

(a) **Underdose of insulin due insulin pump failure**

An underdose of insulin due to an insulin pump failure should be assigned 996.57, Mechanical complication due to insulin pump, as the principal or first listed code, followed by the appropriate diabetes mellitus code based on documentation.

(b) **Overdose of insulin due to insulin pump failure**

The principal or first listed code for an encounter due to an insulin pump malfunction resulting in an overdose of insulin, should also be 996.57, Mechanical complication due to insulin pump, followed by code 962.3, Poisoning by insulins and antidiabetic agents, and the appropriate diabetes mellitus code based on documentation.

4. **Chapter 4: Diseases of Blood and Blood Forming Organs (280-289)**

Reserved for future guideline expansion

5. **Chapter 5: Mental Disorders (290-319)**

Reserved for future guideline expansion

6. **Chapter 6: Diseases of Nervous System and Sense Organs (320-389)**

Reserved for future guideline expansion

7. **Chapter 7: Diseases of Circulatory System (390-459)**

   a. **Hypertension**

   Hypertension Table

   The Hypertension Table, found under the main term, "Hypertension", in the Alphabetic Index, contains a complete listing of all conditions due to or associated with hypertension and classifies them according to malignant, benign, and unspecified.

   1) **Hypertension, Essential, or NOS**

      Assign hypertension (arterial) (essential) (primary) (systemic) (NOS) to category code 401 with the appropriate fourth digit to indicate malignant (.0), benign (.1), or unspecified (.9). Do not use either .0 malignant or .1 benign unless medical record documentation supports such a designation.

   2) **Hypertension with Heart Disease**

      Heart conditions (425.8, 429.0-429.3, 429.8, 429.9) are assigned to a code from category 402 when a causal relationship is stated (due to hypertension) or implied (hypertensive). Use an additional code from category 428 to identify the type of heart failure in those patients with heart failure. More than one code from category 428 may be assigned if the patient has systolic or diastolic failure and congestive heart failure.

      The same heart conditions (425.8, 429.0-429.3, 429.8, 429.9) with hypertension, but without a stated casual relationship, are coded separately. Sequence according to the circumstances of the admission/encounter.

3)   Hypertensive Renal Disease with Chronic Renal Failure

Assign codes from category 403, Hypertensive renal disease, when conditions classified to categories 585-587 are present. Unlike hypertension with heart disease, ICD-9-CM presumes a cause-and-effect relationship and classifies renal failure with hypertension as hypertensive renal disease.

4)   Hypertensive Heart and Renal Disease

Assign codes from combination category 404, Hypertensive heart and renal disease, when both hypertensive renal disease and hypertensive heart disease are stated in the diagnosis. Assume a relationship between the hypertension and the renal disease, whether or not the condition is so designated. Assign an additional code from category 428, to identify the type of heart failure. More than one code from category 428 may be assigned if the patient has systolic or diastolic failure and congestive heart failure.

5)   Hypertensive Cerebrovascular Disease

First assign codes from 430-438, Cerebrovascular disease, then the appropriate hypertension code from categories 401-405.

6)   Hypertensive Retinopathy

Two codes are necessary to identify the condition. First assign the code from subcategory 362.11, Hypertensive retinopathy, then the appropriate code from categories 401-405 to indicate the type of hypertension.

7)   Hypertension, Secondary

Two codes are required: one to identify the underlying etiology and one from category 405 to identify the hypertension. Sequencing of codes is determined by the reason for admission/encounter.

8)   Hypertension, Transient

Assign code 796.2, Elevated blood pressure reading without diagnosis of hypertension, unless patient has an established diagnosis of hypertension. Assign code 642.3x for transient hypertension of pregnancy.

9)   Hypertension, Controlled

Assign appropriate code from categories 401-405. This diagnostic statement usually refers to an existing state of hypertension under control by therapy.

10) Hypertension, Uncontrolled

Uncontrolled hypertension may refer to untreated hypertension or hypertension not responding to current therapeutic regimen. In either case, assign the appropriate code from categories 401-405 to designate the stage and type of hypertension. Code to the type of hypertension.

11) Elevated Blood Pressure

For a statement of elevated blood pressure without further specificity, assign code 796.2, Elevated blood pressure reading without diagnosis of hypertension, rather than a code from category 401.

b. Cerebral infarction/stroke/cerebrovascular accident (CVA)

The terms stroke and CVA are often used interchangeably to refer to a cerebral infarction. The terms stroke, CVA, and cerebral infarction NOS are all indexed to the default code 434.91, Cerebral artery occlusion, unspecified, with infarction. Code 436, Acute, but ill-defined, cerebrovascular disease, should not be used when the documentation states stroke or CVA.

c. Postoperative cerebrovascular accident

A cerebrovascular hemorrhage or infarction that occurs as a result of medical intervention is coded to 997.02, Iatrogenic cerebrovascular infarction or hemorrhage. Medical record documentation should clearly specify the cause- and-effect relationship between the medical intervention and the cerebrovascular accident in order to assign this code. A secondary code from the code range 430-432 or from a code from subcategories 433 or 434 with a fifth digit of "1" should also be used to identify the type of hemorrhage or infarct.

This guideline conforms to the use additional code note instruction at category 997. Code 436, Acute, but ill-defined, cerebrovascular disease, should not be used as a secondary code with code 997.02.

d. Late Effects of Cerebrovascular Disease

1) Category 438, Late Effects of Cerebrovascular disease

Category 438 is used to indicate conditions classifiable to categories 430-437 as the causes of late effects (neurologic deficits), themselves classified elsewhere. These "late effects" include neurologic deficits that persist after initial onset of conditions classifiable to 430-437. The neurologic deficits caused by cerebrovascular disease may be present from the onset or may arise at any time after the onset of the condition classifiable to 430-437.

2) **Codes from category 438 with codes from 430-437**

Codes from category 438 may be assigned on a health care record with codes from 430-437, if the patient has a current cerebrovascular accident (CVA) and deficits from an old CVA.

3) **Code V12.59**

Assign code V12.59 (and not a code from category 438) as an additional code for history of cerebrovascular disease when no neurologic deficits are present.

Chapter 8: Diseases of Respiratory System (460-519)

a. **Chronic Obstructive Pulmonary Disease [COPD] and Asthma**

1) **Conditions that comprise COPD and Asthma**

The conditions that comprise COPD are obstructive chronic bronchitis, subcategory 491.2, and emphysema, category 492. All asthma codes are under category 493, Asthma. Code 496, Chronic airway obstruction, not elsewhere classified, is a nonspecific code that should only be used when the documentation in a medical record does not specify the type of COPD being treated.

2) **Acute exacerbation of chronic obstructive bronchitis and asthma**

The codes for chronic obstructive bronchitis and asthma distinguish between uncomplicated cases and those in acute exacerbation. An acute exacerbation is a worsening or a decompensation of a chronic condition. An acute exacerbation is not equivalent to an infection superimposed on a chronic condition, though an exacerbation may be triggered by an infection.

3) **Overlapping nature of the conditions that comprise COPD and asthma**

Due to the overlapping nature of the conditions that make up COPD and asthma, there are many variations in the way these conditions are documented. Code selection must be based on the terms as documented. When selecting the correct code for the documented type of COPD and asthma, it is essential to first review the index, and then verify the code in the tabular list. There are many instructional notes under the different COPD subcategories and codes. It is important that all such notes be reviewed to assure correct code assignment.

4) Acute exacerbation of asthma and status asthmaticus

An acute exacerbation of asthma is an increased severity of the asthma symptoms, such as wheezing and shortness of breath. Status asthmaticus refers to a patient's failure to respond to therapy administered during an asthmatic episode and is a life threatening complication that requires emergency care. If status asthmaticus is documented by the provider with any type of COPD or with acute bronchitis, the status asthmaticus should be sequenced first. It supersedes any type of COPD including that with acute exacerbation or acute bronchitis. It is inappropriate to assign an asthma code with 5th digit 2, with acute exacerbation, together with an asthma code with 5th digit 1, with status asthmatics. Only the 5th digit 1 should be assigned.

b. Chronic Obstructive Pulmonary Disease [COPD] and Bronchitis

1) Acute bronchitis with COPD

Acute bronchitis, code 466.0, is due to an infectious organism. When acute bronchitis is documented with COPD, code 491.22, Obstructive chronic bronchitis with acute bronchitis, should be assigned. It is not necessary to also assign code 466.0. If a medical record documents acute bronchitis with COPD with acute exacerbation, only code 491.22 should be assigned. The acute bronchitis included in code 491.22 supersedes the acute exacerbation. If a medical record documents COPD with acute exacerbation without mention of acute bronchitis, only code 491.21 should be assigned.

9. Chapter 9: Diseases of Digestive System (520-579)

Reserved for future guideline expansion

10. Chapter 10: Diseases of Genitourinary System (580-629)

Reserved for future guideline expansion

11. Chapter 11: Complications of Pregnancy, Childbirth, and the Puerperium (630-677)

a. General Rules for Obstetric Cases

1) Codes from chapter 11 and sequencing priority

Obstetric cases require codes from chapter 11, codes in the range 630-677, Complications of Pregnancy, Childbirth, and the Puerperium. Chapter 11 codes have sequencing priority over codes from other chapters. Additional codes from other chapters may be used in conjunction with chapter 11 codes to further specify conditions. Should the provider document that the pregnancy is incidental to the encounter, then code V22.2 should be used in place of any chapter 11 codes. It is the provider's responsibility to state that the condition being treated is not affecting the pregnancy.

2) Chapter 11 codes used only on the maternal record

Chapter 11 codes are to be used only on the maternal record, never on the record of the newborn.

3) Chapter 11 fifth-digits

Categories 640-648, 651-676 have required fifth-digits, which indicate whether the encounter is antepartum, postpartum and whether a delivery has also occurred.

4) Fifth-digits, appropriate for each code

The fifth-digits, which are appropriate for each code number, are listed in brackets under each code. The fifth-digits on each code should all be consistent with each other. That is, should a delivery occur all of the fifth-digits should indicate the delivery.

b. Selection of OB Principal or First-listed Diagnosis

1) Routine outpatient prenatal visits

For routine outpatient prenatal visits when no complications are present codes V22.0, Supervision of normal first pregnancy, and V22.1, Supervision of other normal pregnancy, should be used as the first-listed diagnoses. These codes should not be used in conjunction with chapter 11 codes.

2) Prenatal outpatient visits for high-risk patients

For prenatal outpatient visits for patients with high-risk pregnancies, a code from category V23, Supervision of high-risk pregnancy, should be used as the principal or first-listed diagnosis. Secondary chapter 11 codes may be used in conjunction with these codes if appropriate.

3) Episodes when no delivery occurs

In episodes when no delivery occurs, the principal diagnosis should correspond to the principal complication of the pregnancy, which necessitated the encounter. Should more than one complication exist, all of which are treated or monitored, any of the complications codes may be sequenced first.

4) When a delivery occurs

When a delivery occurs, the principal diagnosis should correspond to the main circumstances or complication of the delivery. In cases of cesarean delivery, the selection of the principal diagnosis should correspond to the reason the cesarean delivery was performed unless the reason for admission/encounter was unrelated to the condition resulting in the cesarean delivery.

5) Outcome of delivery

An outcome of delivery code, V27.0-V27.9, should be included on every maternal record when a delivery has occurred. These codes are not to be used on subsequent records or on the newborn record.

c. Fetal Conditions Affecting the Management of the Mother

1) Codes from category 655

Known or suspected fetal abnormality affecting management of the mother, and category 656, Other fetal and placental problems affecting the management of the mother, are assigned only when the fetal condition is actually responsible for modifying the management of the mother, i.e., by requiring diagnostic studies, additional observation, special care, or termination of pregnancy. The fact that the fetal condition exists does not justify assigning a code from this series to the mother's record.

2)   **In utero surgery**

In cases when surgery is performed on the fetus, a diagnosis code from category 655, Known or suspected fetal abnormalities affecting management of the mother, should be assigned identifying the fetal condition. Procedure code 75.36, Correction of fetal defect, should be assigned on the hospital inpatient record.

No code from Chapter 15, the perinatal codes, should be used on the mother's record to identify fetal conditions. Surgery performed in utero on a fetus is still to be coded as an obstetric encounter.

d.   **HIV Infection in Pregnancy, Childbirth and the Puerperium**

During pregnancy, childbirth or the puerperium, a patient admitted because of an HIV-related illness should receive a principal diagnosis of 647.6X, Other specified infectious and parasitic diseases in the mother classifiable elsewhere, but complicating the pregnancy, childbirth or the puerperium, followed by 042 and the code(s) for the HIV-related illness(es).

Patients with asymptomatic HIV infection status admitted during pregnancy, childbirth, or the puerperium should receive codes of 647.6X and V08.

e.   **Current Conditions Complicating Pregnancy**

Assign a code from subcategory 648.x for patients that have current conditions when the condition affects the management of the pregnancy, childbirth, or the puerperium. Use additional secondary codes from other chapters to identify the conditions, as appropriate.

f.   **Diabetes mellitus in pregnancy**

Diabetes mellitus is a significant complicating factor in pregnancy. Pregnant women who are diabetic should be assigned code 648.0x, Diabetes mellitus complicating pregnancy, and a secondary code from category 250, Diabetes mellitus, to identify the type of diabetes.

Code V58.67, Long-term (current) use of insulin, should also be assigned if the diabetes mellitus is being treated with insulin.

g. **Gestational diabetes**

Gestational diabetes can occur during the second and third trimester of pregnancy in women who were not diabetic prior to pregnancy. Gestational diabetes can cause complications in the pregnancy similar to those of pre-existing diabetes mellitus. It also puts the woman at greater risk of developing diabetes after the pregnancy. Gestational diabetes is coded to 648.8x, Abnormal glucose tolerance. Codes 648.0x and 648.8x should never be used together on the same record.

Code V58.67, Long-term (current) use of insulin, should also be assigned if the gestational diabetes is being treated with insulin.

h. **Normal Delivery, Code 650**

1) **Normal delivery**

Code 650 is for use in cases when a woman is admitted for a full-term normal delivery and delivers a single, healthy infant without any complications antepartum, during the delivery, or postpartum during the delivery episode. **Code 650 is always a principal diagnosis. It is not to be used if any other code from chapter 11 is needed to describe a current complication of the antenatal, delivery, or perinatal period. Additional codes from other chapters may be used with code 650 if they are not related to or are in any way complicating the pregnancy.**

2) **Normal delivery with resolved antepartum complication**

Code 650 may be used if the patient had a complication at some point during her pregnancy, but the complication is not present at the time of the admission for delivery.

3) **V27.0, Single liveborn, outcome of delivery**

V27.0, Single liveborn, is the only outcome of delivery code appropriate for use with 650.

i. **The Postpartum and Peripartum Periods**

1) **Postpartum and peripartum periods**

The postpartum period begins immediately after delivery and continues for six weeks following delivery. The peripartum period is defined as the last month of pregnancy to five months postpartum.

2) Postpartum complication

A postpartum complication is any complication occurring within the six-week period.

3) Pregnancy-related complications after 6 week period

Chapter 11 codes may also be used to describe pregnancy-related complications after the six-week period should the provider document that a condition is pregnancy related.

4) Postpartum complications occurring during the same admission as delivery

Postpartum complications that occur during the same admission as the delivery are identified with a fifth digit of "2." Subsequent admissions/encounters for postpartum complications should be identified with a fifth digit of "4."

5) Admission for routine postpartum care following delivery outside hospital

When the mother delivers outside the hospital prior to admission and is admitted for routine postpartum care and no complications are noted, code V24.0, Postpartum care and examination immediately after delivery, should be assigned as the principal diagnosis.

6) Admission following delivery outside hospital with postpartum conditions

A delivery diagnosis code should not be used for a woman who has delivered prior to admission to the hospital. Any postpartum conditions and/or postpartum procedures should be coded.

j. Code 677, Late effect of complication of pregnancy

1) Code 677

Code 677, Late effect of complication of pregnancy, childbirth, and the puerperium is for use in those cases when an initial complication of a pregnancy develops a sequelae requiring care or treatment at a future date.

2)   After the initial postpartum period

This code may be used at any time after the initial postpartum period.

3)   Sequencing of Code 677

This code, like all late effect codes, is to be sequenced following the code describing the sequelae of the complication.

k.   Abortions

1)   Fifth-digits required for abortion categories

Fifth-digits are required for abortion categories 634-637. Fifth-digit 1, incomplete, indicates that all of the products of conception have not been expelled from the uterus. Fifth-digit 2, complete, indicates that all products of conception have been expelled from the uterus prior to the episode of care.

2)   Code from categories 640-648 and 651-659

A code from categories 640-648 and 651-659 may be used as additional codes with an abortion code to indicate the complication leading to the abortion.

Fifth digit 3 is assigned with codes from these categories when used with an abortion code because the other fifth digits will not apply. Codes from the 660-669 series are not to be used for complications of abortion.

3)   Code 639 for complications

Code 639 is to be used for all complications following abortion. Code 639 cannot be assigned with codes from categories 634-638.

4)   Abortion with Liveborn Fetus

When an attempted termination of pregnancy results in a liveborn fetus assign code 644.21, Early onset of delivery, with an appropriate code from category V27, Outcome of Delivery. The procedure code for the attempted termination of pregnancy should also be assigned.

5)   Retained Products of Conception following an abortion

Subsequent admissions for retained products of conception following a spontaneous or legally induced abortion are assigned the appropriate code from category 634, Spontaneous abortion, or 635 Legally induced abortion, with a fifth digit of "1" (incomplete). This advice is appropriate even when the patient was discharged previously with a discharge diagnosis of complete abortion.

12. Chapter 12: Diseases Skin and Subcutaneous Tissue (680-709)

Reserved for future guideline expansion

13. Chapter 13: Diseases of Musculoskeletal and Connective Tissue (710-739)

Reserved for future guideline expansion

14. Chapter 14: Congenital Anomalies (740-759)

a. Codes in categories 740-759, Congenital Anomalies

Assign an appropriate code(s) from categories 740-759, Congenital Anomalies, when an anomaly is documented. A congenital anomaly may be the principal/first listed diagnosis on a record or a secondary diagnosis. Use additional secondary codes from other chapters to specify conditions associated with the anomaly, if applicable. Codes from Chapter 14 may be used throughout the life of the patient. If a congenital anomaly has been corrected, a personal history code should be used to identify the history of the anomaly.

For the birth admission, the appropriate code from category V30, Liveborn infants, according to type of birth should be sequenced as the principal diagnosis, followed by any congenital anomaly codes, 740-759.

15. Chapter 15: Newborn (Perinatal) Guidelines (760-779)

For coding and reporting purposes the perinatal period is defined as birth through the 28th day following birth. The following guidelines are provided for reporting purposes. Hospitals may record other diagnoses as needed for internal data use.

a. General Perinatal Rules

1) Chapter 15 Codes

They are __never__ for use on the maternal record. Codes from Chapter 11, the obstetric chapter, are never permitted on the newborn record. Chapter 15 code may be used throughout the life of the patient if the condition is still present.

2)   **Sequencing of perinatal codes**

Generally, codes from Chapter 15 should be sequenced as the principal/first-listed diagnosis on the newborn record, with the exception of the appropriate V30 code for the birth episode, followed by codes from any other chapter that provide additional detail. The "use additional code" note at the beginning of the chapter supports this guideline. If the index does not provide a specific code for a perinatal condition, assign code 779.89, Other specified conditions originating in the perinatal period, followed by the code from another chapter that specifies the condition. Codes for signs and symptoms may be assigned when a definitive diagnosis has not been established.

3)   **Birth process or community acquired conditions**

If a newborn has a condition that may be either due to the birth process or community acquired and the documentation does not indicate which it is, the default is due to the birth process and the code from Chapter 15 should be used. If the condition is community-acquired, a code from Chapter 15 should not be assigned.

4)   **Code all clinically significant conditions**

All clinically significant conditions noted on routine newborn examination should be coded. A condition is clinically significant if it requires:
- clinical evaluation; or
- therapeutic treatment; or
- diagnostic procedures; or
- extended length of hospital stay; or
- increased nursing care and/or monitoring; or
- has implications for future health care needs

Note: The perinatal guidelines listed above are the same as the general coding guidelines for "additional diagnoses", except for the final point regarding implications for future health care needs. **Codes should be assigned for conditions that have been specified by the provider as having implications for future health care needs. Codes from the perinatal chapter should not be assigned unless the provider has established a definitive diagnosis.**

b.   Use of codes V30-V39

When coding the birth of an infant, assign a code from categories V30-V39, according to the type of birth. A code from this series is assigned as a principal diagnosis, and assigned only once to a newborn at the time of birth.

c.   Newborn transfers

If the newborn is transferred to another institution, the V30 series is not used at the receiving hospital.

d.   Use of category V29

1)   Assigning a code from category V29

Assign a code from category V29, Observation and evaluation of newborns and infants for suspected conditions not found, to identify those instances when a healthy newborn is evaluated for a suspected condition that is determined after study not to be present. Do not use a code from category V29 when the patient has identified signs or symptoms of a suspected problem; in such cases, code the sign or symptom.

A code from category V29 may also be assigned as a principal code for readmissions or encounters when the V30 code no longer applies. Codes from category V29 are for use only for healthy newborns and infants for which no condition after study is found to be present.

2)   V29 code on a birth record

A V29 code is to be used as a secondary code after the V30, Outcome of delivery, code.

e.   Use of other V codes on perinatal records

V codes other than V30 and V29 may be assigned on a perinatal or newborn record code. The codes may be used as a principal or first-listed diagnosis for specific types of encounters or for readmissions or encounters when the V30 code no longer applies.

See Section I.C.18 for information regarding the assignment of V codes.

f.   Maternal Causes of Perinatal Morbidity

Codes from categories 760-763, Maternal causes of perinatal morbidity and mortality, are assigned only when the maternal condition has actually affected the fetus or newborn. The fact that the mother has an associated medical condition or experiences some complication of pregnancy, labor or delivery does not justify the routine assignment of codes from these categories to the newborn record.

g. **Congenital Anomalies in Newborns**

For the birth admission, the appropriate code from category V30, Liveborn infants according to type of birth, should be used, followed by any congenital anomaly codes, categories 740-759. **Use additional secondary codes from other chapters to specify conditions associated with the anomaly, if applicable.**

Also, see Section I.C.14 for information on the coding of congenital anomalies.

h. **Coding Additional Perinatal Diagnoses**

1) **Assigning codes for conditions that require treatment**

Assign codes for conditions that require treatment or further investigation, prolong the length of stay, or require resource utilization.

2) **Codes for conditions specified as having implications for future health care needs**

Assign codes for conditions that have been specified by the provider as having implications for future health care needs.

Note: This guideline should not be used for adult patients.

3) **Codes for newborn conditions originating in the perinatal period**

Assign a code for newborn conditions originating in the perinatal period (categories 760-779), as well as complications arising during the current episode of care classified in other chapters, only if the diagnoses have been documented by the responsible provider at the time of transfer or discharge as having affected the fetus or newborn.

i. **Prematurity and Fetal Growth Retardation**

Providers utilize different criteria in determining prematurity. A code for prematurity should not be assigned unless it is documented. The 5th digit assignment for codes from category 764 and subcategories 765.0 and 765.1 should be based on the recorded birth weight and estimated gestational age.

A code from subcategory 765.2, Weeks of gestation, should be assigned as an additional code with category 764 and codes from 765.0 and 765.1 to specify weeks of gestation as documented by the provider in the record.

j. Newborn sepsis

Code 771.81, Septicemia [sepsis] of newborn, should be assigned with a secondary code from category 041, Bacterial infections in conditions classified elsewhere and of unspecified site, to identify the organism. It is not necessary to use a code from subcategory 995.9, Systemic inflammatory response syndrome (SIRS), on a newborn record. A code from category 038, Septicemia, should not be used on a newborn record. Code 771.81 describes the sepsis.

16. Chapter 16: Signs, Symptoms and Ill-Defined Conditions (780-799)

Reserved for future guideline expansion

17. Chapter 17: Injury and Poisoning (800-999)

a. Coding of Injuries

When coding injuries, assign separate codes for each injury unless a combination code is provided, in which case the combination code is assigned. Multiple injury codes are provided in ICD-9-CM, but should not be assigned unless information for a more specific code is not available. These codes are not to be used for normal, healing surgical wounds or to identify complications of surgical wounds.

The code for the most serious injury, as determined by the provider and the focus of treatment, is sequenced first.

1) Superficial injuries

Superficial injuries such as abrasions or contusions are not coded when associated with more severe injuries of the same site.

2) Primary injury with damage to nerves/blood vessels

When a primary injury results in minor damage to peripheral nerves or blood vessels, the primary injury is sequenced first with additional code(s) from categories 950-957, Injury to nerves and spinal cord, and/or 900-904, Injury to blood vessels. When the primary injury is to the blood vessels or nerves, that injury should be sequenced first.

b. **Coding of Fractures**

The principles of multiple coding of injuries should be followed in coding fractures. Fractures of specified sites are coded individually by site in accordance with both the provisions within categories 800-829 and the level of detail furnished by medical record content. Combination categories for multiple fractures are provided for use when there is insufficient detail in the medical record (such as trauma cases transferred to another hospital), when the reporting form limits the number of codes that can be used in reporting pertinent clinical data, or when there is insufficient specificity at the fourth-digit or fifth-digit level. More specific guidelines are as follows:

1) **Multiple fractures of same limb**

Multiple fractures of same limb classifiable to the same three-digit or four-digit category are coded to that category.

2) **Multiple unilateral or bilateral fractures of same bone**

Multiple unilateral or bilateral fractures of same bone(s) but classified to different fourth-digit subdivisions (bone part) within the same three-digit category are coded individually by site.

3) **Multiple fracture categories 819 and 828**

Multiple fracture categories 819 and 828 classify bilateral fractures of both upper limbs (819) and both lower limbs (828), but without any detail at the fourth-digit level other than open and closed type of fractures.

4) **Multiple fractures sequencing**

Multiple fractures are sequenced in accordance with the severity of the fracture. The provider should be asked to list the fracture diagnoses in the order of severity.

c. **Coding of Burns**

Current burns (940-948) are classified by depth, extent and by agent (E code). Burns are classified by depth as first degree (erythema), second degree (blistering), and third degree (full-thickness involvement).

1) **Sequencing of burn codes**

Sequence first the code that reflects the highest degree of burn when more than one burn is present.

2) **Burns of the same local site**

Classify burns of the same local site (three-digit category level, 940-947) but of different degrees to the subcategory identifying the highest degree recorded in the diagnosis.

3) Non-healing burns

Non-healing burns are coded as acute burns.
Necrosis of burned skin should be coded as a non-healed burn.

4) Code 958.3, Posttraumatic wound infection

Assign code 958.3, Posttraumatic wound infection, not elsewhere classified, as an additional code for any documented infected burn site.

5) Assign separate codes for each burn site

When coding burns, assign separate codes for each burn site. Category 946 Burns of Multiple specified sites, should only be used if the location of the burns are not documented. Category 949, Burn, unspecified, is extremely vague and should rarely be used.

6) Assign codes from category 948, Burns

Burns classified according to extent of body surface involved, when the site of the burn is not specified or when there is a need for additional data. It is advisable to use category 948 as additional coding when needed to provide data for evaluating burn mortality, such as that needed by burn units. It is also advisable to use category 948 as an additional code for reporting purposes when there is mention of a third-degree burn involving 20 percent or more of the body surface.

In assigning a code from category 948:

> Fourth-digit codes are used to identify the percentage of total body surface involved in a burn (all degree).

> Fifth-digits are assigned to identify the percentage of body surface involved in third-degree burn.

> Fifth-digit zero (0) is assigned when less than 10 percent or when no body surface is involved in a third-degree burn.

> Category 948 is based on the classic "rule of nines" in estimating body surface involved: head and neck are assigned nine percent, each arm nine percent, each leg

18 percent, the anterior trunk 18 percent, posterior trunk 18 percent, and genitalia one percent. Providers may change these percentage assignments where necessary to accommodate infants and children who have proportionately larger heads than adults and patients who have large buttocks, thighs, or abdomen that involve burns.

7) Encounters for treatment of late effects of burns

Encounters for the treatment of the late effects of burns (i.e., scars or joint contractures) should be coded to the residual condition (sequelae) followed by the appropriate late effect code (906.5-906.9). A late effect E code may also be used, if desired.

8) Sequelae with a late effect code and current burn

When appropriate, both a sequelae with a late effect code, and a current burn code may be assigned on the same record **(when both a current burn and sequelae of an old burn exist).**

d. Coding of Debridement of Wound, Infection, or Burn

Excisional debridement involves an excisional debridement (surgical removal or cutting away), as opposed to a mechanical (brushing, scrubbing, washing) debridement.

For coding purposes, excisional debridement **is assigned to code 86.22.**

Nonexcisional debridement is assigned to **code 86.28.**

e. Adverse Effects, Poisoning and Toxic Effects

The properties of certain drugs, medicinal and biological substances or combinations of such substances, may cause toxic reactions. The occurrence of drug toxicity is classified in ICD-9-CM as follows:

1) Adverse Effect

When the drug was correctly prescribed and properly administered, code the reaction plus the appropriate code from the E930-E949 series. Codes from the E930-E949 series must be used to identify the causative substance for an adverse effect of drug, medicinal and biological substances, correctly prescribed and properly administered. The effect, such as tachycardia, delirium, gastrointestinal hemorrhaging, vomiting, hypokalemia, hepatitis, renal failure, or respiratory failure, is

coded and followed by the appropriate code from the
E930-E949 series.

Adverse effects of therapeutic substances correctly prescribed
and properly administered (toxicity, synergistic reaction, side
effect, and idiosyncratic reaction) may be due to (1) differences
among patients, such as age, sex, disease, and genetic factors,
and (2) drug-related factors, such as type of drug, route of
administration, duration of therapy, dosage, and bioavailability.

2) Poisoning

(a) Error was made in drug prescription

Errors made in drug prescription or in the
administration of the drug by provider, nurse, patient,
or other person, use the appropriate poisoning code
from the 960-979 series.

(b) Overdose of a drug intentionally taken

If an overdose of a drug was intentionally taken or
administered and resulted in drug toxicity, it would be
coded as a poisoning (960-979 series).

(c) Nonprescribed drug taken with correctly prescribed and properly administered drug

If a nonprescribed drug or medicinal agent was taken in
combination with a correctly prescribed and properly
administered drug, any drug toxicity or other reaction
resulting from the interaction of the two drugs would be
classified as a poisoning.

(d) Sequencing of poisoning

When coding a poisoning or reaction to the improper
use of a medication (e.g., wrong dose, wrong substance,
wrong route of administration) the poisoning code is
sequenced first, followed by a code for the
manifestation. If there is also a diagnosis of drug abuse
or dependence to the substance, the abuse or
dependence is coded as an additional code.

**See Section I.C.3.a.6.b. if poisoning is the result of
insulin pump malfunctions and Section I.C.19 for
general use of E-codes.**

3) Toxic Effects

(a)   **Toxic effect codes**

When a harmful substance is ingested or comes in contact with a person, this is classified as a toxic effect. The toxic effect codes are in categories 980-989.

(b)   **Sequencing toxic effect codes**

A toxic effect code should be sequenced first, followed by the code(s) that identify the result of the toxic effect.

(c)   **External cause codes for toxic effects**

An external cause code from categories E860-E869 for accidental exposure, codes E950.6 or E950.7 for intentional self-harm, category E962 for assault, or categories E980-E982, for undetermined, should also be assigned to indicate intent.

18.   Classification of Factors Influencing Health Status and Contact with Health Service (Supplemental V01-V84)

Note: The chapter specific guidelines provide additional information about the use of V codes for specified encounters.

a.   Introduction

ICD-9-CM provides codes to deal with encounters for circumstances other than a disease or injury. The Supplementary Classification of Factors Influencing Health Status and Contact with Health Services (V01.0 - V84.8) is provided to deal with occasions when circumstances other than a disease or injury (codes 001-999) are recorded as a diagnosis or problem.

There are four primary circumstances for the use of V codes:

1)   A person who is not currently sick encounters the health services for some specific reason, such as to act as an organ donor, to receive prophylactic care, such as inoculations or health screenings, or to receive counseling on health related issues.

2)   A person with a resolving disease or injury, or a chronic, long-term condition requiring continuous care, encounters the health care system for specific aftercare of that disease or injury (e.g., dialysis for renal disease; chemotherapy for malignancy; cast change). A diagnosis/symptom code should be used whenever

a current, acute, diagnosis is being treated or a sign or symptom is being studied.

3) Circumstances or problems influence a person's health status but are not in themselves a current illness or injury.

4) Newborns, to indicate birth status

b. **V codes use in any healthcare setting**

V codes are for use in any healthcare setting. V codes may be used as either a first listed (principal diagnosis code in the inpatient setting) or secondary code, depending on the circumstances of the encounter. Certain V codes may only be used as first listed, others only as secondary codes. See Section I.C.18.e, **V Code Table.**

c. **V Codes indicate a reason for an encounter**

They are not procedure codes. A corresponding procedure code must accompany a V code to describe the procedure performed.

d. **Categories of V Codes**

1) **Contact/Exposure**

Category V01 indicates contact with or exposure to communicable diseases. These codes are for patients who do not show any sign or symptom of a disease but have been exposed to it by close personal contact with an infected individual or are in an area where a disease is epidemic. These codes may be used as a first listed code to explain an encounter for testing, or, more commonly, as a secondary code to identify a potential risk.

2) **Inoculations and vaccinations**

Categories V03-V06 are for encounters for inoculations and vaccinations. They indicate that a patient is being seen to receive a prophylactic inoculation against a disease. The injection itself must be represented by the appropriate procedure code. A code from V03-V06 may be used as a secondary code if the inoculation is given as a routine part of preventive health care, such as a well-baby visit.

3) **Status**

Status codes indicate that a patient is either a carrier of a disease or has the sequelae or residual of a past disease or condition. This includes such things as the presence of prosthetic or mechanical devices resulting from past treatment.

A status code is informative, because the status may affect the course of treatment and its outcome. A status code is distinct from a history code. The history code indicates that the patient no longer has the condition.

A status code should not be used with a diagnosis code from one of the body system chapters, if the diagnosis code includes the information provided by the status code. For example, code V42.1, Heart transplant status, should not be used with code 996.83, Complications of transplanted heart. The status code does not provide additional information. The complication code indicates that the patient is a heart transplant patient.

The status V codes/categories are:

V02   Carrier or suspected carrier of infectious diseases
           Carrier status indicates that a person harbors the specific organisms of a disease without manifest symptoms and is capable of transmitting the infection.

V08   Asymptomatic HIV infection status
           This code indicates that a patient has tested positive for HIV but has manifested no signs or symptoms of the disease.

V09   Infection with drug-resistant microorganisms
           This category indicates that a patient has an infection that is resistant to drug treatment. Sequence the infection code first.

V21   Constitutional states in development

V22.2   Pregnant state, incidental
           This code is a secondary code only for use when the pregnancy is in no way complicating the reason for visit. Otherwise, a code from the obstetric chapter is required.

V26.5x   Sterilization status

V42   Organ or tissue replaced by transplant

V43   Organ or tissue replaced by other means

V44   Artificial opening status

V45   Other postsurgical states

V46   Other dependence on machines

V49.6   Upper limb amputation status

V49.7   Lower limb amputation status

V49.81   Postmenopausal status

V49.82   Dental sealant status

V49.83   Awaiting organ transplant status

V58.6   Long-term (current) drug use

This subcategory indicates a patient's continuous use of a prescribed drug (including such things as aspirin therapy) for the long-term treatment of a condition or for prophylactic use. It is not for use for patients who have addictions to drugs.

V83   Genetic carrier status

Genetic carrier status indicates that a person carries a gene, associated with a particular disease, which may be passed to offspring who may develop that disease. The person does not have the disease and is not at risk of developing the disease.

V84   Genetic susceptibility status

Genetic susceptibility indicates that a person has a gene that increases the risk of that person developing the disease.

Note: Categories V42-V46, and subcategories V49.6, V49.7 are for use only if there are no complications or malfunctions of the organ or tissue replaced, the amputation site or the equipment on which the patient is dependent. These are always secondary codes.

4)   **History (of)**

There are two types of history V codes, personal and family. Personal history codes explain a patient's past medical condition that no longer exists and is not receiving any treatment, but that has the potential for recurrence, and therefore may require continued monitoring. The exceptions to this general rule are category V14, Personal history of allergy to medicinal agents, and subcategory V15.0, Allergy, other than to medicinal agents. A person who has had an allergic episode to a substance or food in the past should always be considered allergic to the substance.

Family history codes are for use when a patient has a family member(s) who has had a particular disease that causes the patient to be at higher risk of also contracting the disease.

Personal history codes may be used in conjunction with follow-up codes and family history codes may be used in conjunction with screening codes to explain the need for a test or procedure. History codes are also acceptable on any medical record regardless of the reason for visit. A history of an illness, even if no longer present, is important information that may alter the type of treatment ordered.

The history V code categories are:

V10   Personal history of malignant neoplasm
V12   Personal history of certain other diseases
V13   Personal history of other diseases
       Except: V13.4, Personal history of arthritis, and V13.6, Personal history of congenital malformations. These conditions are life-long so are not true history codes.
V14   Personal history of allergy to medicinal agents
V15   Other personal history presenting hazards to health
       Except: V15.7, Personal history of contraception.
V16   Family history of malignant neoplasm
V17   Family history of certain chronic disabling diseases
V18   Family history of certain other specific diseases
V19   Family history of other conditions

5)   **Screening**

Screening is the testing for disease or disease precursors in seemingly well individuals so that early detection and treatment can be provided for those who test positive for the disease. Screenings that are recommended for many subgroups in a population include: routine mammograms for women over 40, a fecal occult blood test for everyone over 50, an amniocentesis to rule out a fetal anomaly for pregnant women over 35, because the incidence of breast cancer and colon cancer in these subgroups is higher than in the general population, as is the incidence of Down's syndrome in older mothers.

The testing of a person to rule out or confirm a suspected diagnosis because the patient has some sign or symptom is a diagnostic examination, not a screening. In these cases, the sign or symptom is used to explain the reason for the test.

A screening code may be a first listed code if the reason for the visit is specifically the screening exam. It may also be used as an additional code if the screening is done during an office visit for other health problems. A screening code is not necessary if the screening is inherent to a routine examination, such as a pap smear done during a routine pelvic examination.

Should a condition be discovered during the screening then the code for the condition may be assigned as an additional diagnosis.

The V code indicates that a screening exam is planned. A procedure code is required to confirm that the screening was performed.

The screening V code categories:
V28   Antenatal screening
V73-V82   Special screening examinations

6)   Observation

There are two observation V code categories. They are for use in very limited circumstances when a person is being observed for a suspected condition that is ruled out. The observation codes are not for use if an injury or illness or any signs or symptoms related to the suspected condition are present. In such cases the diagnosis/symptom code is used with the corresponding E code to identify any external cause.

The observation codes are to be used as principal diagnosis only. The only exception to this is when the principal diagnosis is required to be a code from the V30, Live born infant, category. Then the V29 observation code is sequenced after the V30 code. Additional codes may be used in addition to the observation code but only if they are unrelated to the suspected condition being observed.

The observation V code categories:
V29   Observation and evaluation of newborns for
           suspected condition not found
           For the birth encounter, a code from category V30
           should be sequenced before the V29 code.
V71   Observation and evaluation for suspected condition
           not found

7)   Aftercare

Aftercare visit codes cover situations when the initial treatment of a disease or injury has been performed and the patient requires continued care during the healing or recovery phase, or for the long-term consequences of the disease. The aftercare V code should not be used if treatment is directed at a current, acute disease or injury, the diagnosis code is to be used in these cases. Exceptions to this rule are codes V58.0, Radiotherapy, and V58.1, Chemotherapy. These codes are to be first listed, followed by the diagnosis code when a patient's encounter is solely to receive radiation therapy or chemotherapy for the treatment of a neoplasm. Should a patient receive both chemotherapy and radiation therapy during the same encounter code V58.0 and V58.1 may be used together on a record with either one being sequenced first.

The aftercare codes are generally first listed to explain the specific reason for the encounter. An aftercare code may be used as an additional code when some type of aftercare is provided in addition to the reason for admission and no diagnosis code is applicable. An example of this would be the closure of a colostomy during an encounter for treatment of another condition.

Certain aftercare V code categories need a secondary diagnosis code to describe the resolving condition or sequelae, for others, the condition is inherent in the code title.

Additional V code aftercare category terms include, fitting and adjustment, and attention to artificial openings.

Status V codes may be used with aftercare V codes to indicate the nature of the aftercare. For example code V45.81, Aortocoronary bypass status, may be used with code V58.73, Aftercare following surgery of the circulatory system, NEC, to indicate the surgery for which the aftercare is being performed. Also, a transplant status code may be used following code V58.44, Aftercare following organ transplant, to identify the organ transplanted. A status code should not be used when the aftercare code indicates the type of status, such as using V55.0, Attention to tracheostomy with V44.0, Tracheostomy status.

The aftercare V category/codes:

V52	Fitting and adjustment of prosthetic device and implant
V53	Fitting and adjustment of other device
V54	Other orthopedic aftercare
V55	Attention to artificial openings
V56	Encounter for dialysis and dialysis catheter care
V57	Care involving the use of rehabilitation procedures
V58.0	Radiotherapy
V58.1	Chemotherapy
V58.3	Attention to surgical dressings and sutures
V58.41	Encounter for planned post-operative wound closure

V58.42	Aftercare, surgery, neoplasm
V58.43	Aftercare, surgery, trauma
V58.44	**Aftercare involving organ transplant**
V58.49	Other specified aftercare following surgery
V58.7x	Aftercare following surgery
V58.81	Fitting and adjustment of vascular catheter
V58.82	Fitting and adjustment of non-vascular catheter
V58.83	Monitoring therapeutic drug
V58.89	Other specified aftercare

8)   Follow-up

The follow-up codes are used to explain continuing surveillance following completed treatment of a disease, condition, or injury. They imply that the condition has been fully treated and no longer exists. They should not be confused with aftercare codes that explain current treatment for a healing condition or its sequelae. Follow-up codes may be used in conjunction with history codes to provide the full picture of the healed condition and its treatment. The follow-up code is sequenced first, followed by the history code.

A follow-up code may be used to explain repeated visits. Should a condition be found to have recurred on the follow-up visit, then the diagnosis code should be used in place of the follow-up code.

The follow-up V code categories:
V24	Postpartum care and evaluation
V67	Follow-up examination

9)   Donor

Category V59 is the donor codes. They are used for living individuals who are donating blood or other body tissue. These codes are only for individuals donating for others, not for self donations. They are not for use to identify cadaveric donations.

10)   Counseling

Counseling V codes are used when a patient or family member receives assistance in the aftermath of an illness or injury, or when support is required in coping with family or social problems. They are not necessary for use in conjunction with a diagnosis code when the counseling component of care is considered integral to standard treatment.

The counseling V categories/codes:

V25.0   General counseling and advice for contraceptive management

V26.3   Genetic counseling

V26.4   General counseling and advice for procreative management

V61   Other family circumstances

V65.1   Person consulted on behalf of another person

V65.3   Dietary surveillance and counseling

V65.4   Other counseling, not elsewhere classified

11) Obstetrics and related conditions

See Section I.C.11., the Obstetrics guidelines for further instruction on the use of these codes.

V codes for pregnancy are for use in those circumstances when none of the problems or complications included in the codes from the Obstetrics chapter exist (a routine prenatal visit or postpartum care). Codes V22.0, Supervision of normal first pregnancy, and V22.1, Supervision of other normal pregnancy, are always first listed and are not to be used with any other code from the OB chapter.

The outcome of delivery, category V27, should be included on all maternal delivery records. It is always a secondary code.

V codes for family planning (contraceptive) or procreative management and counseling should be included on an obstetric record either during the pregnancy or the postpartum stage, if applicable.

Obstetrics and related conditions V code categories:

V22   Normal pregnancy

V23   Supervision of high-risk pregnancy
Except: V23.2, Pregnancy with history of abortion. Code 646.3, Habitual aborter, from the OB chapter is required to indicate a history of abortion during a pregnancy.

V24   Postpartum care and evaluation

V25   Encounter for contraceptive management
Except V25.0x (See Section I.C.18.d.11, Counseling)

V26   Procreative management
Except V26.5x, Sterilization status, V26.3 and V26.4 (See Section I.C.18.d.11., Counseling)

V27   Outcome of delivery

V28 Antenatal screening
   (See Section I.C.18.d.6., Screening)

12) Newborn, infant and child

See Section I.C.15, the Newborn guidelines for further instruction on the use of these codes.

Newborn V code categories:
V20 Health supervision of infant or child
V29 Observation and evaluation of newborns for suspected condition not found (See Section I.C.18.d.7, Observation).
V30-V39 Liveborn infant according to type of birth

13) Routine and administrative examinations

The V codes allow for the description of encounters for routine examinations, such as, a general check-up, or, examinations for administrative purposes, such as, a pre-employment physical. The codes are for use as first listed codes only, and are not to be used if the examination is for diagnosis of a suspected condition or for treatment purposes. In such cases the diagnosis code is used. During a routine exam, should a diagnosis or condition be discovered, it should be coded as an additional code. Pre-existing and chronic conditions and history codes may also be included as additional codes as long as the examination is for administrative purposes and not focused on any particular condition.

Pre-operative examination V codes are for use only in those situations when a patient is being cleared for surgery and no treatment is given.

The V codes categories/code for routine and administrative examinations:

V20.2 Routine infant or child health check
   Any injections given should have a corresponding procedure code.
V70 General medical examination
V72 Special investigations and examinations
   Except V72.5 and V72.6

14) Miscellaneous V codes

The miscellaneous V codes capture a number of other health care encounters that do not fall into one of the other categories.

Certain of these codes identify the reason for the encounter, others are for use as additional codes that provide useful information on circumstances that may affect a patient's care and treatment.

Miscellaneous V code categories/codes:

V07	Need for isolation and other prophylactic measures
V50	Elective surgery for purposes other than remedying health states
V58.5	Orthodontics
V60	Housing, household, and economic circumstances
V62	Other psychosocial circumstances
V63	Unavailability of other medical facilities for care
V64	Persons encountering health services for specific procedures, not carried out
V66	Convalescence and Palliative Care
V68	Encounters for administrative purposes
V69	Problems related to lifestyle

15)   Nonspecific V codes

Certain V codes are so non-specific, or potentially redundant with other codes in the classification, that there can be little justification for their use in the inpatient setting. Their use in the outpatient setting should be limited to those instances when there is no further documentation to permit more precise coding. Otherwise, any sign or symptom or any other reason for visit that is captured in another code should be used.

Nonspecific V code categories/codes:

V11	Personal history of mental disorder
	A code from the mental disorders chapter, with an in remission fifth-digit, should be used.
V13.4	Personal history of arthritis
V13.6	Personal history of congenital malformations
V15.7	Personal history of contraception
V23.2	Pregnancy with history of abortion
V40	Mental and behavioral problems
V41	Problems with special senses and other special functions
V47	Other problems with internal organs
V48	Problems with head, neck, and trunk
V49	Problems with limbs and other problems

Exceptions:

V49.6	Upper limb amputation status
V49.7	Lower limb amputation status
V49.81	Postmenopausal status

V49.82   Dental sealant status

V49.83   Awaiting organ transplant status

V51   Aftercare involving the use of plastic surgery

V58.2   Blood transfusion, without reported diagnosis

V58.9   Unspecified aftercare

V72.5   Radiological examination, NEC

V72.6   Laboratory examination

Codes V72.5 and V72.6 are not to be used if any sign or symptoms, or reason for a test is documented. See Section IV.K. and Section IV.L. of the Outpatient guidelines.

<u>**V Code Table**</u>
<u>Items in bold indicate a change from the October 2003 table</u>
<u>Items underlined have been moved within the table since October 2003</u>

FIRST LISTED: V codes/categories/subcategories which are only acceptable as
             principal/first listed.
Codes:
V22.0   Supervision of normal first pregnancy
V22.1   Supervision of other normal pregnancy
V46.12   **Encounter for respirator dependence during power failure**
V56.0   <u>Extracorporeal dialysis</u>
V58.0   Radiotherapy
V58.1   Chemotherapy
             V58.0 and V58.1 may be used together on a record with either one being
             sequenced first, when a patient receives both chemotherapy and radiation
             therapy during the same encounter code.

Categories/Subcategories:
V20   Health supervision of infant or child
V24   Postpartum care and examination
V29   Observation and evaluation of newborns for suspected condition not found
             Exception: A code from the V30-V39 may be sequenced before the V29 if it
                    is the newborn record.
V30-V39   Liveborn infants according to type of birth
V59   Donors
V66   Convalescence and palliative care
             Exception: V66.7 Palliative care
V68   Encounters for administrative purposes
V70   General medical examination
             Exception: V70.7 Examination of participant in clinical trial
V71   Observation and evaluation for suspected conditions not found
V72   Special investigations and examinations
             Exceptions:
             V72.5 Radiological examination, NEC
             V72.6 Laboratory examination

FIRST OR ADDITIONAL: V code categories/subcategories which may be either
principal/first listed or additional codes
Codes:
V43.22   Fully implantable artificial heart status
V49.81   Asymptomatic postmenopausal status (age-related) (natural)
V70.7   Examination of participant in clinical trial

Categories/Subcategories:
V01   Contact with or exposure to communicable diseases
V02   Carrier or suspected carrier of infectious diseases
V03-06   Need for prophylactic vaccination and inoculations
V07   Need for isolation and other prophylactic measures
V08   Asymptomatic HIV infection status

V10	Personal history of malignant neoplasm
V12	Personal history of certain other diseases
V13	Personal history of other diseases
	Exception:
	V13.4 Personal history of arthritis
	V13.69 Personal history of other congenital malformations
V16-V19	Family history of disease
V23	Supervision of high-risk pregnancy
V25	Encounter for contraceptive management
V26	Procreative management
	Exception: V26.5 Sterilization status
V28	Antenatal screening
V45.7	Acquired absence of organ
V50	Elective surgery for purposes other than remedying health states
V52	Fitting and adjustment of prosthetic device and implant
V53	Fitting and adjustment of other device
V54	Other orthopedic aftercare
V55	Attention to artificial openings
V56	Encounter for dialysis and dialysis catheter care
	Exception: V56.0 Extracorporeal dialysis
V57	Care involving use of rehabilitation procedures
V58.3	Attention to surgical dressings and sutures
V58.4	Other aftercare following surgery
<u>V58.6</u>	<u>Long-term (current) drug use</u>
V58.7	Aftercare following surgery to specified body systems, not elsewhere classified
V58.8	Other specified procedures and aftercare
V61	Other family circumstances
V63	Unavailability of other medical facilities for care
V65	Other persons seeking consultation without complaint or sickness
V67	Follow-up examination
V69	Problems related to lifestyle
V73-V82	Special screening examinations
V83	Genetic carrier status

ADDITIONAL ONLY: V code categories/subcategories which may only be used as additional codes, not principal/first listed

Codes:

V13.61	Personal history of hypospadias
V22.2	Pregnancy state, incidental
V49.82	Dental sealant status
V49.83	**Awaiting organ transplant status**
V66.7	Palliative care

Categories/Subcategories:

V09	Infection with drug-resistant microorganisms

V14	Personal history of allergy to medicinal agents
V15	Other personal history presenting hazards to health
	Exception: V15.7 Personal history of contraception
V21	Constitutional states in development
V26.5	Sterilization status
V27	Outcome of delivery
V42	Organ or tissue replaced by transplant
V43	Organ or tissue replaced by other means
	Exception: V43.22 Fully implantable artificial heart status
V44	Artificial opening status
V45	Other postsurgical states
	Exception: Subcategory V45.7 Acquired absence of organ
V46	Other dependence on machines
	Exception: V46.12 Encounter for respirator dependence during power failure
V49.6x	Upper limb amputation status
V49.7x	Lower limb amputation status
V60	Housing, household, and economic circumstances
V62	Other psychosocial circumstances
V64	Persons encountering health services for specified procedure, not carried out
V84	**Genetic susceptibility to disease**

NONSPECIFIC CODES AND CATEGORIES:

V11	Personal history of mental disorder
V13.4	Personal history of arthritis
V13.69	Personal history of congenital malformations
V15.7	Personal history of contraception
V40	Mental and behavioral problems
V41	Problems with special senses and other special functions
V47	Other problems with internal organs
V48	Problems with head, neck, and trunk
V49	Problems with limbs and other problems
	Exceptions:
	V49.6 Upper limb amputation status
	V49.7 Lower limb amputation status
	V49.81 Postmenopausal status (age-related) (natural)
	V49.82 Dental sealant status
	V49.83 Awaiting organ transplant status
V51	Aftercare involving the use of plastic surgery
V58.2	Blood transfusion, without reported diagnosis
V58.5	Orthodontics
V58.9	Unspecified aftercare
V72.5	Radiological examination, NEC
V72.6	Laboratory examination

19. Supplemental Classification of External Causes of Injury and Poisoning (E-codes, E800-E999)

Introduction: These guidelines are provided for those who are currently collecting E codes in order that there will be standardization in the process. If your institution plans to begin collecting E codes, these guidelines are to be applied. The use of E codes is supplemental to the application of ICD-9-CM diagnosis codes. E codes are never to be recorded as principal diagnoses (first-listed in non-inpatient setting) and are not required for reporting to CMS.

External causes of injury and poisoning codes (E codes) are intended to provide data for injury research and evaluation of injury prevention strategies. E codes capture how the injury or poisoning happened (cause), the intent (unintentional or accidental; or intentional, such as suicide or assault), and the place where the event occurred.

Some major categories of E codes include:
> transport accidents
> poisoning and adverse effects of drugs, medicinal substances and biologicals
> accidental falls
> accidents caused by fire and flames
> accidents due to natural and environmental factors
> late effects of accidents, assaults or self injury
> assaults or purposely inflicted injury
> suicide or self inflicted injury

These guidelines apply for the coding and collection of E codes from records in hospitals, outpatient clinics, emergency departments, other ambulatory care settings and provider offices, and nonacute care settings, except when other specific guidelines apply.

a. General E Code Coding Guidelines

1) Used with any code in the range of 001-V84.8

An E code may be used with any code in the range of 001-V84.8, which indicates an injury, poisoning, or adverse effect due to an external cause.

2) Assign the appropriate E code for all initial treatments

Assign the appropriate E code for the initial encounter of an injury, poisoning, or adverse effect of drugs, **not for subsequent treatment.**

3) Use the full range of E codes

Use the full range of E codes to completely describe the cause, the intent and the place of occurrence, if applicable, for all injuries, poisonings, and adverse effects of drugs.

4) **Assign as many E codes as necessary**

Assign as many E codes as necessary to fully explain each cause. If only one E code can be recorded, assign the E code most related to the principal diagnosis.

5) **The selection of the appropriate E code**

The selection of the appropriate E code is guided by the Index to External Causes, which is located after the alphabetical index to diseases and by Inclusion and Exclusion notes in the Tabular List.

6) **E code can never be a principal diagnosis**

An E code can never be a principal (first listed) diagnosis.

7) **External cause code(s) with systemic inflammatory response syndrome (SIRS)**

An external cause code(s) may be used with codes 995.93, Systemic inflammatory response syndrome due to noninfectious process without organ dysfunction, and 995.94, Systemic inflammatory response syndrome due to noninfectious process with organ dysfunction, if trauma was the initiating insult that precipitated the SIRS. The external cause(s) code should correspond to the most serious injury resulting from the trauma. The external cause code(s) should only be assigned if the trauma necessitated the admission in which the patient also developed SIRS. If a patient is admitted with SIRS but the trauma has been treated previously, the external cause codes should not be used.

b. **Place of Occurrence Guideline**

Use an additional code from category E849 to indicate the Place of Occurrence for injuries and poisonings. The Place of Occurrence describes the place where the event occurred and not the patient's activity at the time of the event.

Do not use E849.9 if the place of occurrence is not stated.

c. Adverse Effects of Drugs, Medicinal and Biological Substances Guidelines

1) Do not code directly from the Table of Drugs

Do not code directly from the Table of Drugs and Chemicals. Always refer back to the Tabular List.

2) Use as many codes as necessary to describe

Use as many codes as necessary to describe completely all drugs, medicinal or biological substances.

3) If the same E code would describe the causative agent

If the same E code would describe the causative agent for more than one adverse reaction, assign the code only once.

4) If two or more drugs, medicinal or biological substances

If two or more drugs, medicinal or biological substances are reported, code each individually unless the combination code is listed in the Table of Drugs and Chemicals. In that case, assign the E code for the combination.

5) When a reaction results from the interaction of a drug(s)

When a reaction results from the interaction of a drug(s) and alcohol, use poisoning codes and E codes for both.

6) If the reporting format limits the number of E codes

If the reporting format limits the number of E codes that can be used in reporting clinical data, code the one most related to the principal diagnosis. Include at least one from each category (cause, intent, place) if possible.

If there are different fourth digit codes in the same three digit category, use the code for "Other specified" of that category. If there is no "Other specified" code in that category, use the appropriate "Unspecified" code in that category.

If the codes are in different three digit categories, assign the appropriate E code for other multiple drugs and medicinal substances.

7) Codes from the E930-E949 series

Codes from the E930-E949 series must be used to identify the causative substance for an adverse effect of drug, medicinal and biological substances, correctly prescribed and properly administered. The effect, such as tachycardia, delirium, gastrointestinal hemorrhaging, vomiting, hypokalemia, hepatitis, renal failure, or respiratory failure, is coded and followed by the appropriate code from the E930-E949 series.

d. Multiple Cause E Code Coding Guidelines

If two or more events cause separate injuries, an E code should be assigned for each cause. The first listed E code will be selected in the following order:

E codes for child and adult abuse take priority over all other E codes. See Section I.C.19.e., Child and Adult abuse guidelines

E codes for terrorism events take priority over all other E codes except child and adult abuse

E codes for cataclysmic events take priority over all other E codes except child and adult abuse and terrorism.

E codes for transport accidents take priority over all other E codes except cataclysmic events and child and adult abuse and terrorism.

The first-listed E code should correspond to the cause of the most serious diagnosis due to an assault, accident, or self-harm, following the order of hierarchy listed above.

e. Child and Adult Abuse Guideline

1) Intentional injury

When the cause of an injury or neglect is intentional child or adult abuse, the first listed E code should be assigned from categories E960-E968, Homicide and injury purposely inflicted by other persons, (except category E967). An E code from category E967, Child and adult battering and other maltreatment, should be added as an additional code to identify the perpetrator, if known.

2) Accidental intent

In cases of neglect when the intent is determined to be accidental E code E904.0, Abandonment or neglect of infant and helpless person, should be the first listed E code.

f. Unknown or Suspected Intent Guideline

1) If the intent (accident, self-harm, assault) of the cause of an injury or poisoning is unknown

If the intent (accident, self-harm, assault) of the cause of an injury or poisoning is unknown or unspecified, code the intent as undetermined E980-E989.

2) If the intent (accident, self-harm, assault) of the cause of an injury or poisoning is questionable

If the intent (accident, self-harm, assault) of the cause of an injury or poisoning is questionable, probable or suspected, code the intent as undetermined E980-E989.

g. Undetermined Cause

When the intent of an injury or poisoning is known, but the cause is unknown, use codes: E928.9, Unspecified accident, E958.9, Suicide and self-inflicted injury by unspecified means, and E968.9, Assault by unspecified means.

These E codes should rarely be used, as the documentation in the medical record, in both the inpatient outpatient and other settings, should normally provide sufficient detail to determine the cause of the injury.

h. Late Effects of External Cause Guidelines

1) Late effect E codes

Late effect E codes exist for injuries and poisonings but not for adverse effects of drugs, misadventures and surgical complications.

2) Late effect E codes (E929, E959, E969, E977, E989, or E999.1)

A late effect E code (E929, E959, E969, E977, E989, or E999.1) should be used with any report of a late effect or sequela resulting from a previous injury or poisoning (905-909).

3) Late effect E code with a related current injury

A late effect E code should never be used with a related current nature of injury code.

4) Use of late effect E codes for subsequent visits

Use a late effect E code for subsequent visits when a late effect of the initial injury or poisoning is being treated. There is no late effect E code for adverse effects of drugs. Do not use a late effect E code for subsequent visits for follow-up care (e.g., to assess healing, to receive rehabilitative therapy) of the injury or poisoning when no late effect of the injury has been documented.

i. Misadventures and Complications of Care Guidelines

1) Code range E870-E876

Assign a code in the range of E870-E876 if misadventures are stated by the provider.

2) Code range E878-E879

Assign a code in the range of E878-E879 if the provider attributes an abnormal reaction or later complication to a surgical or medical procedure, but does not mention misadventure at the time of the procedure as the cause of the reaction.

j. Terrorism Guidelines

1) Cause of injury identified by the Federal Government (FBI) as terrorism

When the cause of an injury is identified by the Federal Government (FBI) as terrorism, the first-listed E-code should be a code from category E979, Terrorism. The definition of terrorism employed by the FBI is found at the inclusion note at E979. The terrorism E-code is the only E-code that should be assigned. Additional E codes from the assault categories should not be assigned.

2) Cause of an injury is suspected to be the result of terrorism

When the cause of an injury is suspected to be the result of terrorism a code from category E979 should not be assigned. Assign a code in the range of E codes based circumstances on the documentation of intent and mechanism.

3) Code E979.9, Terrorism, secondary effects

Assign code E979.9, Terrorism, secondary effects, for conditions occurring subsequent to the terrorist event. This code should not be assigned for conditions that are due to the initial terrorist act.

4)   Statistical tabulation of terrorism codes

For statistical purposes these codes will be tabulated within the category for assault, expanding the current category from E960-E969 to include E979 and E999.1.

Section II. Selection of Principal Diagnosis

The circumstances of inpatient admission always govern the selection of principal diagnosis. The principal diagnosis is defined in the Uniform Hospital Discharge Data Set (UHDDS) as "that condition established after study to be chiefly responsible for occasioning the admission of the patient to the hospital for care."

The UHDDS definitions are used by hospitals to report inpatient data elements in a standardized manner. These data elements and their definitions can be found in the July 31, 1985, Federal Register (Vol. 50, No, 147), pp. 31038-40.

Since that time the application of the UHDDS definitions has been expanded to include all non-outpatient settings (acute care, short term, long term care and psychiatric hospitals; home health agencies; rehab facilities; nursing homes, etc).

In determining principal diagnosis the coding conventions in the ICD-9-CM, Volumes I and II take precedence over these official coding guidelines. (See Section I.A., Conventions for the ICD-9-CM).

The importance of consistent, complete documentation in the medical record cannot be overemphasized. Without such documentation the application of all coding guidelines is a difficult, if not impossible, task.

A. Codes for symptoms, signs, and ill-defined conditions

Codes for symptoms, signs, and ill-defined conditions from Chapter 16 are not to be used as principal diagnosis when a related definitive diagnosis has been established.

B. Two or more interrelated conditions, each potentially meeting the definition for principal diagnosis.

When there are two or more interrelated conditions (such as diseases in the same ICD-9-CM chapter or manifestations characteristically associated with a certain disease) potentially meeting the definition of principal diagnosis, either condition may be sequenced first, unless the circumstances of the admission, the therapy provided, the Tabular List, or the Alphabetic Index indicate otherwise.

C. Two or more diagnoses that equally meet the definition for principal diagnosis

In the unusual instance when two or more diagnoses equally meet the criteria for principal diagnosis as determined by the circumstances of admission, diagnostic workup and/or therapy provided, and the Alphabetic Index, Tabular List, or another coding guidelines does not provide sequencing direction, any one of the diagnoses may be sequenced first.

D. Two or more comparative or contrasting conditions.

In those rare instances when two or more contrasting or comparative diagnoses are documented as "either/or" (or similar terminology), they are coded as if the diagnoses were confirmed and the diagnoses are sequenced according to the circumstances of the admission. If no further determination can be made as to which diagnosis should be principal, either diagnosis may be sequenced first.

E. A symptom(s) followed by contrasting/comparative diagnoses

When a symptom(s) is followed by contrasting/comparative diagnoses, the symptom code is sequenced first. All the contrasting/comparative diagnoses should be coded as additional diagnoses.

F. Original treatment plan not carried out

Sequence as the principal diagnosis the condition, which after study occasioned the admission to the hospital, even though treatment may not have been carried out due to unforeseen circumstances.

G. Complications of surgery and other medical care

When the admission is for treatment of a complication resulting from surgery or other medical care, the complication code is sequenced as the principal diagnosis. If the complication is classified to the 996-999 series and the code lacks the necessary specificity in describing the complication, an additional code for the specific complication should be assigned.

H. Uncertain Diagnosis

If the diagnosis documented at the time of discharge is qualified as "probable", "suspected", "likely", "questionable", "possible", or "still to be ruled out", code the condition as if it existed or was established. The bases for these guidelines are the diagnostic workup, arrangements for further workup or observation, and initial therapeutic approach that correspond most closely with the established diagnosis.

Note: This guideline is applicable only to short-term, acute, long-term care and psychiatric hospitals.

Section III. Reporting Additional Diagnoses

GENERAL RULES FOR OTHER (ADDITIONAL) DIAGNOSES

For reporting purposes the definition for "other diagnoses" is interpreted as additional conditions that affect patient care in terms of requiring:

> clinical evaluation; or
> therapeutic treatment; or

diagnostic procedures; or
extended length of hospital stay; or
increased nursing care and/or monitoring.

The UHDDS item #11-b defines Other Diagnoses as "all conditions that coexist at the time of admission, that develop subsequently, or that affect the treatment received and/or the length of stay. Diagnoses that relate to an earlier episode which have no bearing on the current hospital stay are to be excluded." UHDDS definitions apply to inpatients in acute care, short-term, long term care and psychiatric hospital setting. The UHDDS definitions are used by acute care short-term hospitals to report inpatient data elements in a standardized manner. These data elements and their definitions can be found in the July 31, 1985, Federal Register (Vol. 50, No, 147), pp. 31038-40.

Since that time the application of the UHDDS definitions has been expanded to include all non—outpatient settings (acute care, short term, long term care and psychiatric hospitals; home health agencies; rehab facilities; nursing homes, etc).

The following guidelines are to be applied in designating "other diagnoses" when neither the Alphabetic Index nor the Tabular List in ICD-9-CM provide direction. The listing of the diagnoses in the patient record is the responsibility of the attending provider.

A. Previous conditions

If the provider has included a diagnosis in the final diagnostic statement, such as the discharge summary or the face sheet, it should ordinarily be coded. Some providers include in the diagnostic statement resolved conditions or diagnoses and status-post procedures from previous admission that have no bearing on the current stay. Such conditions are not to be reported and are coded only if required by hospital policy.

However, history codes (V10-V19) may be used as secondary codes if the historical condition or family history has an impact on current care or influences treatment.

B. Abnormal findings

Abnormal findings (laboratory, x-ray, pathologic, and other diagnostic results) are not coded and reported unless the provider indicates their clinical significance. If the findings are outside the normal range and the **attending** provider has ordered other tests to evaluate the condition or prescribed treatment, it is appropriate to ask the provider whether the abnormal finding should be added.

Please note: This differs from the coding practices in the outpatient setting for coding encounters for diagnostic tests that have been interpreted by a provider.

C. Uncertain Diagnosis

If the diagnosis documented at the time of discharge is qualified as "probable", "suspected", "likely", "questionable", "possible", or "still to be ruled out", code the condition as if it existed or was established. The bases for these guidelines are the diagnostic workup, arrangements for further workup or observation, and initial therapeutic approach that correspond most closely with the established diagnosis. **Note: This guideline is applicable only to short-term, acute, long-term care and psychiatric hospitals.**

Section IV. Diagnostic Coding and Reporting Guidelines for Outpatient Services

These coding guidelines for outpatient diagnoses have been approved for use by hospitals/ providers in coding and reporting hospital-based outpatient services and provider-based office visits.

Information about the use of certain abbreviations, punctuation, symbols, and other conventions used in the ICD-9-CM Tabular List (code numbers and titles), can be found in Section IA of these guidelines, under "Conventions Used in the Tabular List." Information about the correct sequence to use in finding a code is also described in Section I.

The terms encounter and visit are often used interchangeably in describing outpatient service contacts and, therefore, appear together in these guidelines without distinguishing one from the other.

Though the conventions and general guidelines apply to all settings, coding guidelines for outpatient and provider reporting of diagnoses will vary in a number of instances from those for inpatient diagnoses, recognizing that:

The Uniform Hospital Discharge Data Set (UHDDS) definition of principal diagnosis applies only to inpatients in acute, short-term, long-term care **and psychiatric** hospitals.

Coding guidelines for inconclusive diagnoses (probable, suspected, rule out, etc.) were developed for inpatient reporting and do not apply to outpatients.

A. Selection of first-listed condition

In the outpatient setting, the term first-listed diagnosis is used in lieu of principal diagnosis.

In determining the first-listed diagnosis the coding conventions of ICD-9-CM, as well as the general and disease specific guidelines take precedence over the outpatient guidelines.

Diagnoses often are not established at the time of the initial encounter/visit. It may take two or more visits before the diagnosis is confirmed.

The most critical rule involves beginning the search for the correct code assignment through the Alphabetic Index. Never begin searching initially in the Tabular List as this will lead to coding errors.

B. Codes from 001.0 through V84.8

The appropriate code or codes from 001.0 through V84.8 must be used to identify diagnoses, symptoms, conditions, problems, complaints, or other reason(s) for the encounter/visit.

C. Accurate reporting of ICD-9-CM diagnosis codes

For accurate reporting of ICD-9-CM diagnosis codes, the documentation should describe the patient's condition, using terminology which includes specific diagnoses as well as symptoms, problems, or reasons for the encounter. There are ICD-9-CM codes to describe all of these.

D. Selection of codes 001.0 through 999.9

The selection of codes 001.0 through 999.9 will frequently be used to describe the reason for the encounter. These codes are from the section of ICD-9-CM for the classification of diseases and injuries (e.g. infectious and parasitic diseases; neoplasms; symptoms, signs, and ill-defined conditions, etc.).

E. Codes that describe symptoms and signs

Codes that describe symptoms and signs, as opposed to diagnoses, are acceptable for reporting purposes when a diagnosis has not been established (confirmed) by the provider. Chapter 16 of ICD-9-CM, Symptoms, Signs, and Ill-defined conditions (codes 780.0 - 799.9) contain many, but not all codes for symptoms.

F. Encounters for circumstances other than a disease or injury

ICD-9-CM provides codes to deal with encounters for circumstances other than a disease or injury. The Supplementary Classification of factors Influencing Health Status and Contact with Health Services (V01.0- V84.8) is provided to deal with occasions when circumstances other than a disease or injury are recorded as diagnosis or problems.

G. Level of Detail in Coding

1.   ICD-9-CM codes with 3, 4, or 5 digits

ICD-9-CM is composed of codes with either 3, 4, or 5 digits. Codes with three digits are included in ICD-9-CM as the heading of a category of codes that may be further subdivided by the use of fourth and/or fifth digits, which provide greater specificity.

2. Use of full number of digits required for a code

A three-digit code is to be used only if it is not further subdivided. Where fourth-digit subcategories and/or fifth-digit subclassifications are provided, they must be assigned. A code is invalid if it has not been coded to the full number of digits required for that code. See also discussion under Section I.b.3., General Coding Guidelines, Level of Detail in Coding.

H. ICD-9-CM code for the diagnosis, condition, problem, or other reason for encounter/visit

List first the ICD-9-CM code for the diagnosis, condition, problem, or other reason for encounter/visit shown in the medical record to be chiefly responsible for the services provided. List additional codes that describe any coexisting conditions. **In some cases the first-listed diagnosis may be a symptom when a diagnosis has not been established (confirmed) by the physician.**

I. "Probable", "suspected", "questionable", "rule out", or "working diagnosis"

Do not code diagnoses documented as "probable", "suspected," "questionable," "rule out," or "working diagnosis". Rather, code the condition(s) to the highest degree of certainty for that encounter/visit, such as symptoms, signs, abnormal test results, or other reason for the visit. **Please note:** This differs from the coding practices used by **short-term, acute care, long-term care and psychiatric** hospitals.

J. Chronic diseases

Chronic diseases treated on an ongoing basis may be coded and reported as many times as the patient receives treatment and care for the condition(s)

K. Code all documented conditions that coexist

Code all documented conditions that coexist at the time of the encounter/visit, and require or affect patient care treatment or management. Do not code conditions that were previously treated and no longer exist. However, history codes (V10-V19) may be used as secondary codes if the historical condition or family history has an impact on current care or influences treatment.

L. Patients receiving diagnostic services only

For patients receiving diagnostic services only during an encounter/visit, sequence first the diagnosis, condition, problem, or other reason for encounter/visit shown in the medical record to be chiefly responsible for the outpatient services provided during the encounter/visit. Codes for other diagnoses (e.g., chronic conditions) may be sequenced as additional diagnoses.

For outpatient encounters for diagnostic tests that have been interpreted by a physician, and the final report is available at the time of coding, code any confirmed or definitive diagnosis(es) documented in the interpretation. Do not code related signs and symptoms as additional diagnoses.

Please note: This differs from the coding practice in the hospital inpatient setting regarding abnormal findings on test results.

M. Patients receiving therapeutic services only

For patients receiving therapeutic services only during an encounter/visit, sequence first the diagnosis, condition, problem, or other reason for encounter/visit shown in the medical record to be chiefly responsible for the outpatient services provided during the encounter/visit. Codes for other diagnoses (e.g., chronic conditions) may be sequenced as additional diagnoses.

The only exception to this rule is that when the primary reason for the admission/encounter is chemotherapy, radiation therapy, or rehabilitation, the appropriate V code for the service is listed first, and the diagnosis or problem for which the service is being performed listed second.

N. Patients receiving preoperative evaluations only

For patients receiving preoperative evaluations only, sequence **first** a code from category V72.8, Other specified examinations, to describe the pre-op consultations. Assign a code for the condition to describe the reason for the surgery as an additional diagnosis. Code also any findings related to the pre-op evaluation.

O. Ambulatory surgery

For ambulatory surgery, code the diagnosis for which the surgery was performed. If the postoperative diagnosis is known to be different from the preoperative diagnosis at the time the diagnosis is confirmed, select the postoperative diagnosis for coding, since it is the most definitive.

P. Routine outpatient prenatal visits

For routine outpatient prenatal visits when no complications are present, codes V22.0, Supervision of normal first pregnancy, **or** V22.1, Supervision of other normal pregnancy, should be used as **the** principal diagnosis. These codes should not be used in conjunction with chapter 11 codes.

Index

(continued)

(continued)

(continued)

(continued)

(continued)

AHIMA Certification:
Your Valuable Career Asset

AHIMA offers a variety of credentials whether you're just starting out in the health information management (HIM) field, are an advanced coding professional, or play an important privacy or security role at your facility. Employers are looking for your commitment to the field and a certain competency level. AHIMA credentials help you stand out from the crowd of resumés.

✔ Registered Health Information Administrator (RHIA)/Registered Health Information Technician (RHIT)

✔ Certified Coding Associate (CCA), entry-level

✔ Certified Coding Specialist (CCS), advanced

✔ Certified Coding Specialist—Physician-based (CCS-P), advanced

✔ Certified in Healthcare Privacy (CHP)

✔ Certified in Healthcare Security (CHS), offered by HIMSS through AHIMA

In recent AHIMA-sponsored research groups, healthcare executives and recruiters cited three reasons for preferring credentialed personnel:

1. Assurance of current knowledge through continued education

2. Possession of field-tested experience

3. Verification of base level competency

AHIMA is a premier organization for HIM professionals, with more than 50,000 members nationwide. AHIMA certification carries a strong reputation for quality—the requirements for our certification are rigorous.

AHIMA exams are computer-based and available throughout the year.

Make the right move...pair your degree and experience with AHIMA certification to maximize your career possibilities.

For more information on AHIMA credentials and how to sit for the exams, you can either visit our Web site at www.ahima.org/certification, send an e-mail to **certdept@ahima.org,** or call **(800) 335-5535.**

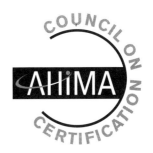

Look for These Quality AHIMA Publications at Bookstores, Libraries and Online

Applying Inpatient Coding Skills under Prospective Payment

Basic CPT/HCPCS Coding

Basic ICD-9-CM Coding

The Best of In Confidence

Calculating and Reporting Healthcare Statistics

Clinical Coding Workout: Practice Exercises for Skill Development

Coding and Reimbursement for Outpatient Care

CPT/HCPCS Coding and Reimbursement for Physician Services

Documentation for Acute Care

Documentation for Ambulatory Care

Documentation and Reimbursement for Behavioral Healthcare Services

Documentation and Reimbursement for Long-term Care (book and CD)

Documentation and Reimbursement for Home Care and Hospice Programs

Effective Management of Coding Services

Electronic Health Record

Health Information Management

Health Information Management Technology

Health Information Management Compliance (book and CD)

HIPAA in Practice

ICD-9-CM Diagnostic Coding and Reimbursement for Physician Services

ICD-9-CM Diagnostic Coding for Long-Term Care and Home Care

ICD-10-CM and ICD-10-PCS Preview (book and CD)

Quality and Performance Improvement in Healthcare

More Information

Textbook details and easy ordering are available online at **www.ahima.org/store.**
For textbook content questions, contact **publications@ahima.org,** and
for sales information contact **info@ahima.org** or **(800) 335-5535.**

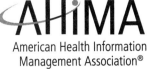

Kick Your Future into High Gear Today by Joining AHIMA!

The American Health Information Management Association (AHIMA), the name you can trust in quality healthcare education, has represented the interests of HIM professionals since 1928.

We have been at the forefront of change in healthcare, anticipating trends, preparing for the future, and advancing careers. AHIMA membership affords you a vast array of resources including:

- **HIM Body of Knowledge**
- **Leadership Opportunities**
- **Latest Industry Information**
- **New Certifications**
- **Continuing Education**
- **An Award-Winning Journal**
- **Advocacy**

This list just touches on the benefits of AHIMA membership. To learn more about the benefits of membership or how to renew you membership, just visit **www.ahima.org/membership**, or call **(800) 335-5535**.

There is no better time to join than today

Fill out an online application at **www.ahima.org/membership,** or call **(800) 335-5535** for more information.

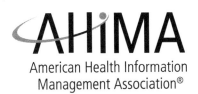

American Health Information
Management Association®